I0492210

NATURAL
BIRTH SECRETS

An Insider's Guide on How to Give Birth Holistically,
Healthfully, and Safely, and Love the Experience!

Second Edition

NATURAL
BIRTH SECRETS

An Insider's Guide on How to Give Birth Holistically,
Healthfully, and Safely, and Love the Experience!

Second Edition

Anne Margolis, CNM, LM, MSN, BSN, RNC

#1 INTERNATIONAL BESTSELLING AUTHOR

NATURAL BIRTH SECRETS

An Insider's Guide How to Give Birth Holistically, Healthfully
and Safely, and Love the Experience!
Copyright © 2020 by Anne Margolis, CNM, LM, MSN, BSN, RNC

All rights reserved. No part of this publication may be reproduced, distributed or transmitted in any form or by any means, including via photocopying, recording, or other electronic or mechanical methods, without the prior written permission of the publisher, except in the case of brief quotations embodied in critical reviews and certain other noncommercial uses permitted by copyright law. For permission requests, write to the publisher, addressed: "Attention: Permissions Coordinator".

Limit of Liability Disclaimer: The information contained in this book is for information purposes only and may not apply to your situation. The author, publisher, distributor, and provider provide no warranty about the content or accuracy of content enclosed. Information provided is subjective. Keep this in mind when reviewing this guide.

Although the author and publisher have made every effort to ensure that the information in this book was correct at press time, the author and publisher do not assume and hereby disclaim any liability to any party for any loss, damage, or disruption caused by errors or omissions, whether such errors or omissions result from negligence, accident, or any other cause.

This book is not intended as a substitute for medical advice. The reader should regularly consult a midwife or physician in matters relating to their health and particularly with respect to any symptoms that may require diagnosis or medical attention.

Website: *www.homesweethomebirth.com*

Ordering Information: Quantity sales. Special discounts are available on multiple purchases by corporations, associations, and others.

For details, contact the "Special Sales Department" at the address above.

- 1st edition, 2018
- 2nd Edition, 2020
Book Layout: © 2020 EvolveGlobalPublishing.com
ISBN: (Paperback) 978-1-64871-315-6
ISBN: (Hardcover) 978-1-64871-316-3
ISBN-10: (Amazon Print) 1720818800
ISBN-13: (Amazon Print) 978-1720818809
ISBN: (Smashwords) 9780463817636
ASIN: (Amazon Kindle) B07HB545SC

This book is available on Barnes & Noble, Kobo, Apple iBooks (digital)

TABLE OF CONTENTS

Want to learn more or have more questions?

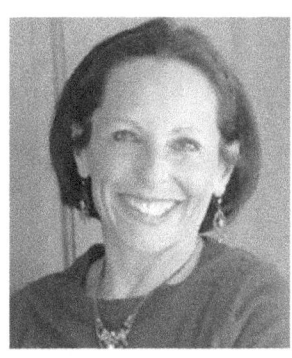

Anne loves helping mamas have the best journey to birth possible. She also loves helping people heal their inner stress, wounds, and suffering, and reclaim their joy - rebirth themselves.

Anne will answer common questions she is often asked as a holistic midwife, on video, which are supplements to watch in adjunct to the Natural Birth Secrets book.

Grab Your Free Book Bonuses below:
https://homesweethomebirth.com/nbsbookbonus

About Anne's Credentials:

- Bachelors in Nursing from the University of Pennsylvania
- Degree in Nurse-Midwifery from the Frontier School of Midwifery and Family Nursing
- Masters in Nursing from Case Western Reserve University.
- Licensed Midwife in New York
- Certified by the American Midwifery Certification Board
- Prenatal, Postpartum and Restorative yoga teacher training from Yoga Garden of San Francisco - Yoga Alliance Certified
- Yoga teacher training from Nosara Yoga Institute - Yoga Alliance Certified
- Completed the Spirit Junkie Masterclass Level One and Two

Training with Gabrielle Bernstein
- Mastery and Creation Course Graduate of Mama Gena's School of Womanly Arts
- Certified Clarity Breathwork Practitioner - Completed Levels One Through Five
- Licensed Femme! Teacher

WHAT OTHERS SAY ABOUT ANNE AND HER WORK

❝ *My homebirth was the beginning of the journey that led me to my dharma. It was an experience of transcendental ecstasy. Anne Margolis was my incredible midwife. She is practical, science-based, and vastly experienced, but most importantly, she's an awakened woman here to light the path to your most joyful self. Anne is the incredible midwife who taught me, through this process, how to midwife my own patients' rebirth experience.*

Her own educational course is a deep but manageable dive into her accumulated wisdom, packaged for your journey. Forget your childbirth class, and take steps to your most empowering experience. If you are thinking about conception, pregnant, or love someone who is, take it from me that her wisdom is life-changing."

—Yours in the truth, Kelly Brogan, MD

"I want to thank you for your online course. Because of it, I was able to do a home waterbirth in Nicaragua where it is not common at all. I live abroad, so it was my dream to have a natural birth in my home. Little did I know there are no doulas or certified midwives in the country. Your course helped me through it!

My father-in-law, who is an OBGYN in Brazil that only does cesareans, so he'd never done a home or natural birth, caught the baby. What a special moment for the family! Thank you again for the knowledge I was able to achieve online!"

—Brittany S., Nicaragua

"*Michael and I want to sincerely thank you for being the best midwife I had hoped for. You immediately made us feel comfortable and confident in our choice to have a homebirth. I also feel fortunate from the successful outcome of my birth experience. Close friends of mine who had very similar circumstances during labor ALL went to surgery. That shows me the confidence you have in our bodies and your amazing skills to help people birth naturally. For that, I am truly grateful. I am so happy with my choices and that you were there to guide me through it all.*"

—Much love and hugs, Lisa and Michael

"*I wanted to say thank you for making my homebirth a possibility. It almost seemed like it wasn't going to happen, with all of our obstacles, but I am so happy it did. You are absolutely amazing and so inspiring!*

Thank you for all your dedication and support in honoring women's holistic health choices. From answering my questions, my mom's questions, my husband's questions—to labor and birth prep—your support, encouragement, telling me to follow and listen to my body, not telling me to push, suggesting the warm compress, and all of the herbal and nutritional support and information were invaluable. Thank you!

I've had a wonderful postpartum period, and I'm sure one of the biggest reasons is the care I received from you. I really cannot thank you enough! I hope I can express the gratitude I have for you and your practice."

—Lots of love, Angeline

"*You are an absolutely amazing midwife. My experience with you is unforgettable. During pregnancy, I enjoyed getting care and valuable information about my child's development and emotional support. You bring a lot of positive energy into the world! Thank you! There are not enough words to express my gratitude to you.*"

—Marina

"Your course and videos are riveting—both my husband and I could not stop watching ... and we are the grandparents! So informative, realistic, reassuring, wise, loving, and inspiring. I've gifted the course to my daughter-in-law who is finding it unbiased, deeper, clearer, and more encouraging than the other classes she was told to take. Anne, your 'delivery' is fantastic!"

—Susan Sparkman

"My four childbirth experiences were among the most pivotal, transformative, empowering instances in my life. They shape who I am today and how I relate to the world, and I don't underestimate Anne's role in giving me that gift. Her support and wisdom made a lasting impact on me for the way I face challenges when they arise."

—Julie D.

"I am so happy to have chosen you to care for me. I would recommend you to anyone having a baby. You are very caring, thorough, and professional. I knew I was in good hands with you. I get emotional thinking about the outstanding care you gave me and my family. We were so blessed. Words cannot explain how grateful I am. Thank you for all your love and support. This was one of the best experiences of my life. I have very beautiful memories, and I'm grateful to have you as a part of them. You are fantastic at what you do. Thanks again for everything."

—With lots of love, Erin

"I signed up for Anne's "Love Your Birth" class online, and it's been a hugely important part of my pregnancy, and I dearly wanted to share about this and Anne's view on pregnancy in our country at this time. If you or someone you love is having a baby, LOVE YOUR BIRTH is a fantastic program to participate in."

— Dr. Christine Schaffner, Naturopathic Physician

"I can't tell you how amazing it was to see you yesterday. You bring such a warm comfortable joy and energy with you it's really hard to put into words. I couldn't be any happier that you are with us on this journey!!

I really cannot express how grateful I am for you, Anne. Thank you for being an inspiration and for encouraging/validating me throughout my pregnancy and labor, and especially offering to travel here so I could have a most amazing home birth. I have so much respect, admiration, and love for you—talk to you soon!

I want everyone to know how great you are.

Anne's online birthing class is perfect for every mom to educate, calm nerves and ROCK their birth! Anne is amazingly knowledgeable and can answer any question you may have. She also makes herself easily available to you.

Because of Anne, I had tricks and tips that have helped tremendously!!

Thanks Anne!"

— OurBrokenCompass Vlog

"After taking Anne's online birthing class, I feel full of useful knowledge, healthy perspectives, and natural birth encouragement! Anne has an outstanding job of identifying what women need to know & hear. I'm thrilled about the wonderful words, lessons, and resources Anne has equipped me with during my pregnancy! Thank you for the wonderful work you do!!!

— Maggie Lilley

"Watching this course feels like you're having long talks with a dear but very knowledgeable friend. The course helped me keep my thoughts in line when there are so many things we don't have control of in life, and it helped me feel more confident by getting educated in areas where I had little. There is a lot of information, which is great for a first time pregnancy. Anne is delightful and really knows her stuff. She helped me feel more prepared and confident for pregnancy and birth. This course is priceless."

— Misty A.

"Anne!! She's a wonderful teacher, no prejudice, calm and thinks of everything. The videos are easy to digest and full of brilliant, empowering information. As a full time mom, I feel that I can take on the world. I CAN DO THIS! I just feel empowered now."

— Chloe JM

"I SO appreciate Anne's course, knowledge and support. I wasn't happy with the options for prenatal classes available to me and I was thrilled to find her site. Thank you Anne for creating this online course! This was my first pregnancy and it was a big part of educating and empowering me through my pregnancy and home birth. Highly recommended!"

— @terrikretai

"This course not only prepared me for childbirth, but also for motherhood and beyond. It was so much more than how to approach labor and delivery and really tapped into the mind, heart, spirit and body for the full journey. It helped me discuss things with my partner that I did not even know needed to be discussed. I feel like a true team now that we've taken the course and discussed the workbook. I was so afraid we may not be on the same page and this course kept us on track! The information I've received is priceless. Thank you."

— Lindsay R.

"Eight months ago we met and I was a little worried but determined to have a homebirth. Eventually, our dream came true, and our sweet baby came into the world peacefully and lovingly at home.

Some people tell me we were fortunate, but I know we were fortunate because we were also very well prepared, from spending priceless hours with you during pregnancy. For us, those hours were designed and allowed the beautiful event of birth to become what it was. Now its time to thank you Anne for all the amazing work you did with us preparing us for the most important event in our life so far.

You were so patient with us discussing again and again possible complications that concerned us, explaining interventions and ways to overcome these possibilities.

You were so thorough and serious about the health and wellbeing of me and my baby, offering vast knowledge and experience not only with the "medical" aspect of things, but also with nutrition, supplements, and offering reading material on every possible issue that came along.

Most of all you educated us to become people who can choose out of knowledge. I don't know where else we could get this information, encouragement and stability along the process. The more I try to get into the details with what you have provided us, the more I understand I will not be able to do that, because it was so much.

I will not say it was impossible to do a home birth without you, but I will say that what we received was above and beyond any expectation we have ever had, and that you were an inseparable part of the wonderful results!

We haven't mentioned your extraordinary personality, a combination of beauty, kindness, warmth, empathy as well as sharpness, intelligence and strength. You are a real gift to this world and we are very fortunate to find you and have your guidance and support. Thank you from the bottom of our hearts. Please save a spot for next time!"

— Love you very much, Michal

"I just wanted to thank you for all you have done. I couldn't have chosen better support! Your knowledge, experience, and kind heart helped to make my pregnancy and birth a wonderful experience. I feel so blessed to have had such a great birth and you are part of that. My baby entered the world in a pretty amazing way. She was born in the comfort of her own home, surrounded by her family, close friends and two amazing women who helped her come into the world safely and naturally.

Nothing in the world compares to that incredible experience and I am so thankful to be able to look back on it as my girl grows. Your kind words and encouragement really helped. Thank you for being a part of such a special time in my life. I am forever grateful! I can't put into words how much you have helped and what a difference you have made. You will forever bring a smile to our faces."

— Thank you, Ashley

"My experience with you Anne was amazing from start to finish. The appointments during pregnancy were beyond thorough, and any questions I had between appointments were answered by you directly and promptly. The level of care I received is incomparable to any other physician that I 've met. I just wanted to thank you for helping me bring our beautiful daughter into this world, the best way we knew how. Anne, you changed our lives in so many ways...including getting my very skeptical mother on board for this very special journey.

After just 4 hours of labor, we gave birth to our beautiful baby girl in the comfort of our own home. It was truly a beautiful experience and a moment that we will always cherish. We can't thank you enough for guiding us through this journey. You are truly an amazing person. I would absolutely recommend you to anyone I care about and would absolutely choose to journey to birth with you again."

— Love, Leah and Chris

"This is long overdue in saying thank you and great appreciations!!!! From my initial phone call answered by your enthusiasm to your compassionate phone calls in the colic first few weeks, I am simply so appreciative to you. I think sooooo often of the compassionate care I received from you both prenatally and postnatally and think you are a healer of an ancient order.

Energetically, you are healing this world and making birth a sacred rite again in a world where it is chronically devalued. You are doing sacred work and making the world change one birth at a time. You are so awesome. Most women don't know how they can be treated in pregnancy, labor, and birth. I don't know if mere words can express the energy of this idea in my heart.

I can't wait to get pregnant again and have your energy and passion guard my pregnancy and birth. From the bottom of my heart, I am so appreciative and grateful to connect with you. Thank you for doing your work in such a powerful, honorable and empowering manner."

— In gratitude, reverence and great love, Jill W

"I just wanted to reach out to send you a personal thank you message. I love YOU. You have been present for so much of my pregnancy journey and have always sent nothing but love. I want you to know how deeply it means to me, that I am truly grateful and that I send ALL MY LOVE back to you always."

— Nikkee

"Words can't begin to thank you for all you did for our family! We were so blessed to have found you and we are so appreciative of all your help and care throughout my pregnancy and birth. You provided such a peaceful 9 months and 6 days! ;0). I can honestly say my birth was one of the most amazing experiences of my life and you were an integral part of it all. May you be blessed in the service you provide for women and their children. I look forward to a future of more pregnancies with you!"

— Love and blessings, Emily and Aaron

This book is dedicated to women, their partners, and their

babies ... in this current generation, and in future generations.

It is dedicated to my children and their children, their children's

children, and beyond. It is dedicated to doing what I can to

improve pregnancy, birth, and postpartum experiences and

outcomes to restore vibrant health, humanity, and celebration to

the peak life experience of having a baby.

Anne Margolis

ACKNOWLEDGMENTS

I want to thank my own dear beloved babies, now grown, who were my greatest of gifts and teachers. I want to thank my husband, Jay, for really being there with me always—a rooted, sturdy, and giving tree through the thick and thin of it all; devoted, adoring, and so very proud. I could not have been such a busy midwife and raised four kids without his huge help, unshakable stability, and loving support.

I want to thank the thousands of moms, babies, and families I have been blessed and honored to help over all these years—I have learned more from you than any academic training or professor, no matter how prestigious.

I have had many role models of ideal holistic maternity and newborn care, whose books I have read and continuously recommend, whose many workshops and conferences I attended—from renowned midwife, Ina May Gaskin, to my dear friend and colleague, Karen Strange, to esteemed obstetricians/gynecologists, Dr. Michel Odent, Dr. Marsden Wagner, Dr. Christiane Northrup, and family physician, Dr. Sarah Buckley.

I want to thank sister midwives and birth professionals in my area for their love, guidance, and support—for always being there for me at all hours. A special thank you to two special colleagues and friends: Debra Pascale Bonaro, for all she is doing for mothers and babies, and for including me and my clients in her Orgasmic Birth documentary; and Sister Goddess Sheila Kamera Hay for also inspiring and empowering women to birth with pleasure and have an ecstatic experience.

I must acknowledge beloved OB/GYN Dr. David Kliot who brought me into his doctor-midwife team practice as a new graduate midwife. His practice *was an example of true collaboration between physicians, midwives, and expert hospital maternity care—where he stood for women to have vaginal breech and twin births, and vaginal births after cesarean (VBAC) in a climate that was becoming less and less supportive, where all women benefited from midwifery, no matter their risk.*

I also have enormous gratitude for dear Dr. Andrew Garber—my long-term collaborative obstetrician and perinatologist, whose kindness and advocacy was always there for me and my clients, along with his medical and surgical expertise. He encouraged me and my homebirth midwifery care for healthy women having healthy pregnancies, but reassured us all that he was there if needed. He told my clients that I was one of his favorite midwives, which always touched me deeply. I told them the feeling was mutual. I also want to thank wonderful pediatrician, Dr. Kenneth Zatz, for his ongoing support of my practice and for being a haven for families who give birth at home with midwives.

I am forever grateful to the infinite being that created and runs the world for our ultimate good—even when we don't understand the hows and whys, who has given me many gifts, blessings, miracles, and immense hardships and challenges that made me who I am today.

—Anne Margolis

FOREWORD

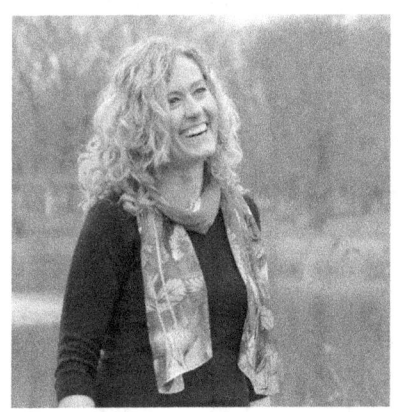

I remember being in your shoes—excited, scared, and overwhelmed. I wanted to have a healthy pregnancy and create the birth I desired for me and my baby. There are so many options out there, even more than when I was pregnant, and what you read can truly shape or change your views—releasing fear or, unfortunately, increasing fear. Much of the available information today can result in "prenatal scare and not care." However, you deserve evidence-based information delivered with care and respect to prepare you for pregnancy, birth, and parenthood with love.

You have come to the right place to find the care and information you need from an experienced and wise midwife whom I have known for over 20 years. Having supported hundreds of births as a doula myself, many at home, at birth centers, and in hospitals around the world, I have a unique view of birth. I appreciate the wise midwives who are keeping the sacred gateway of birth safe and supporting birth-givers and their families to experience the joy, love, and pleasure that is available in childbirth. Sadly, this is not the mainstream paradigm of birth. Midwives like Anne are unique guardians or "lifeguards" at birth—encouraging women to move and find their own rhythm and positions with birth—only intervening when necessary to keep a woman and her baby safe.

Many providers have been trained in a fear-based model, seeing everything as an emergency waiting to happen. Rather than waiting and supporting natural birth, women are expected to birth on their backs, making birth longer and harder with added precautions and technology. Humans can't labor and birth easily when they don't feel safe and private, but instead feel watched and measured at every moment. Anne's gentle presence at more than a 1,000 births has provided her with the wisdom to truly know and understand what is needed to have a gentle natural birth, something I am sad to say many experienced providers will never know, as the only births they see are modified with synthetic hormones, interventions, and IV drips, thus disturbing nature's design. So, instead of an easier, joyful, and pleasurable birth, many of our hospital environments and practices actually put women in a state of stress that slows their ability to open to birth and creates more pain.

I remember the first births I attended as a doula with Anne. I will always remember how safe my clients felt and how warm and gentle she was in her care of them. The lights were dim, music played, and her words, touch, and gentle listening encircled us all with her trust of birth. Years later, when a client offered to have their birth filmed for my documentary Orgasmic Birth: The Best-Kept Secret, I was thrilled to learn Anne was their midwife, as I knew she understood the ways to support and protect the intimate, sensuous, and pleasurable opportunities birth provides, having had her own "orgasmic births." Now, Anne will provide you with all of the care and wisdom that you need to have an orgasmic birth too! I am honored to call Anne part of our Orgasmic Birth family—a friend and colleague who brings joy and pleasure to birth and life!

The term "orgasmic birth" is often misinterpreted. Elizabeth Davis and I, in our book Orgasmic Birth: Your Guide to a Safe, Satisfying, and Pleasurable Birth Experience, define "orgasmic birth" as "broad enough to include those who describe birth as ecstatic and specific enough to give voice to those who actually feel the contractions of orgasm and climax at the moment of delivery. Many of our interviewees spoke of astounding pressure and sensation in the vagina as birth approached, followed by a flood of release and emotion as the baby emerged. Whenever a woman can look back on these moments with joy, when the physical and emotional aspects of birth are fully experienced." With this new definition of "orgasmic birth"—I hope you can agree that an "orgasmic birth" is within your reach as you are holding the guide in your hands full of Natural Birth Secrets!

If you are considering becoming pregnant or are pregnant, Anne Margolis's Natural Birth Secrets provides you with Anne's 22-plus years of midwifery wisdom and guidance for body, mind, and spirit. From enhancing fertility, creating health with nutrition, yoga, meditation, breathwork, and visualization practices, you will have the information you need to create a solid foundation to enjoy and grow during your pregnancy. But health is not enough!

Our complicated, highly medicalized maternity care system takes time to navigate to create the safest and most satisfying environment for you to welcome your baby into your arms gently, with love. Too many people don't ask questions and turn their body and their baby over to medicine that serves us when we are ill, but does not always have the best record of keeping healthy and safe mothers and babies.

The same technology that can save a life, when overused without a compelling benefit, puts you and your baby at risk of complications. It is up to you to understand your options and speak up, as you are the best advocate for yourself and your baby. Anne's years of experience as a home-birth midwife will provide an inside look at hospitals and the US culture of birth, and guide you to ask questions and trust your intuition to create a birth plan for a safe, satisfying birth experience.

As a childbirth educator, DONA doula trainer, and doula myself—my heart sings as Anne speaks about the importance of a "good" comprehensive evidence-based childbirth class that includes pleasure and the beneficial role and value of doulas.

As Anne explains the doula's role, "It's having a personal coach so that you have the healthiest, most wonderful experience possible. All successful professional athletes, performers, and most leading businesses and entrepreneurs also have a coach of some sort. This is doula love." Anne continues to list the many benefits of having a doula, their role, training, and how midwives and doulas are perfect together. I have been blessed to attend births as a doula with Anne, so I know firsthand how well we work together creating a circle of support where each person feels safe to move and open to birth and parenthood.

You may wonder why there is a section in this book on vaginal birth after cesarean (VBAC) if you are pregnant for the first time. With a 31% cesarean birth rate in the US, your risk of cesarean is an average of one in three people. At some hospitals, that risk is even higher as there are facilities with cesarean rates over 40%, and in some countries, it's 70% to 80%. Your hospital's, and more importantly, your caregiver's rate of cesarean birth is the percentage of risk that you too will have a cesarean. A cesarean rate in hospitals of 10% to 15% has been documented as providing the most benefits and lowest risk of overuse of major abdominal surgery. Anne has a cesarean rate of 5%, as she offers a range of skills that greatly lower your risk of needing a cesarean, and when needed, it is done gently, with dignity and love. Preparing for and understanding your options around gentle cesarean birth, should you need a cesarean, as well as understanding the safety of VBAC is important as there is a great deal of mis- or dis-information around cesarean birth and VBAC.

Knowledge is power. Don't let anyone take your power away in birth. Anne provides you the power to understand your options, so you will be part of decision-making—a key component to people who feel empowered by their birth. When has allowing others to make decisions about your body and wellbeing served you? Most birth trauma comes when people don't feel heard, when things are done to you in childbirth without your input, and sometimes without your permission. Anne is offering you a gift that will guide you to create a sacred birth memory that you will treasure all your life. When you give birth in your power, you will open up access to pleasure with the hormones of love and joy, and this is how you have what I call an "orgasmic birth"!

I remember my first pregnancy. I spent so much time thinking about birth and so little about postpartum. That is the one thing about my childbirth experience I wish I could change. I wish I knew and understood more about my changing body postpartum and had knowledge and tips to help me prepare to breastfeed; I would have asked for more support. I wish someone had talked to me about postpartum sex. Stumbling through postpartum, feeling ashamed, thinking that I was the only one with a roller coaster of emotions, unsure about why my body looked and felt this way, I wish I had Anne's guidance then, as I would have been so much more prepared. My feelings would have been validated, and I would have felt less afraid, as I would have been prepared to navigate the journey from maidenhood to motherhood.

Childbirth is an opportunity to tap into your intuitive wisdom and discover your inner strength and power. When you give birth with your choices and you trust your body, your baby, and your birth, then you will gain a power that will transform you on every level, which is what nature intended for us—to be strong mothers contributing to our families and communities. I know it sounds overused, but childbirth is a moment that will change who you are in ways you can't imagine. I know that my first birth truly changed my life and set me on my path to help all parents understand what birth has to offer. It's not just a day—it is a day that has the opportunity to heal us, to fill us with love, and in doing so, to create healthy relationships and families that our world desperately needs.

Natural Birth Secrets takes you from conception to parenthood and will provide you with the secrets to creating a powerful, passionate, pleasurable, natural birth in any setting, while at the same time learning how to avoid the overuse of technology and birth trauma that too many people are facing today. If you have had a difficult, challenging, or traumatic birth, Anne will guide you to healing. As we are human, healing is always available to us.

Whether it's your first baby or your tenth, each birth is a journey into the unknown through the ancient rite of passage of bringing a new life into the world. You have a gift before you to prepare to give birth mindfully, with love, gently, using the wisdom and techniques that midwives have passed down for generations; wisdom that Anne has put together in this book for you! The secrets are in the pages that follow. May you be inspired as I was to read on, to take the heroic journey of preparing to give birth in your power, with knowledge, support, love, and pleasure.

—Debra Pascali-Bonaro, director of the award-winning documentary "Orgasmic Birth: The Best Kept Secret," author, international speaker, DONA doula trainer, Lamaze childbirth educator, and creatrix of Pain to Power Online Childbirth Classes and Pleasure Essentials
www.OrgasmicBirth.com
www.PaintoPowerChildbirth.com

Anne Margolis

PREFACE

Pregnancy is a time of profound transition. Who you are, as you go through this rite of passage into motherhood, will never be the same. This being that you are gestating will expand your heart in love beyond your imagination. This expanded capacity to love and feel will bless you by intensifying the rainbow of emotions you can experience on any given day, at any given moment. Motherhood is not for the faint of heart—it can be challenging, exhausting, endless, AND joyful, exciting, fun, momentous, and deeply fulfilling, all at the same time.

How can you handle that? How do you prepare for such an experience? By becoming connected to your deep feminine wisdom, that raw primal power that resides within each of us that can guide us in every instance toward our deepest truth and intuition.

Birth is the transition point, the apex of this rite of passage into motherhood, but it is truly just the warmup, preparing us for the marathon of motherhood. Consciously preparing for birth—mind, body, and soul—yields many gifts that flow beyond the moment of birth and right into motherhood. I want every woman to know this and embrace this about labor and birth, rather than wish this rite of passage away, numb it, or bypass it completely. There are gifts for you here that will serve you and your child for the rest of your lives.

How can you unlock these gifts? Through expanding your consciousness about what is possible! By finding yourself a guide, someone who has been there, who can show you the glorious peaks and valleys, hold your hand when you get scared, and answer any questions along the way.

Oh, how I wish I had Anne Margolis at my side when I was pregnant with my first child! I knew I wanted a midwife and said as much to my husband who assured me it was fine, as long as she worked in the "best hospital" with the "best doctor." That was my first introduction to the politics of birth and the divisions between traditional prenatal care and midwifery care.

We stumbled our way through that birth as I bowed to societal and familial pressures rather than honor my own truth. I believe strongly that you get the birth you need, and this first traumatic birth experience activated me, impelled me to find another way.

When we finally did hire a midwife to attend the birth of our second child, we didn't share that information with many of our friends and family as we didn't want to expose ourselves to their fear and judgment about what that meant. There is so much misconception and fear-mongering around what it means to give birth, which is only augmented when it comes to giving birth naturally and midwifery care. What is safe and what isn't?

There is no one better to dispel that fear than Anne Margolis, who has attended the births of more than 1,000 healthy babies over the 22-plus years of her midwifery practice. Anne's rate of interventions for her birthing mamas is astoundingly low, with her cesarean section rate at 5%. Compare that to the national average of 30-40%! Anne's career as a midwife is a testament to the fact that honoring a woman's body and her processes leads to better (and ultimately safer) outcomes.

From that starting point, we can talk about pleasure—the amount of joy, empowerment, and transformation that can occur for a woman in birth. My second birth was a reclamation of my relationship with my desires, my own body, and my deep feminine wisdom. Rather than feeling victimized and powerless, as I did after my first birth, I glowed after my second. I felt healthy, vibrant, beautiful, and sexy.

For my third birth, I decided to prepare for pleasure. In every book I had ever read about natural birth, there was always one line, one sentence, in a 200-300-page book, that said something along the lines of "some women experience ecstasy, bliss, and even orgasm when they give birth." I wanted to know what that was about and prepared for this on every level.

I danced through that labor and the experience left me higher than I've ever been in my life. Even though I had been preparing for pleasure, this birth took me to heights of ecstasy that I never knew possible. Afterward, I turned to my husband and said, "I don't understand. Why didn't I know it could be this good? Why doesn't every woman know?" Thus, began my career as an Ecstatic Birth advocate and coach, teaching women how to ENJOY birth and training birth practitioners how to do the same with their clients.

Anne Margolis, my dear friend, colleague, and co-conspirator, is a visionary and leader in this field. Having experienced pleasurable birth firsthand, she was inspired to become a midwife and has been supporting others in having amazing birth experiences ever since. In stepping out with this book and her online course, Anne is making her years of wisdom and experience available to so many more women. What a gift!

This book will not only provide mothers-to-be with invaluable information to empower them in birthing their babies, but will raise the collective consciousness around natural birth and midwifery care. Anne writes, "Let me help you have the most exquisite birth experience of your life." Oooo, yes, mama! Ecstasy, joy, and empowerment are well within reach with this book in your hands. Read it well and allow Anne's wisdom to guide you through to the other side!

—In love and pleasure, Sheila Kamara Hay
http://ecstatic-birth.com/

ABOUT THE AUTHOR

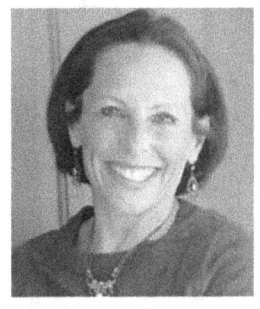

Anne Margolis is a Licensed Certified Nurse Midwife, Licensed Femme! Teacher, Certified Clarity Breathwork Practitioner, and Yoga Teacher and practitioner. In her family line, Anne is a third-generation guide to mamas birthing babies. Anne has helped thousands of families in her 24+ year midwifery practice and has personally ushered the births of over 1,000 healthy babies into the world. She has also guided countless human beings to heal from emotional pain, inner stress, and trauma, and to tap into their strength and power, live fully and vibrantly, and reclaim their radiance, joyfulness, calm, and overall sense of wellbeing.

Anne is a mother of four. She has midwifed her own daughters as they had each of their babies. As a holistic certified nurse-midwife, Clarity Breathwork practitioner, and yoga teacher who has helped thousands, she wishes she had access to the tools that she has now for her earlier births.

Anne knows what it's like to give birth using both conventional and alternative methods, and she wants women to know that it is absolutely possible to have an amazing experience, no matter what you choose. Whether you go natural, need medicine, or require interventions, she will meet you right where you are to guide you towards an epic, empowering experience that you will cherish for a lifetime.

Through her online childbirth course "Love Your Birth," her online and in-person midwifery for pregnancy and postpartum support consultations, her birth professional mentoring, her holistic gynecology, Clarity Breathwork offerings, and Femme! experience offerings, Anne infuses wisdom, compassion, inspiration, and joy into the entire process of women's healthcare—from teen-aged years to menopause. Anne also facilitates incredible healing and wellness for both men and women of all ages. Anne is now part of a wonderful team of holistic midwives that attends births in a supportive mother-baby friendly hospital birthing center.

Anne is a two-time number one national and international best-selling author with this book and also Trauma Release Formula: The Revolutionary Step-by-Step Program for Eliminating Effects of Childhood Abuse, Trauma, Emotional Pain, and Crippling Inner Stress, to Living in Joy Without Drugs or Therapy. Anne's work, insights, and advice have been featured on TV shows and movies, including four episodes of A Baby Story on TLC Discovery Channel, the award-winning feature documentary Orgasmic Birth, and The Human Longevity Project. She has been interviewed for multiple local, national, and international radio programs, shows, and podcasts. Anne has also been a featured speaker and expert panelist at distinguished events for Weil-Cornell School of Medicine, the University of Pennsylvania School of Nursing, RCC State University of New York School of Nursing, Birthnet Association of Childbirth Professionals, and Hudson Valley Birth Network, to name a few.

Anne's Clarity Breathwork and Femme! healing movement workshops have been hosted at several yoga studios and wellness centers, including the conscious, high vibration, and transformational community at The Assemblage in New York City. Anne is a proud founding member of The Health and Wellness Business Association, which was created to promote initiatives that support better collaboration, interaction, and ethical business practices within the health and wellness business community.

Anne has midwifed mamas and babies for over two decades and guides individuals to birth themselves as healthy and whole human beings capable of immense joy and inner peace. Her clients describe her as "passionate," "sensitive," "big-hearted," and a "playful ball of light." When she's not helping mamas around the world, you can find her doing yoga (anywhere and everywhere), dancing, taking or facilitating powerful growth and healing workshops, traveling, enjoying family time, and watching historical dramas and comedies.

Learn more by visiting Anne's website: *www.HomeSweetHomeBirth.com*

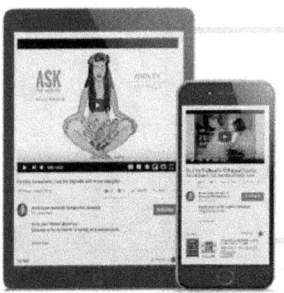

Want to learn more or have more questions?

Grab your free Book Bonuses below:
https://homesweethomebirth.com/nbsbookbonus

Anne Margolis

Benefiting from This Book

Throughout this book, you will find references to articles and ideas about natural healthy living, pregnancy, childbirth, and postpartum. The more you are empowered to learn, the healthier and happier an experience you will have. You are a warrior or you love someone who is—so take your time learning these lessons and developing your own plan for the best pregnancy to birth and mamahood possible.

INTRODUCTION

An Insider's Guide on How to Give Birth Holistically, Healthfully, and Safely, and Love the Experience!

Natural Birth Secrets offers a unique approach on how to have the most healthy, deeply positive, empowered, and joyful journey through pregnancy, birth, and becoming a mom postpartum.

Whether you have visions of a cozy home water birth, giving birth in a birth center free of pain meds and intervention, or a hospital birth with the latest technology and emergency care access just in case, this book provides the ultimate pregnancy-to-postpartum training, so you can be prepared from an emotional, physical, and spiritual perspective to relax into birth and mamahood with optimal wellbeing, excitement, and ease.

This comprehensive training will help you find your center and feel balanced, strong, relaxed, and calm within yourself during this special rite of passage into mamahood in the midst of all the chaos of life along the way. It will help you tune in to your deepest desires and create joy and pleasure in your pregnancy, birth, and new life as a mom—to take you and your family higher.

The insights in this book come from my learning, training, and support of thousands of women, babies, and their families from over twenty years in my private practice, locally, and around the world where I've worked to improve maternity and newborn care and experiences by empowering women and their families to speak up.

These are my insider's secrets to increase your likelihood of avoiding health issues, high rates of risky medical and surgical interventions, and serious complications, including birth trauma for you and your baby, so that you can have the birth of your dreams.

I honor the billions of strong women who have found their strength and birthed—the majority at home, naturally—since the beginning of time. Billions. This is something for you to remember in labor, to encourage and empower yourself!

When I see my exam table with its oven-mitt-covered stirrups, I often wonder to myself, "How many warriors have been here?" because women are warriors. Period. No matter where and how they birthed, whether they had babies or not, women are warriors. In all these years, I have met so many amazing women, women who have faced and dealt with a range of serious life challenges, many who grew, birthed, fed, and raised little humans, and those who were unable to get pregnant or carry their pregnancies. I am awed by these warrior women who found their strength at times when it seemed impossible, and those are the women I have been blessed to know and learn from.

Warriors are not born, and they are not made ... Warriors create themselves through trial and error, mistakes and limitations, pain and suffering, being upside down, wide open and vulnerable–and that is strength. Warriors get up and try again in spite of all of it.

"Strength doesn't come from what you can do. It comes from overcoming the things you thought you couldn't."

—Rikki Rogers

We, women, are stronger than we know, and we find that out when we have to. And once we tap into that power, we birth our babies, we handle the challenges, we birth ourselves ... each and every day, with the little hardships and the mountains that seem impossible to climb ... until we do.

"Behind every man stands no woman. There is no greater man than the man that can acknowledge the woman standing right next to him."

—Rachel Wolchin

Women rock! Mothers rock! We are strong because we had to be, wiser because we learned through our powerful experiences, always doing our best with what we know, have faced, and are facing. We are admirable warriors of honor because we stayed the course, did not give up despite the challenges and struggles and had the courage to plow forward regardless of our fears.

Our blessings are that we have a fan club—the little ones we grow within us, birth, nurture and take care of, who adore us without caring about the mess, the laundry, our to-do lists. They are the little ones we adopt or foster. They are the people we deeply care for, some who are and others who are not our babies. We are beautiful to them no matter how we look or dress. We are perfect for them even when we make mistakes. They want our time and loving attention more than any material gift.

I would love women to be treated and to treat themselves like the goddesses they are. This book should support you and all women in our goddess journeys of life.

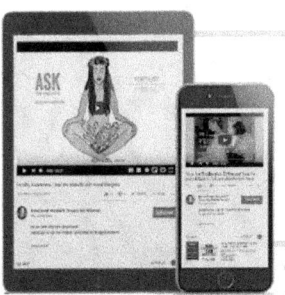

Want to learn more or have more questions?

Grab your free Book Bonuses below:
https://homesweethomebirth.com/nbsbookbonus

Getting Pregnant Naturally

Anne Margolis

Preparing for Pregnancy

There are so many things to consider when preparing for pregnancy.

Every mama wants to give her baby the best possible start in life. Preparing for pregnancy will enhance your own health for fertility success and set you up to provide a healthy environment for your baby.

But, where do you start?

Taking a natural, holistic approach to preparing for pregnancy includes optimizing your diet, supplements, physical movement, and state-of-mind, as well as minimizing toxic exposures, especially from cleaning and body care products, and where you spend most of your time. This is a less invasive, less expensive, and much healthier approach for both mama and baby before even considering the standard fertility treatments.

Eating for a Healthy Pregnancy

When preparing for pregnancy, it's best to eat a wide variety of fresh, whole, mostly plant-based foods and adequate protein. Your plate should be beautiful and colorful with plenty of varied vegetables, fruits, whole grains, beans, and some nuts and seeds, all of which are seasoned with fresh herbs and spices. Look for the following:

Organic. Free of toxic chemicals and pesticides that can damage fetal development—this is the best option for produce. Use the Dirty Dozen as a basic guide when eating out or traveling when organic options are limited. These foods are to be eaten organic or, otherwise, avoided altogether.

Local. Choosing local typically means the food is at the peak of freshness, which ensures the likelihood of it maintaining more nutritional integrity.

Colorful. A variety of colorful fruits and vegetables provides differing nutrients. Make sure you're eating a full spectrum of color to get a well-rounded diet.

Unprocessed. Foods with chemical additives, preservatives, artificial sweeteners, food coloring, and genetic modification are void of nourishment and can negatively affect your health and your baby's. If food comes in packaging with ingredients you do not recognize, it's probably not the best option.

Sugar-Free. Cane sugar is damaging to your and your baby's cells. It causes blood sugar imbalances, inflammation, and disrupts gut flora. It negatively impacts your pregnancy and how you feel physically and emotionally. Sugar is found in almost all processed food. Even white flours and simple starches act like sugar in your body. Look out for marketing tricks, like using four or five different types of sweeteners so manufacturers don't have to list a kind of sugar as the first ingredient. Stick with natural sugars like what's found in fruit. If you must add a sweetener, pure raw honey or maple syrup is better.

Gluten-Free & Dairy-Free. Most women feel best when they are dairy and gluten-free. Try removing them from your diet for a month and see if you feel better in your mind and body, if you gain more energy or clarity. Many who feel better off cow dairy can tolerate organic, grass-fed goat or sheep dairy products. Some feel best also off soy and corn.

Hormone-Free & Antibiotic-Free. Whenever possible, select the highest-quality, pastured, grass-fed, organic meats and animal products, including wild fish from non-polluted waters. If the animal food you're eating was treated with hormones and antibiotics, your body and baby will be affected by that. And consider that most farm animals are fed genetically modified (GMO) corn and feed that was highly sprayed with pesticides. Animals that are free to move in the sunshine and graze in green pastures, as they did for thousands of years before the modernization of the farming industry, produce the healthiest meat, dairy, and eggs for human consumption.

Healthy Fats. Your body needs plenty of high-quality fat, especially when preparing for pregnancy. Ideally, eat wild Alaskan or Norwegian salmon and other freshwater fish at least twice per week, as well as plenty of nuts, seeds, and healthy oils. Use organic, cold pressed extra virgin olive oil on cold foods (like for salad dressing) and light sautéing, and organic, cold-pressed, unrefined coconut oil or organic grass-fed clarified butter like ghee for cooking at higher temperatures. Stay away from unhealthy partially hydrogenated refined vegetable oils and trans fats.

Hydration. Don't forget to drink plenty of fresh spring or filtered water throughout the day. Work your way up to half your body weight in ounces. For example, if you weigh 150 pounds, drink 75 ounces of water daily.

Preparing for Pregnancy with Supplements

In a perfect world, we would get all the nutrients we need from our food. But, with today's industrialization of food and depleted soils, that has become virtually impossible. Additionally, the standard American diet is empty of needed nutrition, and even those of us with the best intentions do not eat all of what is needed for our own health or our body's healthy when pregnant. The supplements you need when preparing for pregnancy depend on your specific situation.

However, there are a few supplements that every woman should take daily. I take them myself and recommend them to all my clients. Following this supplement protocol has blessed me with feeling wonderfully vital and blessed with rarely getting sick, even when a bug is going around my house. To find out more, read the chapter on "Nutritional Best Practices for Mom."

My online dispensary is a convenient way for you to purchase my hand-picked, professional-grade, whole-food supplements and other natural health products at discount. Ordering is simple as it is by category (supplements are listed in the prenatal and multivitamin sections), and the products will be shipped directly to your home or work within a few days.

Exercise for a Healthy Pregnancy and Beyond

Movement is another important aspect of preparing for pregnancy. When you have a strong, agile, and flexible body, not only are you able to provide a better prenatal home for a baby, it will minimize aches and pains along the way, reduce inner stress, help in labor, and aid in postpartum recovery. The right exercise can also get your body ready to ease your baby into a perfect birthing position.

Ultimately, the best exercise is that which you enjoy, so that you stick with it. Vary doing the exercise activities that you love, and incorporate exercise into your life consistently to decrease any overall feelings of stress. Here are some types of movement to consider:

- **Brisk Walking.** This is a great place to start if you're someone who currently isn't getting much exercise. Begin with a leisurely 15 to 20-minute walk every day, and build up to 45 to 60 minutes at a faster pace. Walk outside when you can, and try hiking in beautiful places.
- **Yoga.** Yoga will not only strengthen your body and make you more flexible, but it's also been known to decrease stress and enhance your overall wellbeing. There are tremendous health benefits to regular yoga practice, covered more in the chapter "Yoga for Pregnancy and Labor." There are even fertility yoga classes out there, designed with just this topic in mind! I teach private and small group yoga classes, including yoga workshops for pregnancy and labor, as well as postpartum, which can be done locally or on Skype.
- **Dance.** Dancing is such a great way to keep healthy and active! It is so much fun and provides a direct path to feeling awesome without realizing you are also getting a fabulous workout. It relieves stress, helps you feel and move emotions, and creates happiness for yourself and your baby. This is because both stress

hormones, as well as happy love hormones, pass through the placenta to the baby ... and both are contagious to those around you. Dancing also helps you tap into your sensual or sassy sexy, which is beneficial in pregnancy, labor, and life! Dancing, like labor, uses gravity and asymmetrical movements, which helps to ease a baby down and out through a wider birth canal. Start by taking dance classes, but you can also just turn on the music and dance like no one is watching. I give small group and private healing movement workshops called Femme!, which offer a wonderful experience for both men and women to move freely, get primal, and release and move through a full range of emotions to African drumming.

- **Weight-Training.** If you are not called to yoga or dance, then back, arm, leg, and core weight-training exercises also help align your body and provide great preparation for the uneven weight of pregnancy. Squatting helps prepare for delivery.
- **Pilates.** Pilates has a strong emphasis on core conditioning and is also great for mamas-to-be. Core strength prevents common issues like lower back pain and even helps to keep a baby in a good head-down position in the last few months of pregnancy.
- **Swimming.** It gets you outside, connected to nature, and immersed in healing waters that soothe the soul. Swimming and water aerobics are great ways to be active. In advancing pregnancy, swimming relieves common aches and discomforts, and pregnant women love the sense of weightlessness they feel in the water.

If you're someone who currently has an intense workout regimen and are having trouble conceiving, consider dialing it back to a lower intensity. Otherwise, moderately moving your body and being active each day is the way to go.

Tapping into Mindfulness and Joy

Reducing inner stress and living in joy is central to preparing for pregnancy. Inner stress can actually prevent pregnancy. Many of us recognize that we have grown out of alignment with our true natural being, and it's time to get back to our original design ... get back in touch with the cyclic nature of our human bodies, our minds, our hearts, and our spirits. The thoughts we think and the perspective we carry while preparing for pregnancy are incredibly influential.

Find ways to slow down, unplug, be outside in nature more, and enjoy the journey. Make sure you are well-rested and getting seven to eight hours of sleep each night. Practice saying no to anything that is really not necessary, and doesn't bring you calm and pleasure during this time. Explore ways to bring joy back into the things that aren't optional. Stay as much as possible in the present moment, one moment, one breath at a time. Practice mindfulness—anchoring into what is going on around you and the sensations within you in the now. When you regularly practice mindfulness, it can transform your life and will benefit your labor immensely.

Having a daily practice of breathwork and meditation will help you to master the ability to relax yourself. Please see the chapter "Meditation, Breathwork, and Visualization: for more details. Consider journaling and creating any form of art to tap into your creative capacity, and help your body keep a calm and joyful state. Decide to live a glorious life. Dress and treat yourself like the goddess you are. Focus on what you have to be grateful for and all the blessings in your life. Connect more in community with those you love and those who inspire you. Clear your body of trapped emotional pain, trauma, and internal stress, and transform self-limiting beliefs and thought patterns with Clarity Breathwork. Turn negative thoughts into positive affirmations; for example, My body is strong and healthy for pregnancy or I am the perfect age to become a mother. Empowering, uplifting thoughts are usually the opposite of and truer than the false stories (i.e., limiting beliefs) we typically tell ourselves.

Acupuncture is a great way to relax, balance and clear blocked flow of your life force energy, and has the added bonus of hormone regulation and improved ovarian function. Many women who had some initial trouble conceiving often get pregnant after receiving acupuncture by a practitioner with expertise in fertility. I have seen it used in conjunction with routine infertility treatments and have seen successful pregnancies even after several failed IVF attempts.

We've discussed a lot of lifestyle factors here. Some might be big changes for you. Don't let them overwhelm you. Unless you have health issues that necessitate otherwise, I'm a huge fan of the 80-20 rule. Spend 80% of your efforts on achieving optimal habits and allow yourself the freedom to enjoy the other 20% without guilt.

Fertility Awareness

Learn the signs of fertility, so you can make sure you have intercourse during the small window of time when you are likely to conceive. Doing so results in the most accurate estimation of pregnancy dating, and you will even know when you are pregnant before you can take a pregnancy test. This is key, and it will also provide helpful information as to the causes of difficulties should you need professional guidance. The next two chapters look at this all-important subject: fertility awareness and methods. Once you learn it, then relax and enjoy the ride.

Additional Resources

- *wellnessmama.com*—"an online resource for women and moms who want to live a healthier life ... fact-checked by [an] editorial and research team and reviewed by medical advisors for accuracy." Her Paleo recipes are excellent.
- *ireadlabelsforyou.com*—a wonderful, trusted resource for well-researched, safe, non-toxic products for your body and home, so you can make empowered, informed decisions for yourself and your family when creating a healthy household and life.
- *thehealthyhomeeconomist.com*—a practical and researched-based resource for optimal health and wellness and green living.
- *ewg.org*—"a non-profit, non-partisan organization dedicated to protecting human health and the environment ... to empower people to live healthier lives in a healthier environment ... with breakthrough research and education."

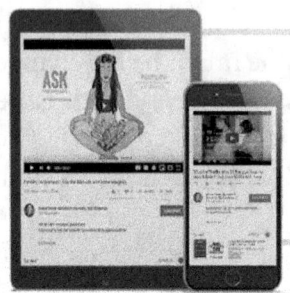

Want to learn more or have more questions?

Grab your free Book Bonuses below:
https://homesweethomebirth.com/nbsbookbonus

The Natural Fertility Method (System)

The greatest gift a woman is endowed with is the ability to carry a life inside of her womb. She dreams of being a mom and wants everything to go as planned. Fertility is the ability to conceive a child, then carry it to term, and it is empowering to understand the process along the way. Natural pregnancy and childbirth, therefore, begin with an understanding of fertility and an awareness of how the process flows from conception to birth and beyond.

We will begin with the obvious first step of understanding, which is getting pregnant. As we move through the chapters, I will be giving you valuable advice based on the methods I have successfully used over the years that assist in the beautiful and natural process of bringing a baby into the world.

Getting Pregnant Naturally

The first step is to know your menstrual cycles and signs of fertility. The Fertility Awareness Method is used to increase your chances of getting pregnant and in some cases to prevent pregnancy. When you have an accurate estimate of your due date, this helps to prevent unnecessary or risky interventions, like induction for postdates when you are not at term.

It has many other benefits too. For instance, it provides you with knowledge of your own body's normal functioning, so you can embrace your symptoms as signs of health without feeling dirty, shame, or embarrassment. With this method, you can know when you are ovulating–without an ovulation kit. You can also know you are "probably pregnant" without a pregnancy test.

By keeping track of your cycles, you can better detect when something is off–from gynecologic and urinary tract infections to hormonal imbalances or cervical problems. It helps you and your healthcare provider figure out issues behind infertility and prevents its false diagnosis when you are just missing the narrow fertile window. In turn, this saves you from invasive and costly diagnostic and treatment procedures. It also significantly reduces the chances of unplanned pregnancy, which accounts for the majority of pregnancies!

Debunking Fertility Myths

Let's begin by debunking the myth: *most women are fertile on day 14 of their cycle*. While it is true that some women are, most are not. We must remember that we all have different cycles ranging on average from 24 to 36 days, and sometimes longer. On top of that, our cycles change over time and depending on what is happening in our lives at that moment. Travel, stress, illness and health issues, medications, sudden weight changes, and even working nightshifts can all bring changes to our cycles. In fact, the same woman could be fertile on day 14 on one month, and in the next month, it may be day 16 or 20, for example. There is much variation in the time between the last period and ovulation, but once ovulation occurs, there is a finite length of time (usually 12 to 16 days) before the next period, unless you get pregnant. Think about fertility not as a "day", but rather a period of time when you ovulate and make the most cervical fluid.

The cervical fluid keeps sperm alive longer and enables them to travel way up into your fallopian tubes to fertilize the egg(s); it also makes intercourse so much more enjoyable, for both you and your partner. You will notice that your vagina is moist, wet, lubricated, and supple; and it is no wonder that some women have higher sexual arousal around the time of ovulation. Remember, inherent within the incredible divine wisdom of mother nature, a healthy woman's body is perfectly designed to make healthy babies and populate the world.

Fertility awareness does require you to make observations about your body on a daily basis and record your observations on a chart or journal of some sort, but it is free, safe, and effective for healthy women when used correctly, without the risks, side effects, and problems associated with other methods of birth control or fertility enhancement.

When Are Women Most Fertile?

As a woman, you are most fertile during your peak day of wetness. That is, the last day you produce the most cervical fluid, which usually happens the day before or day that you ovulate. You are also fertile several days before that, as soon as you start producing cervical fluid. During this peak day, you will also notice a change in your "basal body" temperature, and after ovulation, it stays elevated until your next period or through your pregnancy.

This is where you will need your basal body oral thermometer like Daysy, so you can have a good handle on what your body temperature is during the time you are most fertile. It's not like you have a fever, but rather you'll notice that your temperature rises slightly above your baseline.

There are other signs of fertility, but *knowing your dates and cervical fluid are most critical.* This helps you know approximately when you "may" get pregnant, so you can try to get pregnant or refrain from sex to prevent getting pregnant. For additional protection against pregnancy, you may want to use an alternate form of contraception, like a condom or diaphragm and unscented spermicide during the nine to ten days of possible conception.

The sperm can live up to five days in the cervical fluid while the egg has a very short lifespan–at max 12 to 24 hours. Therefore, it is possible to have intercourse one day but not get pregnant until you ovulate several days later.

To learn more about your cycles and signs of fertility, observe what your body is doing and keep track of (a record) your cycles by charting them. Remember, the process of natural pregnancy and birth is a beautiful time, but the more you are educated about it all, the healthier and easier it will be.

Resources

There are many FREE online programs for cycle charting, such as *tcoyf. com*, and a wonderful book on the topic, *Taking Charge of Your Fertility: The Definitive Guide to Natural Birth Control, Pregnancy Achievement, and Reproductive Health* by Toni Weschler.

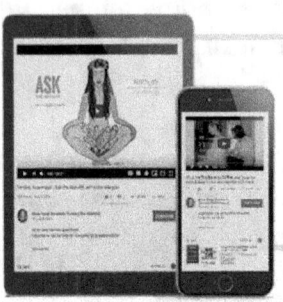

Want to learn more or have more questions?

Grab your free Book Bonuses below:
https://homesweethomebirth.com/nbsbookbonus

The Fertility Awareness Method

Here we are going to get into the entire process of getting pregnant naturally in more detail. Whether you are looking to conceive or prevent pregnancy, getting to know your body will help empower you to take more control of your reproduction and embrace and promote your own optimal health and sexuality. Fertility awareness begins with charting your cycle dates, fertility signs, and your peak fertile days, so you can either conceive or prevent pregnancy. You will note what symptoms are normal for you, along with your typical cyclic changes, so you can also be aware of when something is off. Let's begin learning how to chart your monthly cycle.

What You Will Need

- Pencil and ruler if you like charting using paper
- You can work directly on the online fertility charting programs or practice by printing out several of the charts from Toni Weschler's *Taking Charge of Your Fertility*
- Calendar
- Basal body oral thermometer—NOT any other type, such as a digital thermometer or those applied to the ears or forehead. A highly recommended BBT product is Daysy, that comes with an app to make the tracking much easier.
- Watch

Fertility Awareness Method

The more you chart and practice paying close attention to the clues your body gives you, the better the odds are that you'll achieve your goals. It is done by charting the dates your cyclical symptoms occur and tracking your cervical fluid and your basal body temperatures. It includes noting the following as well: when you have sexual intercourse and any significant life events that may impact your cervical fluid, your temperature, or the length of time between your period and when you ovulate. You can also record other cyclic symptoms you experience.

It is so empowering to know your body before you get pregnant!

Step One

Choose a day in the week you want to begin charting. It is easiest to start on the first day of your period, which is cycle day one. Each subsequent day, you record on the chart "M" for menses or "P" for period bleeding, and the characteristics of the vaginal discharge and cervical fluid you note on the other days. The number of days goes up until you get your period again, and then you start another chart, on day one for the first day of bleeding; or, the number of days of no menses increases because, for example, you are pregnant. Once pregnancy is confirmed you do not need to continue charting.

Charting during breastfeeding is resumed when your cycles return postpartum. How to chart your cycles when breastfeeding and not cycling, as well as when experiencing a variety of other reproductive health issues, are covered in the book Take Charge of Your Fertility by Toni Weschler.

Here are your instructions:

1. Use an online fertility chart or app like Daysy, or print out the fertility chart from this site: *http://www.tcoyf.com/wp-content/uploads/charts/TCOYF%20Pregnancy%20Chart%20-%20Classic%20(F)%20With%20Examples.pdf*

2. **Record the cycle day in the box corresponding to date** "cycle day." For example, if your period begins July 26, you will write "1" in that box. The next day, July 27, is your cycle day "2," and so on.

3. **Check your vaginal and cervical fluid** by looking and feeling it a few times each day when you go to the bathroom, using your thumb and index fingers. This is done by swiping or gently inserting your index finger into your vaginal opening, or looking at and touching the discharge on your underwear or the tissue you used to wipe. Then put the index and thumb together and separate them. What do you see? Or don't see?

4. **Record your observations**, the characteristics of your vaginal discharge—dry, sticky, moist, creamy, wet, stretchy, egg white. Place the appropriate initial in the box under the corresponding cycle day.

5. **On the wet days**, you can note and record the increasing peak wetness sensations by coloring in more squares each progressive day or in a way you can understand.

To Record Your Basal Body Temperature

- Before you get out of bed on each morning (begin after your period has ended), place your basal body thermometer under your arm.
- Wait a few minutes for most BBT thermometers, 60 seconds for Daysy, and then remove the thermometer. Read the temperature and record it on the chart. For example, there's one line with only 98s on it. If your temperature is 98.3° F, then you will note the mercury level is three-line measures above 98. Circle or highlight 98.3 on the chart.
- Note the time in the "Time Temp Taken" at the top.

Basal Body Temperature

Basal body temperature (BBT) refers to your internal body temperature before, during, and after you ovulate; it rises significantly from your preovulatory temperature after ovulation due to the increase in progesterone produced by the corpus luteum in your ovary that released the egg. Why is this so important? Temperature changes are a great predictor that you have ovulated. Typically, it is said that you ovulate between the first and third day of your temperature shift.

For women seeking to conceive, consistently elevated BBTs beyond cycle day 16 to 18 can signify you are pregnant. If you did not conceive or had a possible early miscarriage, it will drop back down. The rise in temperature after ovulation is not like a feverish high. Rather, it is a fraction of a degree above your temperature range between each period and ovulation. Typically, your BBT can rise about 0.4 degrees Fahrenheit or 0.2 degrees Celsius higher than your normal BBT on non-ovulation days, but the rise may be slightly less in some cases. What is really important to remember here is that you're charting your temperature, so that you can see the "changes" to better predict ovulation. This is referred to as your biphasic pattern (showing two levels of temperatures).

Next, circle or highlight the dates you have had intercourse, record other symptoms on days related to your cycle, and note anything that may affect your cervical fluid, like lubricant and intercourse, temperature (like an infectious illness or frequent waking in the middle of the night), or unusual events that happen in the time between your period and ovulation (like travel, unusual stress, or sudden weight changes).

When to Have Sex to Get Pregnant or to Avoid Pregnancy?

Women's fertile window is limited, unlike that of men. A woman is only fertile for 12 to 24 hours per cycle (the lifespan of her egg), BUT sperm can live inside a woman's body for up to five days in fertile cervical fluid. The window for possible conception is around six days in total, allowing for the potential lifespan of the sperm. Women have what are called "dry days." These are the days in your cycle that you notice your vulva and vagina are dryer; your discharge is very scant; you become moist only through sexual stimulation, but other than that, your discharge, vulva, and vagina feel drier.

Once you begin to notice your normal vaginal discharge is increasing to include cervical fluid (regardless of sexual stimulation), you're then considered fertile. That is when to time sexual intercourse (this does not take into account health issues) every day or every other day of your wet days, including your peak day of wetness, which indicates imminent ovulation.

- If you have sex six or more days before you ovulate, you will not conceive, especially if on the evening of a dry day.
- If you have sex 24 hours after you ovulate, you're not very likely to conceive.
- If you time it right and have sex three days leading up to and including the day you ovulate, your chances of conception are at their peak. After day two of ovulation, your chances drastically fall.

If you're looking to prevent pregnancy, consider either abstinence or using other forms of barrier and spermacide contraception during the six days of your peak fertile time, plus a few additional days after ovulation to be extra cautious. On average, that means that you should not have unprotected sexual intercourse approximately six days BEFORE you ovulate (during your wet days), and for extra confidence, you should abstain three days after ovulation. So, the evening of the fourth dry day and consecutive rise of your BBT, you are not fertile and pregnancy is highly unlikely from having unprotected sexual intercourse during this time.

To use this method to prevent pregnancy, make sure you chart several cycles and know your fertile and non-fertile times, before relying on it alone.

Additionally, this chart gives you many other characteristics to record and factor into your understanding of your cycles. For example, if you're on IVF, medications, taking supplements and herbs, had any relevant diagnostic or treatment procedures, you can include this relevant information. You can track in this chart if you experience any premenstrual symptoms (PMS) or one-sided low pelvic pain or aching around ovulation. You will also find boxes relating to your cervix. It is an optional assessment to learn what your cervix feels like throughout your cycle. Was it high? Low? Open? Closed?

Once you record several cycles, you will notice a pattern: your range, your normal variations during each cycle and from cycle to cycle. Then you can more easily use this information to get pregnant or prevent pregnancy. You can use this information to know about your reproductive cyclic details and health–like when you ovulate, when you most likely can conceive, when you are probably pregnant, when you may be miscarrying, when you are not fertile, when you did not yet ovulate, when something is not normal for you. Remember, you are most fertile during your wettest days, peak wetness, and on the day of ovulation. Once your basal body temperature rises, you know you have ovulated.

With this knowledge, mamas can TAKE CHARGE OF THEIR FERTILITY to either prevent pregnancy or try to become pregnant, learn when they conceived and know even when they are pregnant before a positive pregnancy test. This is the name of one of my favorite books on the subject, a book I've mentioned a few times already: Toni Weschler's Taking Charge of Your Fertility.

To enhance your fertility, pregnancy, and birth--it also helps to connect with nature and nourish your connection with it. Your body is nature and has its own biological clock. You might want to look into how your body's biological clock relates to the moon cycles (a very interesting study). It helps to connect with the rest of who you are—your heart, your gut, your spirit—and get out of the busy overthinking, worrying, calculating mind that has become way too dependent on man-made, digital precision of industrialized time. Stay present in each precious moment, the only place where life exists. Surrender to what you cannot control of the natural world, and learn ways to relax yourself and tap into a state of inner calm. I love yoga, breathwork, and mindfulness so much because it provides us with tools for doing this.

Determining the Due Date

For mamas who know their date of conception, more details about their cycles, and their past pregnancy history (when they went into labor previously and what the gestational age assessment was of each of their babies), then they can determine a much more accurate due date than basing it solely on the first date of their last period. This is one of many ways mamas can become empowered and proactive.

Most mamas like to count baby's toes and fingers. What about the creases? Abundant creases on the soles of baby's feet are simply one of several signs a baby is "post-term," born in the weeks past the estimated due date, when the baby was ready to be born. It is one of the assessments we use to calculate the new baby's gestational age (how many weeks the baby is in utero).

I marvel how this calculation often differs from standard pregnancy dating. I had a mama in my practice who came to me with her previous four pregnancies. Her previous four babies were born four weeks after her estimated due date had I calculated it based on the first day of her last period alone; but they actually arrived at just the right time, all were evaluated to be term (meaning not late), with minimal foot creases. I used a variety of other assessments, including past history, cycle characteristics, and when she had intercourse, to get a more accurate dating for her latest (fifth) pregnancy.

What Is the Due Date and How Can You More Accurately Help Calculate It to Prevent False Diagnosis of Postdates and Their Associated Risks of Induction?

The estimated due date is just that—an estimate of when a mom and baby of a healthy pregnancy will go into labor. It is an estimate of how many weeks old your fetus is at any stage of your pregnancy, which is important to know, as this impacts your maternity care and the wellbeing of you and your baby. If you go into labor, you and your provider need to know that your baby is term and there are no issues with the baby's gestational age.

For example, if you go into labor at a certain point before your estimated due date, it's critical to know if it is too early for your baby to be born, as your preterm baby would be at increased risk and need intensive care, so efforts would be made to try to stop the labor.

Likewise, if you are past your given due date, in many modern obstetrical practices, in an attempt to avoid the small risks of postdates for babies, risks that increase after 42 weeks, there is a cascade of interventions from frequent testing of fetal wellbeing to induction when you are not really due or ready to labor yet. Postdate pregnancy then can lead to increased stress, more painful, harder labor, the need for anesthesia and other interventions that may culminate in an unplanned cesarean birth. Actually, only 5% of women give birth on their due date, even with the most accurately assessed pregnancy dating. I prefer the language "due month," as most babies come a few weeks before or after that estimated due date—more commonly a week or more after it for first-time mamas.

So, when speaking about due dates and postdates, I like to start with education and prevention during preconception, before a woman gets pregnant. And even if pregnant, we can still do some detective work and might come up with helpful information that can impact a woman's pregnancy dating. I advise women to know their fascinating bodies and menstrual cycles, to track how often their periods come, when they have signs of ovulation, and when they had or did not have intercourse.

I certainly have other date assessment skills I use and other suggestions to help each mama on a more personal level, but these are great places mamas can start. No obstetrical provider or any human can predict when a mama will go into labor. So, one of the great lessons of pregnancy is being okay with not knowing. You might as well enjoy the journey and surrender to a higher intelligence and power over which we are not in control.

In today's times, I do feel compelled to debunk some myths. As I indicated above, the due date is not written in stone. It is an estimate around an average time of when mamas go into labor, plus or minus a few weeks on either side. Although I like referring to the "due month," that has not taken hold in the modern obstetric community, obsessed with measurements. At least we can use it between us and with your extended families, who tend to call you every day after your estimated due date to find out if you had your baby yet.

Yes, now we have the ultrasound to help with estimating the due date. If an ultrasound is done in the first trimester by a practitioner with expertise in pregnancy dating, the accuracy of the estimated due date increases a bit. But not all mamas want a sonogram. And dating sonograms are not always completely accurate, especially when done later in pregnancy. Again, only about 5% of babies are born on their estimated due dates anyway. And it is often miscalculated, if based alone on the first date of the last menstrual period. That date calculation only applies if a mama's cycle comes every 28 days, assuming she ovulated on day 14, and that still could mean the baby could be born on average between 37 and 42 weeks. Healthy term babies can also be born before or after this timeframe.

My pregnancy dating wheel has been with me as long as I can remember. Now it's online. I like the ones that take cycle length and date of conception into consideration. Most women having regular cycles have variation, with sometimes as much as 21 to 45 days between them. And that is normal. There are many factors such as stress, illness, and travel, that can prolong the time between the last period and the next ovulation, but once a woman ovulates, the next period comes close to 14 days later—unless she conceived shortly before or at ovulation.

As a nurse since 1985 and a midwife since 1995, I meet many women who are well informed and know their bodies and histories, and many who are not familiar but are very eager to get empowered and learn more. I have had plenty of women know their exact date of conception from fertility treatments and go into labor weeks before or after their due dates. I have had women who knew exactly when they conceived as they were keeping track, only had intercourse once at or before ovulation. And they gave birth close to the estimated due date.

And I have had women not have a clue about their cycles or when they got pregnant. Each mama and story are different. But more often than realized, modern medicine does not know nearly as much as people might expect.

Oh, the journey of waiting and not knowing when, a journey that has been traveled by billions of women since the beginning of time. It's part of the sacred wonder, including any surprises along the way. Welcome to the Tribe de Mama where we get more and more familiar with nature's own clock. As we realize there is so much we cannot control, we learn to get comfortable with not knowing.

Ready to learn more about this breakthrough method?

Watch my video and get started: *https://homesweethomebirth.com/ nbsbookbonus*

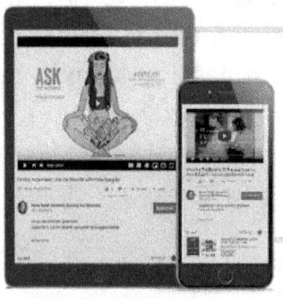

Want to learn more or have more questions?

Grab your free Book Bonuses below:
https://homesweethomebirth.com/nbsbookbonus

A Healthy and Optimal Pregnancy

Three Keys for a Healthy Pregnancy and Birth

With any pregnancy, your hope and deepest desire as a mother is to birth a healthy and beautiful baby, whether you are birthing in a hospital, a freestanding birthing center, or at home. Let's review three keys for improving your chance of having an easier, healthy journey to birth.

Key 1—Maintain a Healthy Physical Wellbeing

Whether you're pregnant or not, there is an almost infinite number of benefits that come with eating fresh, nutritious, and colorful foods, taking supplements, and exercising regularly. Because the next chapter discusses the ideal diet and supplements during pregnancy, we'll look at exercise in this chapter.

Our bodies are meant to move and be active. Exercising throughout all of the trimesters as well as beyond pregnancy creates numerous benefits for you and your unborn baby. Healthy pregnant women are not powerless, but quite capable and strong, and exercise will help you to feed that spirit of strength and vibrancy. If you engage in regular exercise that you enjoy, you will have a more comfortable pregnancy and be less prone to injury. You'll be more able to assume positions that allow for easier active birthing and so you will be more likely to have a shorter, easier labor. You'll also have a quicker recovery, and your body will bounce back faster postpartum.

You may notice more relief from various discomforts like constipation, bloating, swelling, and backaches. You will feel more relaxed and notice an overall sense of wellbeing and energy, even when fatigued. Being active helps maintain a healthy amount of weight gain in pregnancy, stabilize your blood sugar levels, and prevent complications like obesity and gestational diabetes.

If you've exercised consistently throughout your pregnancy, your baby is more likely to have higher Apgar scores (a method to quickly summarize the health of newborns at birth, and the need for emergency help), will transition better outside the womb, and will even develop better cognitive skills in early childhood. Studies have also shown that your baby will be leaner at birth (making them easier to push out) and will be less prone to childhood obesity.

If you are already healthy and active, I encourage you to continue doing the type of exercise you love now that you are pregnant. There are, of course, some exceptions, like extreme and contact sports.

Make it fun! Get 30 to 45 minutes of moderate, varied exercise most days of the week while remaining in tune to your body's needs. This can include muscle-toning and strengthening workouts as well as stretching, aerobics, and dance.

Some types of yoga satisfy all of the above requirements as well. I'm a certified yoga teacher and big proponent of yoga during pregnancy, so much so that you'll find an entire chapter dedicated to it in this book. Yoga is a particularly useful form of exercise for pregnant women because it marries safe movement and breath. It's also a wonderful way to feel more calm, focused, and grounded; essential tools for labor and mamahood.

If you have never exercised before, you can start by taking brisk walks, joining a prenatal yoga, fitness, or dance class, or learning how to swim laps. Vary it up, do what you enjoy and feels fun. On days you can't get out, do an awesome online African dance workout like at Kukuwa Fitness, or home yoga at YogaGlo which both have classes for expecting and postpartum moms as well. Listen to your body, modify your exercise as needed, and maintain a healthy, varied whole-food diet with good hydration. Eating well and exercising regularly will not only keep you and your baby healthy, but your baby will also be in tune with and benefit immensely from the greater amount of energy, inner peace, and positivity that you feel.

Key 2—Reduce Your Stress

Modern life is stressful, and inner stress is definitely not the feeling you want shadowing your pregnancy, your baby's birth, or your mamahood. Take some quiet time with yourself (and your baby) to determine what kind of perspective you're operating from as well as what state of mind you want to impart on your child from as early on as possible in the womb.

Spending energy on the things you can't change—which is most of life—leads to pointless angst and worry. Adopt an attitude of surrender and acceptance for the things over which you have no power. Admittedly, it is not easy to embrace this re-framed way of thinking, but well worth your efforts! And this should not discourage action if it can and does need to be taken.

Instead, focus on what you can change: yourself. You can change and control your attitude, perspective, reactions, choices, and behaviors. This involves a deep and personal look at the thoughts and emotions you host. It takes work but leads to growth that is beyond rewarding and transformative.

Cultivate a spiritual awareness and connection to the magnificent soul within you as it relates to the infinite. Trust that everything happens for your ultimate benefit and growth, even if you don't understand why. Listen to your heart and gut, and live from a place in which what you think, feel, say, and do are in harmony.

Get adequate rest by going to bed at a similar time each night, ideally before 10:00 pm, and aim for seven to eight hours of sleep or more.

Take breaks throughout the day and at least a half-hour power nap in the afternoon. You can also assume a restorative yoga pose like savasana by closing your eyes and quietly focusing only on your breathing. This kind of practice for 20 minutes can be equivalent to two hours of sleep for your body.

Master breathwork, relaxation techniques, and meditation—as addressed in the chapter "Meditation, Breathwork, and Visualization"–to activate your own internal calm.

Beware of over-scheduling yourself. Don't be afraid to ask family and friends for assistance and consider hiring help. Cut down on the non-essential burdens in your life, especially if you feel overwhelmed.

This is all easier said than done, so let your days be filled with what's most important to you and let go of the things that really don't matter. Slow down, just be and fully live your life; don't rush through it.

Monotask rather than multitask! Try to focus on doing one thing at a time with your full attention and make a conscious decision to do fewer tasks each day. Unplug daily by limiting your phone and internet use as well as your screen time. This will not only help you feel better, but also allow you to accomplish more by doing less.

Schedule downtime and guard it fiercely. Do whatever you want as long as it is restful and restorative and has nothing to do with work, chores, being online, or running errands.

Spend quiet time each day to connect to your baby. Talk to your baby. Sing to your baby. Play beautiful music to your baby. Your baby relaxes when you do, and your baby hears and loves these precious moments.

Key 3—Cultivate a Healthy, Supportive Environment

This may be last on the list, but please don't take for granted the value that a fiercely loving support system and environment brings to your pregnancy and childbirth. Uncomfortable, stressful, or even inauthentic surroundings, for example, can surreptitiously raise the discomfort and tension in your body and mind.

A destructive and harmful environment can be just as toxic to your system as any processed or chemically-altered food. Being mindful of your environment can help support your steps for enhancing your wellbeing. In finding the right support system, you'll be adding tremendous value to your experience like finding other like-minded women and partnering with a midwife or doctor that you trust, admire, and whose primary concern is you and your baby.

Women have supported women in community living since the beginning of time. It takes a village to raise a child as well as a new parent. Today, even more importantly, I encourage mamas to create a fortress of positivity around themselves. Hang out with calming, positive, uplifting, empowering, and inspiring people as much as possible. If you do not know any, you can create your own tribe of like-minded mamas—they are out there.

Get off social media and make deeper in-person connections that better nourish your soul. Seek out other women who have a similar outlook regarding holistic health and wellness in pregnancy, labor, birth, breastfeeding, and parenting. Make friends at prenatal yoga class, childbirth class, pregnancy and postpartum support groups, attachment or holistic parenting and babywearing groups, and La Leche League meetings.

If you do not have these resources in your area, create your own. Host a Positive Birth Movement circle, movie screening, or a book reading. Organize a community Blessingway/mother-blessing, a Red Tent event, or a pregnancy day retreat. Create a gathering of pregnant mamas and invite a prenatal henna artist or massage therapist. Do belly casting/art with each other—you name it!

Each one of these tips stands on its own with tremendous value. However, when you combine your healthy eating and exercise habits with your low-stress lifestyle and supportive community, there's no question you'll love your healthier pregnancy and life even more.

Every expectant mother has a right to inner tranquility and a radiant joy.

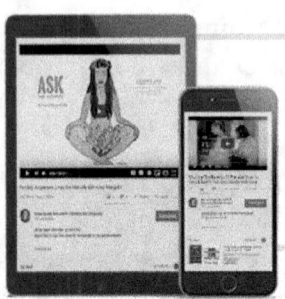

**Want to learn more or
have more questions?**

Grab your free Book Bonuses below:
https://homesweethomebirth.com/nbsbookbonus

Nutritional Best Practices for Mom

Now that we have gone over how to become aware of your cycle and how it impacts your ability to get pregnant, keys to a healthy pregnancy and birth in general, we are going to talk about being pregnant in greater detail. It's the perfect time to wholly dedicate yourself to your health and wellbeing, and doing so will yield lifelong benefits, not only for you but also for your baby and your family. The path is clear, but walking it is up to you. It takes commitment and self-discipline. It might be more expensive to live healthfully, but doing so begets prevention. It's ultimately easier and cheaper than the cost of treating chronic diseases caused by harmful lifestyle habits. It's also especially rewarding to really look and feel your best and improve the quality of all areas of your life.

The decision to take charge of your health can be overwhelming. Make change a little bit at a time rather than all at once. Unless you have health issues that require 100% detoxing, resetting, and healing, consider living by the 80-20 rule, mentioned already in the "Preparing for Pregnancy" chapter. To reiterate, if you can achieve optimal habits 80% of the time, you're doing beautifully! Don't criticize yourself while you go through this transformation. We are all perfectly imperfect, doing our best with what we know and face each day. Instead of criticism, give yourself a hug for doing what you can right now. You just may surprise yourself later when you are able to accomplish more and more. You are welcome to give it your 100%! I have been doing 99% to 100% for many years. Like me, many feel so wonderful living healthfully that they no longer want to live otherwise. Yes, there are things I would never eat or even enjoy as I know too much about what is in it, how I feel afterwards, and how it impacts my health. But, when I go out or travel, I must chose the best of what options are available. Thankfully, many places now have healthy options.

What to Eat: Breaking It Down

Eat mostly a wide variety of fresh, whole, unrefined plant-based foods. They should be the majority of your diet. Ideally, eat organic, locally-grown food, free of chemical fertilizers, pesticides, synthetic additives, preservatives and dyes, artificial sweeteners, processed sugars, refined vegetable oils, and genetic modification. Most women feel their best physically and emotionally on a Paleo-type of diet, which basically means eating whole plant and animal foods, the types that could be obtained through gathering and hunting. It is a diet based on how our ancestors ate for thousands of years, without modern day ailments and chronic disease. Vegan and vegetarian diets are fine if you make sure to get all of what you need from organic foods that are whole and unrefined and that you supplement what you cannot.

I was a vegetarian until I became pregnant, for ethical and what I thought to be health reasons. I will never forget the shocked reactions from my family and friends, the look on my husband's face when he came home from work and I was insisting on meat. I needed meat! I had a craving for schwarma. It is what I once had while backpacking in the countries bordering the Mediterranean Sea. There was no internet then, but he looked in the yellow pages and found a place that became his stop before coming home each evening. Our bodies know what they need, we just need to listen.

Read ingredients and know what you are eating. Your plate should be beautiful and colorful, reflecting an abundance and variety of fresh, unprocessed foods with plenty of vegetables, fruits, whole and sprouted grains, beans, and some nuts and seeds, seasoned with fresh herbs and spices. If you want to add additional sweetener, use raw honey or maple syrup that contain nutritional value without the negative effects of sugar in all its forms. Use Himalayan sea salt to taste, as it is full of health enhancing ionized minerals. Ditch the middle food aisles in supermarkets where the processed items are generally located. For the freshest, top-quality whole-food products, shop at local organic farm stands, farmers markets, food co-ops, and health food stores, which are now online with delivery services. Or better yet, grow your own!

The foods listed below should be proportioned according to your individual needs, but the following is an approximate breakdown.

The Naturally Colorful Plate

The majority of your diet should consist of foods that grow. Each day, eat lots of fresh green, yellow, orange, red, and purple vegetables prepared raw, lightly steamed, sautéed, baked, roasted, or simmered in soup. Include root and sea veggies like radishes, rutabega, parsnips, turnips, kelp, dulse, or sushi nori. Each day, eat four- to five-plus cups of cooked or raw low-carb veggies like zucchini, asparagus, broccoli, cauliflower, green beans, cabbage, pepper, cucumber, or tomatoes. Additionally, eat two-plus cups of uncooked, dark leafy greens like kale, romaine, chard, and spinach, and a side of the high-carb veggies like sweet potatoes, carrots, beets, and winter squash. Get your daily dose of naturally fermented probiotics, in drinks like kombucha and veggies as in kimchi.

Eat two to four servings of fruits daily. Sample serving sizes include one apple, pear, or peach; one small banana; one avocado; one cup of berries. Also include at least a handful of fresh raw or lightly dry-roasted seeds, such as sunflower, pumpkin, and sesame, or nuts, such as coconut, almond, pecan, cashew, hazelnut, pistachio, black walnut, peanut, or two tablespoons of nut butters. Pregnant and nursing women need 75 to 100 grams of protein daily. I suggest one serving at each of your three main meals and with every snack. Servings are approximately the size the of your hand.

If you are eating animal protein, it should ideally be organic, raised without hormones and antibiotics, and free-range to eat their natural diet of grasses and plants that have not been sprayed with chemicals. Basically, this is how animals were traditionally raised before mass production and supermarkets! Today, we have the added benefit of testing animals and their products for infection to ensure they are safe for consumption. Examples include: beef, chicken, duck, Cornish hens, turkey, lamb, wild game like buffalo and venison, liver, pastured eggs (including the yellow and white), and wild-caught fish from non-polluted waters, such as Alaskan or Norwegian salmon. Liver is a superfood loaded with vitamins, minerals and antioxidants, so eat it twice weekly; if you are not a liver fan, a tablespoon of desiccated liver powder can be added to soups, meat, vegetable dishes, casseroles, and stews to boost the nutritional value, and it may be a more palatable option. Again, make sure it is organic and pastured.

Many co-ops and health food stores sell wild-caught fresh fish that has been tested free of many dangerous pollutants. These fish are safe to eat four to five times per week. Fish is one of the ideal animal proteins, loaded with omega three essential fatty acids. Adding a teaspoon of contaminant-free cod liver oil to your soup, salad, cooked food or smoothie is a great way to get some additional omega threes, and fat soluble vitamins D and A; it is very mild tasting, and is often flavored with lemon or herbs like rosemary. There is no limit to eating pastured organic eggs, meat, and poultry—listen to your body and follow its healthy cravings.

If you are eating milk products, use only those that are fresh and organic, ideally from grass-fed animals like goats or sheep. Examples: fresh raw goat/sheep milk, yogurt, kefir, feta, or cheddar, and buffalo mozzarella. These are often available at farm stands, farmers' markets, co-ops, or health food stores. Minimize or avoid cow dairy. Most dairy products at the supermarket, even if organic, have been pasteurized, which is important to kill harmful bacteria and prolong shelf-life from farm to market, but this also destroys key digestive enzymes and nutrients. Raw dairy products in standard markets that have not been pasteurized do carry a risk of certain infections like listeria, which can be serious for babies in the womb, so eating raw dairy needs to be fresh from a farm that tests for such harmful bacteria.

Sources of vegan protein include raw or dry-roasted nuts, nut butters, and nut milks without added sweetener and chemicals, like organic coconut, almond, macadamia, pistachio or hazelnut; seeds and products made from them like tahini; legumes (beans, peas, and lentils) and bean dips like hummus; and 'grains' like quinoa. Minimize soy, unless it's organic, not genetically modified, and is fermented, like tempeh or miso. Other good sources include vegan protein powder, such as rice, pea, and hemp, as well as nutritional yeast. Add two to three tablespoons to fruit/veggie smoothies or hot whole-grain cereal.

Making Sense of Protein Grams

- 3 large eggs = 18 g
- 6 oz salmon = 46 g
- 6 oz chicken = 48 g
- 1 cup of lentils = 18 g
- 1 cup almonds = 20g
- 4 tablespoons of peanut butter = 16 g
- 1 cup quinoa = 8 g
- 3 oz ground beef = 18 g
- 1 cup Greek yogurt = 23 g
- 4 tablespoons of tahini = 10.4 g
- 4 tablespoons of hummus = 4 g

Pregnant women, growing children, breast-feeding women, those with illness, injury, and certain health conditions, like depression, anxiety, mood swings, and low blood sugar need more protein and fat divided over each meal and snacks, and often feel better off gluten, cane sugar, and cow dairy. If you feel well eating grains and are not gluten intolerant, have one serving a day of grains in their whole form, like one slice of sprouted multi-grain bread, a half-cup of cooked oatmeal, or one ounce of dry multigrain cereal. Vary the grains you eat, and don't only eat wheat.

There are many grains to choose from, such as stone-ground or sprouted whole wheat like Ezekiel bread, whole spelt, oats, rye, and barley. Gluten-free options include rice, millet, quinoa, and kasha/buckwheat. You can get gluten-free oats as well. When you combine them with foods such as beans, chickpeas, lentils, split peas, seeds, or nuts, you create a complete protein.

The Importance of Fat in Your Diet

Your body needs a liberal amount of fat, but choose healthy, high-quality fats, which have more omega-three fatty acids than omega-six fatty acids to counteract the modern overexposure to omega-six fatty acids.* Avoid polyunsaturated oils like cottonseed, safflower, sunflower, corn, and soy. Avoid partially hydrogenated fats such as vegetable shortening and margarine as well as refined vegetable oils that have been heated to high temperatures. Use only organic, cold, expeller-pressed oils like extra virgin olive (great for salads and sautéed veggies), coconut oil, and organic pastured clarified butter like ghee (ideally goat) for cooking, baking, and sautéing at high temperatures. Never heat olive oil so high to the point of smoking. Nuts, seeds, and avocados are wonderful sources of fat, but use their oils for cold food only. Storing oils, nuts, and seeds in the fridge preserves their shelf life. If they do not taste or smell good, throw them out, as they have started to oxidize and become carcinogenic.

*Ideally omega-three and six fatty acid intake should be equal in ratio per traditional ancestral diets before there was mass production of foods and supermarkets.

Don't Forget Water

Drink good water and plenty of it. I recommend eight to ten glasses, the equivalent of 64 ounces, thus a half-gallon, daily. Or drink half your body weight in fluid ounces. Good water is spring or well water, full of charge and energy. It has a high reduction potential to detoxify, anti-oxidize free radicals, and hydrate. Obtained fresh from mountain springs or deep in the earth, it is rich in minerals with an alkaline pH and free of chemical pollutants and heavy metals. Since many of us do not live near pure mountain springs and clean wells, the next best option is to drink filtered water, which can be ionized with a Kangen unit. You can install a comprehensive filter like Radiant Life under your kitchen sink or use a portable Clearly Filtered pitcher. Otherwise, fresh glass or stainless steel bottled spring water are great options. To protect your skin, the largest organ of your body, instead of a kitchen sink filter, it is ideal to get an excellent general water filter like Radiant Life filter installed for your home that removes most of the chemicals that come in through the pipes, so that all faucets have pure safe drinking water and to make the water you brush your teeth with and bathe in as pure as possible, without toxic chemicals like chlorine and its gas form that is released with showering.

Ideally, drink mostly in the day, two to three glasses of water at least 20 to 30 minutes before each meal, and a few glasses in between, at least two hours after meals. Have no more than a cup during actual meals, as it dilutes the enzymes needed for digestion and absorption of nutrients. You can add some natural flavor like a slice of lemon, grapefruit, orange, watermelon, cucumber, or mint leaves to taste. But know that pure water is best to hydrate you. Other fluids, like juiced fruits and veggies, even herbal teas, and broths are potentially dehydrating. They are fine to ingest in addition, especially when advised for healing particular issues, but not instead of your recommended daily pure water intake to feel fully and wonderfully hydrated.

How Our World Has Changed

Our ancestors did not take supplements. I often wonder if we are healthier than our ancestors or not. We do know that those communities that followed traditional ancestral diets around the world, did not suffer from chronic diseases of modern times, beginning with the pioneering research done by Dr. Weston A. Price. Modern-day living has benefits, but also comes at great cost to our well-being on so many levels. Although we have more knowledge now, "progress" has had deleterious consequences. As the population increased, consumerism increased, along with the overuse of resources without awareness or concern for the effects, and the world has more pollution now. Industrialization, processing, and pesticides have increased, which adds toxicity to the food that is not as nutrient-dense as it was in the past when we ate from hunting and gathering, small, local farms, and wild-growing produce and gardens.

Organic whole food eating is basically eating real food as it was before it was sprayed with chemicals, highly-processed, and refined. Standard farming practices entail animals being given grains sprayed with unmonitored pesticides to fatten them up cheaply, hormones to boost milk production, and antibiotics to treat infection that develops from overproduction of milk and the inability to be active from confinement. At one time, animals were free to roam pastures, free to eat their natural, varied green diet and use their muscles.

Pasteurization came about to increase the shelf life of dairy, but it destroys the enzymes needed to digest and process milk, as well as its vitamins. The mass production and industrialization of food also messes with the soil, which further contributes to the lessening of essential nutrients it used to have, which made the food nutrient-rich naturally. So much of what is called food now is so refined that its original form is gone. The outer part of grains, for example, is removed and processed down to get white flour, which is basically sugar without the nutrients and fiber. Then they supplement it with synthetic vitamins, help it rise with synthetic yeast that also raises the gluten content, and color it with artificial dyes to make it look more appealing to sell, and add in chemicals to alter it and preservatives so that it lasts longer from factory transport to the supermarket shelves. Most products labeled as "food" found in the middle aisles of typical supermarkets and fast-food restaurants that have ingredients many cannot pronounce, let alone recognize, are loaded with various forms of sugar and unhealthy fats. This has contributed to a wide array of symptoms of dis-ease and multiple health problems from obesity, lactose, casein and gluten intolerance to mental illness, inflammatory conditions, adult-onset diabetes, heart disease, high cholesterol, hypertension, and cancer.

The standard diet is really empty of necessary nutrition and most busy, stressed-out moms in the modern world do not eat all of what is needed for their own health or that of their pregnancy, even if they do try to eat healthfully.

Many articles you read today will mention how we have gotten away from a hands-on lifestyle. We don't grow our own food anymore and have moved into a place of what is convenient and affordable ... at least in the short-term. What people may not realize is the higher cost of eating healthfully today pays off with huge savings from healthier lives and less need for medical care over the long haul.

It's actually a really exciting time right now because we are recognizing that we need to slow down and cultivate a more conscious lifestyle based on mindfulness. It's not just theory anymore, as it's more popular than ever to live a life of awareness. This includes consciously incorporating natural toiletries, cosmetics, and household cleansers into our lives, nourishing ourselves with whole real and pure foods, and removing toxins that can be found in processed foods, beauty and cleaning products.

Many of us recognize that we have grown out of alignment with our true nature and it's time to get back to our original design ... get back in touch with the cyclic nature of our human bodies, our minds, and our spirits, as well as eat foods our bodies are meant to eat.

As written in Gurmukh Kau Khalsa's book, Bountiful, Beautiful, Blissful: Experience the Natural Power of Pregnancy and Birth with Kundalini Yoga and Meditation: "Centripetal energy is the grounding force that makes women the centers of their households. When a woman elevates her life for the better, her entire family benefits because she sets a new level of awareness and clarity in the home. Good nutrition is one of the central pillars of a healthy pregnancy."

Supplements I Recommend

I am often asked what supplements I recommend and why. I like to recommend what I do and do what I recommend. After all, for me to promote a practice or a product, I must believe in and love it. And when I find gold, I like to share it so others can benefit. I have given birth to four babies. I was too nauseous to supplement in the first trimester each time, but when that passed, as far back as I can remember, I was very devoted to eating and living healthfully. And I took my supplements daily. I was blessed with feeling wonderful and having wonderful vitality, and I rarely got sick. I knew my wellbeing had a lot to do with my habits, and my supplements played a huge role. Getting my little ones to supplement as I did was challenging; I was happy when they took to the basics. My husband did not take any supplements, no matter what I said. He just wasn't interested. But he was sick often, and I still remain unsurprised.

I just love to feel awesome, and once I touched that feeling, I wanted to keep it and help others feel their absolute best too.

So, what's my personal supplement magic? I take whole-food, organic supplements from trusted, high-quality, professional-grade companies like Innate Response. I take a multivitamin/mineral combination, vitamin C, D, methylated B complex, calcium, and magnesium. I also take Nordic Naturals or Vital Choice omega-three fatty acids DHA/EPA from wild-caught fish in waters tested free of toxic pollution, evening primrose oil for omega-six fatty acids, and natural immune support supplements. I take these every day, plus superfoods and additional natural remedies as needed periodically. Since I am not pregnant, my recommendations for pregnant women are different. Let's look at those recommendations.

I advise the following whole-food, organic supplements to pregnant mamas. Like what I personally take, I recommend quality, trusted brands like Innate Response, Nordic Naturals, and Vital Choice, but there are plenty of others in my online holistic apothecary, accessible on my website. Here are the supplements I recommend:

- **Prenatal multivitamins with minerals.** For women that aren't pregnant or breastfeeding, the already-mentioned brands above make wonderful multivitamins with minerals. Make sure the 800 to 1,000 mg folic acid and vitamin B12 in the supplement are in the methylated, most absorbable and safe form.
- **Fish oil.** Be sure it is free of pollutants; at least 300 mg each DHA/EPA, one to two times daily.
- **Vitamin D3.** I recommend 1,000 to 2,000 units daily or up to 5,000 units per day if blood levels are low (under 50-70). Take this with the calcium and magnesium supplement.
- **Calcium and magnesium.** Up to 1,200 to 1,500 mg each in divided doses. The amounts I advise are dependent upon diet and lifestyle evaluation.
- **Herbal iron.** As needed, especially with low iron stores (ferritin) and advancing pregnancy. The dose is dependent upon labs and evaluation of symptoms. As a wonderful adjunct

to the supplements, superfoods like powdered or freshly juiced greens can be added to veggies and fruit smoothies. Herbal sources of iron like **nettle** or **yellow dock root** can be made in the form of a drinkable infusion.

- **B-Complex**. I advise 20 to 50 mg, especially to support the stress response, and 1,000 to 5,000 mcg of sublingual methylated B12 if lab levels are below 600 (especially for a vegan or vegetarian, or there are symptoms of deficiency from constipation, trouble sleeping, fatigue and low energy, to anxiety, depression, and neurologic issues).
- **Probiotics**. In addition to eating naturally lactose-fermented foods like pickles, sauerkraut, kimchi, and kombucha, which support your normal gut flora essential for the microbiome and the crucial role that it plays in both physical and mental health, in pregnancy, take additional probiotics. Colon and urogenital-specific, mega-probiotics have been demonstrated to help prevent group B vaginal strep that normally live in the lower intestines. If group B strep grows in the vaginal canal during pregnancy, it can increase the risk of potentially serious newborn infection if exposed in labor/birth. I have had much success with Klaire Labs Therbiotic and Green's First Women's Probiotic that survives obstacles like stomach acid.

When not pregnant, there are other formulas to maintain a healthy balance of good flora. Probiotics boost your immune system, help restore the microbiome after taking antibiotics, and help with intestinal issues and other physical and mental health conditions.

Herbal Infusion

Drink the following herbal infusion daily, which is rich in necessary nutrients and is specifically nourishing for pregnancy, birth, and postpartum:

Place one ounce of dried red raspberry leaf and one ounce of dried nettle leaf in a quart-sized glass canning jar. Fill it with boiling water, cover, and steep for at least two to four hours at room temperature. Strain and place in a covered pitcher.

You can make it in larger quantities and store it in the fridge.

For taste, dilute it with water or steep for less time (but no less than half an hour), add lemon or lime juice, mint leaves, or a teaspoon of honey. Drink one to four cups daily, hot or cold.

Use organic bulk herbs, or you can grow and dry your own.

The Mind-Body Connection

Supplements are meant to provide additional support to a well-rounded diet plan. The thoughts we think and the perspective we carry during pregnancy work with our bodies and what we put into it. Putting good thoughts and positive energy into our minds is a supplement of its own that simply makes your progress that much better.

The 80-20 rule teaches us that there is no such thing as perfection. Every woman that I work with is doing the best she can, and I encourage all women to take this time to slow down, eat mindfully, listen to her body, and take things one step at a time. Any positive choice incorporated is a great one.

For more information, watch my video on supplements : *https://homesweethomebirth.com/nbsbookbonus*

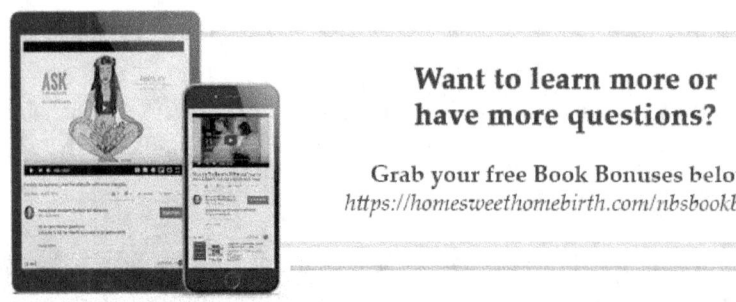

Want to learn more or have more questions?

Grab your free Book Bonuses below:
https://homesweethomebirth.com/nbsbookbonus

Yoga for Pregnancy and Labor

"Most people have no idea how good their body is designed to feel."

—Kevin Trudeau

ountain. Half Moon. Pigeon. Dancer. These are the English words for some well-known "asanas" (or poses) that make up the yoga vocabulary. Most people–especially the uninitiated–equate the practice of yoga with physical exercise. But movement is only the beginning.

Any authentic yogi will tell you that yoga is not just about holding postures and moving the body. A huge component of yoga teaches us to move and breathe consciously with awareness. Breathing in and out sounds like a cliché, doesn't it? The truth is that yoga is partially a practice of breathing. This delivers well-documented and numerous benefits that can be accessed anytime in order to achieve a sense of calm and wellbeing. I'll add to this in the next chapter, where I provide breathwork-specific practices, because breathwork is simply that powerful for pregnant women and mothers.

Pregnant women are often surprised when I encourage them to try yoga prenatally, even if they have never practiced before. They observe their growing bellies and wonder how in the world they could ever bend their bodies into even the most benign of poses. But I tell them that if they have the slightest curiosity, they should check out a prenatal yoga class. As a midwife, I see the difference in laboring women who practice yoga–whether they are advanced veterans or prenatal novices. That difference is often expressed in how a woman breathes, how she moves, how she stays in the present moment and how she copes.

Why is staying in the present moment especially important? Because when a laboring woman is too much in her head, she gets wrapped up with all kinds of thoughts that do her no good–how long has this been going on? When is the baby coming? How many more of these before the baby is born? Can I do this? Whose idea was this, anyway? This worrying thinking uses up precious energy; energy that is required for the 24 or 52 or 4 more sensations to come and for the birthing of her baby. When a woman stays mindful in labor, she copes when she needs to, and she rests when she needs to. That rest–and the ability to reduce her whole body to noodles even if only for a few minutes at a time–will be of tremendous service.

Make no mistake–yoga doesn't make labor all rainbows and candy corn. But it does offer many invaluable benefits. For example, increased flexibility, strength, balance, toning and stamina–all of these things help a woman in labor to have more energy, maintain certain positions for active birthing, and encourage her baby to move down and her body to open.

Let's return to yoga's great teachings around the value of breathing. "Did she actually just say that?" you're asking yourself. "The value of breathing? The value is obvious because it is in staying alive!" But let's put this into the context of labor. Often, when we are anxious or fearful, our fight-or-flight response kicks in, and we either become shallow, rapid breathers, or, even worse, breath-holders. These states do nothing to serve us in labor and can actually gunk up the works.

Yoga practice teaches us to slow and deepen our breathing, which spreads oxygen and "prana" (life force) to every cell in our bodies. When we do this, our brain thanks us, our limbs and digits thank us, our muscles and joints and bones thank us. And most of all, our central nervous system thanks us. When this happens, our heartbeat slows, our blood pressure lowers, our shoulders drop, we experience discomfort less acutely and are showered with serenity. That, my friends, can be helpful on an epic level during labor and delivery!

Childbirth is always unpredictable and how you deal with its challenges remains to be seen. You can't know exactly at any given moment how, from where, or from whom you'll derive comfort. You may have a lot of mobility, or you may not. You may need to lie down, or you may need to pace the hallways. But no matter where you are and no matter what you are doing–your breath is always with you. When you practice yoga, you are able to access this knowledge and be conscious of it at any point during childbirth. The breath is your refuge; it gets you out of your head and into the rest of who you are. It's essentially a one-way ticket to the present moment, just where you need to be in labor and in life. When you get there, you'll experience a sense of awareness that lets you see life clearly. Of course, we can learn lessons from the past and we can plan for the future, but spending too much time in these spaces can sometimes overwhelm us and cause suffering. The mindfulness that yoga teaches offers a way for us to temper the stress and tension that are part of life, and actually embrace it with inner calm and joy. Yes, joy.

Yoga is the gift that keeps on giving! That breathwork will serve you beyond your wildest dreams as you become a parent, and in just about any other situation in which you find yourself. Boss kind of cranky today? Breathe. Your two-year-old has just spilled coffee onto your pocketbook? Breathe. Power went out just as your holiday guests are arriving? Breathe. Your partner comes home and–oblivious to the unfolded laundry, dirty dishes, and the Mount Everest of toys–inquires (while you're nursing the baby) as to why you weren't able to get to the dry cleaners? Breathe.

Will mindful breathing solve all the world's problems? Probably not this week. But it might ameliorate yours. It's an awfully comforting, totally portable, zero-calorie, 100% organic, wildly helpful tool in pregnancy, labor, and in life. You don't need to order it online, and it doesn't require a delivery mechanism. Be good to your lungs, establish a regular yoga practice, get some fresh air on a daily basis, and as the song says, "Just breathe."

Use This Wake-Up Call

As a midwife and a practitioner and teacher of yoga, I have seen many women, once they become pregnant, use this wake-up call to take charge of their health and do what they can to make healthier choices for themselves and their growing families. As these mamas incorporated yoga into their lives, I witnessed even more remarkable improvements in their health, how their practice became a lifesaver for them during childbirth, and how it eased their postpartum recovery and their ability to take on the challenges of caring for their babies with more equanimity and resilience. A healthy life is far beyond eating clean and exercising and taking the whole-food natural supplements I recommended in the previous chapter, although those are important too.

Yoga is an ancient self-help science of optimal health and of the body, mind, heart, and spirit, now demonstrated by much scientific research. I love yoga so much that I want to encourage all to experience how it thoroughly enhances the health of mind and body. Here are some ways regular practice improves your emotions and quality of life:

- Yoga promotes relaxation, peace of mind, and inner calm, which decreases anxiety.
- Yoga makes for a happier, more positive mood and sense of wellbeing, which decreases depression.
- Yoga opens the heart to compassion, and deeper connection with yourself and others, which improves self-awareness and relationships. This also results in increased consciousness of destructive lifestyle patterns and a desire to overcome dysfunctional habits and addictions ... It also allows for better sex.
- Yoga enhances self-esteem, inner emotional strength, resilience, and coping abilities, which help you remain steady with greater equanimity in the face of hardship, drama, bad news, unsettling events, suffering, and life challenges. It can ultimately lead not only to acceptance of much of life that is not in your control, but also to embracing these experiences as gifts, catalysts for change, and personal growth.

- Yoga enhances spiritual connection, no matter your religion, belief system, or faith.
- Yoga leads to improved creativity and can be such fun if done just about anytime, anywhere, such as in the park, by a lake, at the beach, and even with your children.

There are also many physical advantages to yoga, including the following:

- Yoga eases the common discomforts of pregnancy and typically sets you up for a shorter, easier labor and birth, and a quicker, easier postpartum recovery.
- Yoga improves energy and vitality, allowing you to maintain youthfulness. It eases symptoms of menopause too.
- Yoga improves sleep and reduces insomnia.
- Yoga decreases muscle tension, soreness, and actually eases pain due to many chronic conditions.
- Yoga reduces inner stress and the illnesses it causes, which constitute the majority of modern-day conditions.
- Yoga improves muscle strength, function, and tone. It also improves flexibility, balance, coordination, and posture, all of which not only improves athletic performance but also decreases risk of injury.
- Yoga improves the health of bones, muscles, joints, and cartilage, and reduces the risk of problems there, including commonly-affected areas in the back and neck.
- Yoga improves the health of the cardiovascular, circulatory, endocrine, gastrointestinal, and respiratory systems, and decreases the risk of their related diseases.
- Yoga balances the metabolism, helps with weight loss, and leads to healthier eating, self-care, and lifestyle, which reduces health problems linked to obesity and other conditions due to unhealthy habits and addictions.
- Yoga boosts immunity to infection and cancer, and decreases the risk of inflammatory, autoimmune diseases, and allergies.
- Yoga improves focus, memory, attention, and sharpness, which decreases age-related cognitive decline.

Yoga is not a religion, although it can enhance your spiritual connection to your belief system, nor is it just a physical exercise, although that is a wonderful perk. It's not just for those who can do splits and headstands, but it does increase your flexibility and strength on many levels, so you might find yourself doing them one day. It is not just about taking a class either. It can be a part of everything you do on and off the mat! It is also a great way to meet friends and connect to the wonderful community of like-minded others who practice yoga.

Pregnancy is actually a great time to start yoga as you embark on this life-changing journey to become a mother. It is not too late to start, and the more you practice, the more these skills become habitual, so you can easily tap into them in labor or any life challenge.

To learn more about yoga watch my video and get started: *https:// homesweethomebirth.com/nbsbookbonus*

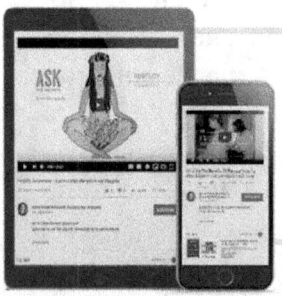

Want to learn more or have more questions?

Grab your free Book Bonuses below:
https://homesweethomebirth.com/nbsbookbonus

MEDITATION, BREATHWORK, AND VISUALIZATION

Here are a few meditative, breathwork, and visualization techniques you can practice regularly in pregnancy and beyond so that you are more prepared and empowered, and can easily tap into them in labor and during any challenge. These techniques will give you immense benefits that are well-researched and widely documented, so much so, they are recommended by cutting-edge integrative healthcare practitioners, and practiced by top athletes, martial artists, warriors, spiritual leaders, healers, and peak performers in a wide variety of professions worldwide. By engaging these techniques in a regular practice, you can learn to activate your own inner calm and minimize the toxic effects of chronic internal stress, increase your focus and concentration, improve your own energy, health, and vitality, and have a more comfortable and easeful labor. They can also aid you to transform your own childbirth experience. Mastering these techniques literally helps you master your own life.

They are simple to do, health-enhancing–especially if you do them often–totally safe, non-toxic, and without unhealthy side effects. They can be done at any time and place. Make these sorts of deep-breathing and breath-awareness practices, along with meditation, visualization, and yoga a regular part of your daily routine.

The Process of Meditating

It is essential for health and wellbeing to periodically take a break to disengage your consciousness from thought and routine activity in order to center and calm yourself, tap into your spiritual self, as well as master your ability to reduce feelings of tension and increase feelings of calm centeredness and balanced grounding. You can begin to do this by taking a "healing interval" to meditate for 10-20 minutes, for 2-3 times per day. Here's how.

Begin meditating by finding a quiet place where you will not be disturbed and set an alarm with a soothing sound, for 3-5 minutes. Sit tall or lie down comfortably, softly close your eyes, and turn your attention inward. Keep your eyes closed and internally focused between your eyebrows (this area is called the "third eye"), or open your eyes and softly gaze at a low, non-moving object or place (like the horizon or where the floor meets the wall). Turn off the mental noise and think and do absolutely nothing. During this time, allow yourself to just BE, breathe, and rest in peaceful stillness without having to DO anything. Allow your mind to be totally immersed in the process of breathing and being. Bring awareness and acceptance not only to your breathing, but also to the sensations you notice and feel in your body. If a thought or emotion comes, notice it, let it be or go, and settle back into your breathing. If you notice your mind wandering as it does–because you have a mind–and you get lost in thought, simply bring your attention back to watch your breath without self-critical judgement. This actually means you are doing it right. Simply be aware of your breathing in all its details, the present moment, and everything that you notice within it.

This is a conscious training of your mind, and like any muscle, it requires regular practice. It is an ongoing practice that changes and evolves as you change and grow. There is no need to control anything. It is kind of like surrendering, letting go of whatever you experience in your mind, body, heart, and spirit–without any interpretation, judgment, reaction, or need to fix anything. Simply watch what is happening within, as a detached witness. This enables you to be mindful in the now, the only place where your life is happening, and is a wonderful way to become present, to get out of your busy thinking mind, and to relax and connect more deeply with yourself and your baby. Staying aware, calm, and present are key to an easier, more meaningful labor and life.

Another form of meditation involves a conscious effort to completely focus your mind's attention on something specific. As above, set a soothing alarm for a few minutes, and take a few moments to get into your meditative state. Then do one of the following, and vary it up each time until you see which resonates most with you to practice regularly:

- With eyes closed, gaze internally towards the tip of your nose or the space between your eyebrows, your "third eye" (even if you cannot see it with your eyes), or with eyes open gaze at a simple object like a candle, or a beautiful natural scene.
- Listen to repetitive 'white noise' sounds like ocean waves, rain, a flowing stream, relaxing chimes, or Gregorian chants.
- Engage in something that requires complete attention and immersion like breathwork exercises, yoga, or creative expression.
- Do rhythmic, repeated movement like dance, walking mindfully, or touching the tips of your fingers in sequence.
- Using objects like mala beads, touch each one while reciting or singing a mantra or yoga sutra. Say chakra syllables, mantras, or simple affirmative words or sounds like "AhhhhhOmmmmmm," "Shhhhhhhh," "Release," "Trust," or "Let go."

Breathwork

Practice breathing exercises 10-20 minutes once or twice per day, like before rising in the morning and before going to sleep at night, and periodically throughout the day, while waiting, traveling, or whenever you feel triggered, upset, stressed, overwhelmed, down, or simply bored. You can even take pauses and do it while eating and engaging in usual activities and chores. Again, practice regularly so breathwork becomes habitual, and you can easily use it when stressed or in labor.

When all is otherwise healthy and well, throughout the breathwork exercises given below, practice embracing, relaxing into, and even magnifying intense sensations without the mental story about them. Can you make friends with sensations of discomfort and pain in your body and/or in your heart, instead of trying to escape, numb, or fight them? Is there something that they can teach you? Allow yourself to fully feel whatever you feel in your body, including the waves of strong emotions that come and go. Get curious about all of their details, including the borders or edges, and the parts of you that feel good or do not have painful sensations. Send breath to any areas of discomfort. Yes, there are remedies to help alleviate pain. But you will be amazed at how effective this practice is and how much it will help you to better cope with your current pain as well as the pain that is an inevitable part of being human. It is the suffering from the pain that is optional, so you can choose not to suffer.

While breathing, be mindful and just observe and release any muscle tension, working your way slowly from head to toe. Next, be mindful of what you are currently seeing, hearing, smelling, feeling, and tasting. Just watch without judgment. This brings you to the present and is wonderfully relaxing. You do this, and you are getting the benefits of both slow, deep breathing, and meditation.

To practice, sit tall with your buttocks perched up on two folded blankets that are against a wall or back of a chair, or you can lie down on a comfortable surface without falling asleep (once you hone these skills, you can do them anywhere). Close your eyes, maintain your gaze between your eyebrows or towards the tip of your nose, or focus on a nonmoving distant object or place with your eyes open.

Try each technique given below for 3-5 minutes by setting a timer so that you move through several cycles. Notice how you feel as you relax into these practices, during and after each exercise. You might like them so much you will continue for longer. Be patient with yourself as you are learning a new skill. Repeat the ones that feel best, as often in the day as you can. Breathwork with extended slow exhales tends to be extremely calming. Alternate nostril and infinity breathing are grounding and emotionally balancing. Rapid forced exhaling through the nose as in the yoga breath of fire, as well as conscious, connected circular breathing with longer inhales is more activating and energizing, but can also lead to great healing and deeper states of relaxation. Choose the technique that helps you the most in each of these various situations.

Here are a variety of breathwork techniques for you to practice:

Breath Awareness

Simply watch the details of your breath without changing or fixing them. Notice the inhale, the exhale, the rise and fall of your chest and belly, the coolness of the air going in, and the warmth of the air going out, and any other associated details. Explore your sensations as you inhale and exhale, what you are currently seeing, hearing, smelling, feeling, and tasting. Just watch without judgment. This brings you to the present and is deliciously relaxing.

Ujjayi Breathing

Practice Ujjayi breathing. This is a wonderful natural tranquilizer and is awesome for yoga, deep relaxation, and labor. Breathe at the pace and depth that feels right for you, by inhaling through your mouth or nose, directing the breath into the back of your throat while slightly constricting it, which makes a sound like ocean waves. It is a calm, slow, and smooth circular version of mild gasping on the inhale and fogging a mirror on the exhale. This is extremely soothing and meditative combined with the benefits of breathwork.

Triangle Breathing

Inhale for a count of three or four, exhale to the same count of three or four, then pause for the same count of three or four while consciously and deeply relaxing your diaphragm muscle of respiration, as well as all other muscles. When breathing in this way, picture the inhale as it goes up the side of a triangle, the exhale as it goes down the other side, and the pause as it travels along the bottom line and third side of the triangle, completing the shape. This breathing entails getting most aligned with your natural relaxed breath rhythm, but doing it consciously is powerful.

Sigh of Relief Exhaling and Yawning

Regularly make or allow yourself to heave a full-body yawn and stretch several times to give yourself a boost of breath, energy, relaxation, stress relief, detoxification, and improve your overall well-being. It is a natural reflex that animals, babies, and children all do until they are cultured to stifle it; and science is beginning to discover its benefits. You can trigger it by wiggling your jaw as you take some inhales. Then just let it happen completely. Also make a practice of periodically sighing, making the noise you need without any inhibition. Take a slow, deep inhale through your nose, drawing your breath deep into your belly and stretching the inhalation to your fullest capacity. The exhale happens naturally. But let it be through your mouth with an audible sigh of relief, consciously releasing and relaxing all tension.

Deeper, Fuller Breathing

Place one hand on your belly and breathe into that hand, paying more attention to the inhale while letting the exhale happen slowly but naturally. Notice the expansion of your belly into your hand and lower back into its surface, behind, or beneath it. Do this for a minute. Next, place your hands around your lower ribs and breathe into your hands. Notice the ribs expand out to the side into your hands for a minute. After this, place a hand on your chest. Notice the rise of your chest into your hand and the expansion of your upper back into the surface, behind, or beneath you for a minute. With your hands by your sides, draw your breath deep down. Expand your pelvic floor and inflate your entire torso like a balloon with each inhale. Then release even deeper on each exhale as you empty your body of breath. Keep it smooth, fluid, and even. This helps you learn deep abdominal breathing, increasing your lung capacity. To further train yourself in this way do abdominal three-part breathing.

Abdominal Three-Part Breathing

This helps you learn deep abdominal breathing, using the maximum capacity of your lungs. Practice abdominal breathing as much as possible so it becomes habitual. This is the ideal form of breathing, as opposed to rapid, shallow breathing. Abdominal breathing is a great way to make your breaths deeper, slower, and more regular, so as to calm the nervous system. To learn, place your hands on your belly and concentrate on breathing into them. Imagine a pump expanding your abdomen and lower back, which causes you to inhale. The pump then releases effortlessly, which causes you to exhale. Continue to exhale slowly while consciously releasing all muscle tension, especially in your jaw and diaphragm, i.e., your breathing muscle. Then there is a natural pause until you need to inhale again.

At first, when breathing in and out, keep the ratio of inhalation and exhalation equal. Inhale slowly through your nose for a count of three. Continue to imagine a pump expanding your abdomen and lower back down to your pelvic floor, causing you to inhale. Allow your ribs to expand with air; then inhale air into your upper chest towards your collarbone and shoulders. Exhale slowly through your mouth for a count of three. Release effortlessly, in the same order you inhaled, returning to baseline: your abdomen, ribs, then upper chest. With each exhalation, try to let go and relax even more.

You can play with counts, using a count of four, maybe even increase to five or six. But keep the count of your inhale the same as the count of your exhale by breathing in a one-to-one ratio. For example, as you are trying to master this, count to three as you inhale, then count to three as you exhale. With practice, you can increase the ratio increments to 4:4, 5:5, or 6:6. Then try pausing for one count between each inhale and exhale. Notice that stillness in between inhalation and exhalation.

Extended Exhale Breathing

Extend or double the exhale. For example, if you are inhaling to a count of three, exhale to a count of six, or if you are inhaling to a count of four, exhale to a count of eight. To take it deeper, imagine the exhale continuing into the pause before the next inhale, while you keep releasing, letting go, and relaxing into the stillness. Stay very still while surrendering even more. If you get to the point that you kind of startle or shake a bit, you know you are in the perfect place, that your body is releasing tension and resetting your nervous system. Your body will know when to begin inhaling again.

Box Breathing

Another great breathing technique that disengages your conscious attention from thought, relaxes the nervous system, and can be done at any time is box breathing. With this exercise, you add a timed pause between each inhalation and exhalation.

Inhale deeply into your belly for a count of three. Hold without tension for a count of six. Exhale to a count of six while consciously relaxing more and more. Hold again without tension for a count of three. You can also see how it feels to inhale, hold, exhale and hold to equal counts of four, for example.

Varied Ratio Breathing

Play with the ratios and counts of inhalation, exhalation, and the pauses in between them. For example, exhale slowly through your mouth with an audible sigh. Inhale slowly through your nose for a count of four, hold for a count of seven, then exhale through your mouth for a count of eight.

Alternate Nostril Breathing

Do this at a pace and depth that is comfortable, with your eyes closed, gazing inward towards the middle of your eyebrows at your "third eye." Place your hand, fingers facing up, by your nose. Occlude your right nostril with your thumb, and inhale through the left nostril. Take your thumb off your right nostril, occlude your left nostril with your pinky finger, then exhale and inhale through your right nostril. Occlude your right nostril with your thumb again as you remove your pinky finger from the left nostril. Exhale then inhale through your left nostril. Repeat for at least three minutes. You can also then play with combining other breathwork techniques while doing this, like pausing for a few counts between inhaling and exhaling, while keeping both nostrils occluded until the next exhale, as well as using, for example, the extended exhale breathing. If your nose is stuffed, you can visualize or imagine breathing in this way.

Forced Exhalation

Another breathing exercise to try is forced exhalation: after a normal breath, try squeezing as much air out as possible, using your intercostal muscles in your chest. Next, allow the breath to come in naturally and deeply, but automatically.

Breath of Fire

This is a powerful breathing exercise to practice five to ten minutes daily to detox, destress, energize your body, and harness your power and strength. You will be amazed how it does that when you are practicing yoga or working out. To start, simply inhale deeply and abdominally, then quickly with an equal inhale-to-exhale ratio, pump air out through your nose with your belly, by engaging your core–like pushing your navel towards your spine. After a few minutes, take a normal breath.

Conscious, Connected Circular Breathing

This is transformational breathing, the kind of breathing that leads to incredible healing, the release of limiting beliefs and habits, and stuck, painful emotions, internal stress or trauma energy. It started in the West with rebirthing and has branched out around the world under a variety of names and styles, like Clarity Breathwork, but the core principles are similar.

In this practice the breath is full and deep, but also circular, flowing and continuous, without pause between inhales and exhales. All breathing is done through the mouth wide open. It is literally aiming to engage all of your respiratory system, so that you inhale 100% of air, "prana" (life-force energy) into your body, enabling the breath to become your medicine.

It is usually done lying down flat or slightly elevated with a bolster, in a comfortable position, for approximately an hour. The inhale is enthusiastic and passionate, with full gusto, deep into your chest and belly, sending air towards the back of your throat, to get take in a deep, long, and slow full-body breath. The exhale is soft, completely passive, without any force, pushing, control, or effort. As you open your mind, body, heart, and soul, and expand to each breath, you also completely relax and go limp, letting go more and more with each exhale. All the while you are staying awake and acutely aware, allowing yourself to go deep and to welcome all sensations and movements that come up as your body processes and releases.

The miracles thousands experience around the globe can come with just one session of this practice, but usually, they happen after a series of sessions. When you can really surrender and relax into the intensity and ride the waves as your body processes, releases, resets, and integrates the wonderfully powerful experience, then you ready yourself for the miracles. Music helps, and many breathworkers have a carefully selected set of songs for the stages of the session or for particular issues that may arise. It is recommended you learn this in a supported group or private sessions before trying on your own. Once you master it, do 100 of these breaths daily. It is life-changing.

A great practice while you are breathing in this way is to state and really visualize your desires as if they are already happening. Aim to keep them pure, direct, to the point, and in the present tense. Examples could be:

- My body knows how to birth my baby.
- I'm safe.
- I'm perfect as I am.
- My life is perfect as it is.
- I'm blessed.
- I'm divine.
- Let go and let G-d.
- Trust.
- I'm grateful.
- I'm joy.
- I'm love.
- I'm calm.
- I've got this.

Create your own mantra as your breathe, and really allow yourself to imagine all the details and sensations of how this new thought feels— what it looks, sounds, smells, tastes, and really feels like.

Don't hesitate to schedule a session with me if you need more guidance with mastering breathwork and experiencing its transformative power.

Be patient with yourself as you are learning a new skill. Repeat the ones that feel best, as often in the day as you can. Choose the breathing technique that helps you the most in a particular situation.

I cover Clarity Breathwork and its power as a healing and transformative modality in greater depth in my book Trauma Release Formula: The Revolutionary Step-by-Step Program for Eliminating Effects of Childhood Abuse, Trauma, Emotional Pain & Crippling Inner Stress to Living in Joy Without Drugs or Therapy. Additional resources include Dr. Ela Manga's book Breathe: Strategizing Energy in the Age of Burnout, and Dr. Andrew Weil's book Breathing: The Master Key to Self Healing. Just Breathe by Dan Brule is an excellent book about all types of breathwork to enhance your wellbeing, including conscious, connected breathwork that facilitates deep transformation and healing, or as he calls it, "spiritual breathing." My other favorite resources for that form of breathwork include Breath Love by Lauren Chelec Cafritz, Breathe Deep, Laugh Loudly: The Joy of Transformational Breathing by Judith Kravitz, as well as the International Breathwork Foundation.

Visualization

Visualization is amazingly effective if you really open your mind, use your imagination, and practice this self-healing skill on a regular basis. Harnessing the power of the mind and its ability to imagine and visualize desired outcomes to heal can promote health, peak performance, and manifest your highest intentions. Visualization has been practiced around the world for thousands of years, and is also now well studied and supported by the scientific literature to be quite effective. I am awed by its power and potential to achieve miraculous results. Renowned surgical oncologist Dr. Bernie Siegel uses forms of this to heal cancer.

Dr. Joe Dispenza teaches thousands around the world with unparalleled success, using the latest scientific research, how to heal a variety of serious chronic diseases and lead more fulfilled lives by the power of creative thought alone. Visualization takes advantage of the fact that a vivid mental imagined experience has a similar effect in the body as an actual one. It is powerful enough to change mental and emotional states, neurological circuitry, genetic expression, hormone production, turn off and on receptor sites and make proteins that are responsible for all bodily functions. The body literally experiences what the mind believes. As in meditation and breathwork, it takes practice, with results dependent on the more you practice and hone your abilities.

In a meditative state, while breathing at a pace and depth that feels most calming for you, you can incorporate a visualization practice that is unique to what you need at that moment. These are only a few examples that have helped many mamas. As with the breathwork, experiment. For example, sit with each one for a few minutes, see what resonates most, then incorporate a few you like best into your regular practice so that you have several to choose from when you need them.

See Your Breath Visualization

You can visualize and literally direct your breath, energy of the spiritual life force, to areas of healing, need, intense sensations, and discomfort. You can direct your breath in various directions to achieve different outcomes.

Muscle Relaxing Visualization

While lying down and breathing deeply, consciously, and progressively, relax each muscle from head to toe. Visualize feeling heavy and limp like a rag doll or like a napping dog or cat. Get heavier and more limp with each exhale.

Phoneline Visualization

To connect with your baby, you can dwell on your feeling of love for your baby. When breathing, you can imagine that feeling growing and expanding. Imagine your inhale going right to your heart center, and then on the exhale, imagine sending that breath, that feeling of love energy, directly to your baby, surrounding your baby. You can give the energy a color if you want. Imagine your baby smiling and basking in the love you are sending. Then visualize a direct impenetrable line of light, color, or energy, connecting your heart with your baby, like a phoneline, always available for connection.

Root Visualization

This visualization practice helps you to feel grounded. If you are standing or seated, imagine roots extending from all points of contact between you and the surface beneath you, extending deep down into the earth center. Inhale breath from your crown, and exhale directing your breath down your spine and out through the roots, which draw you further down and make you heavy. With each exhale your breath extends out through the roots, growing them even further down and spreading out into the earth beneath you. If you are lying down, imagine the breath coming in through the front of your body and the exhale leaving out the back of your body with the same root visual. Feel the pull of gravity down, as the roots wrap around you and hold you secure. Inhale deep into your core, where there is an eternal candle flame, and on the exhale, spread that fire to fill your heart, abdomen, and pelvis.

Golden Light Chakra Visualization

This visualization practice helps you to feel centered. Imagine a straight, sparkling rod of steel, diamond, or golden light extending deep into the earth center, running up your spine, from your sacrum to your crown, and up into the infinite space above. If you are interested in the chakras, see and sense the circular vortexes of energy in their colors around and up your body's center, from the red at your root, then orange at your pelvic area, yellow at your solar plexus, green at your heart space, turquoise at your throat, indigo between your eyebrows, and golden white at your crown just above your head.

Higher Chakra Breathing

There are many ways to breathe up and down through your chakras, but one of my favorites is for connecting you to the higher parts of your being. While breathing through your nose, imagine a light from your heart center traveling up to the area between your eyebrows, or third eye, then traveling back to the heart in an arc or circle as you exhale. Keep this focus for ten to 20 breaths. Then do the same sort of breath, but imagine this light traveling from your throat to your crown chakra about a half-foot above your head as you inhale, and back again on the exhale, following an arc or circle. After another 10-20 breaths, do this from your third eye to what is called your soul star, one to 1.5 feet above your head, with each inhale, and back again with each exhale, for 10-20 breaths.

Spiritual Fortress Visualization

This visualization practice helps you to feel protected. Visualize that as you inhale, you bring into your body a spiritual, healing energy, light, or color from your crown. As you exhale, you direct your breath, that energy, light, or color to fill your entire body, head to toe, and completely surround you like a fortress or eternal spiritual bubble that cannot be broken. Sit in that visual so that you see it, feel it, sense it, know it.

Toxin Release Visualization

This visualization practice helps you to feel cleansed. Inhale from top to bottom or from front to back, a healing color, spiritual energy, or white/golden light that you visualize filling your body. If you are carrying around long-standing anger and rage, for example, exhale all the red fire and loud screams out of your back or any points of contact between you and the ground. If you have chronic sadness, grief, or despair about something that happened a while ago, use the visual of a powerful waterfall or firehose of tears forcefully exiting your body on the exhale. If you have blocks or baggage that weigh you down, use the visual of multiple bricks and heavy rocks exiting your body on the exhale. For the release of all negativity, toxins, beliefs, and habits not serving you, use the visual of black smoke exiting your body on the exhale. Or come up with your own visuals that resonate more with you.

Radiating Sun Visualization

This visualization practice helps you to feel strong and magnificent. Sit tall with the visual of a huge radiating sun, the eternal light of your spirit, filling your heart center, big and huge, extending out in all directions.

Happy Place Visualization

This visualization practice helps you to feel calm and blissful. Imagine yourself in your happy place in all its detail. What does it look like, feel like, sound like, smell like, taste like? Let those feelings take over. Many tend to visualize themselves in a tropical paradise, by the sea, in the mountains, in a cave, floating on a cloud in a blue sky of beauty, by a lake, or in the stillness of the forest. Or, imagine yourself so relaxed that you are like a sleeping cat, a napping dog, or a rag doll–totally surrendered, limp, and released without ANY muscle tension. See any residual tension melt completely, as a tiny piece of ice quickly becomes water on exposure to heat, and watch that water flow down and away from your body.

Infinity Breathing

This visualization helps you feel balanced and deeply relaxed. Imagine an infinity symbol or a sideways figure eight with the middle point of juncture of the two circles between your eyebrows. Do eight cycles of mouth breathing, with your mind's eye watching a beam of light as it travels from the center, around the infinity symbol, inhaling as the light moves up from the middle and exhaling as the light moves down each side. Then do eight cycles of nose breathing, inhaling as it moves up the outer edges of the circles on each side, exhaling as the light moves down towards the center.

Labor-Specific: Wave Visualization

Specifically, for labor, there are some common visualizations that many mamas like to use. Often it helps a mama during childbirth to visualize the waves of the rise and fall of the sensations of labor, like waves of the ocean that rise and fall and come and go. Others like to imagine the surges to be hugs to the baby.

It also helps mamas to visualize during labor the cervix, tightly closed, long, thick, and firm, the entrance to the uterus; and during pushing, the birth canal and the perineum softening and opening like rosebud blossoms opening into a flower. The "ring of fire" commonly referred to when the baby crowns can be seen as a ring of flowers or one big opening lotus or rose flower. What matters is that whatever you are visualizing comforts and helps you.

The most effective visualization for childbirth is to imagine your dream labor and birth, whatever you desire, in all its detail, as if it already happened. Allow yourself to really feel the powerful high energetic vibrational emotions that accompany such an experience. Embody the emotions fully as you did when you were a child. What did you do when you were overflowing with pure joy, freedom, relief, sense of accomplishment, love, gratitude? Do it now, internally.

To learn more, watch my video on breathwork and visualization: *https:// homesweethomebirth.com/nbsbookbonus*

Similar to yoga, regular meditation, breathwork, and visualization practice can make you feel like an active participant in your pregnancy, childbirth, and life experiences–labor and life are not just happening to powerless you; you are present within it, working with it, helping it along, taking positive steps to do what you can to bring your baby into the world with more ease and coping most effectively with whatever comes your way. Through taking responsibility for your own state of mind and wellbeing, by daily practice of meditation, breathwork, and visualization, you are empowering yourself with tools for labor and life's challenges and helping yourself tremendously.

How to Listen to Your Intuition

Learning to listen to your intuition plays a large role in a positive pregnancy experience. I have found that pregnancy is a sacred time, and it's important for women to keep their space sacred throughout the journey. Here are my recommendations for keeping your space sacred, which optimizes your ability to listen to your intuition.

Keep Your Space Sacred

- Create your vision–take some quiet time where you can close your eyes and relax. Take slow deep breaths, releasing on the exhale, and use your mind as a clean slate. Envision on that clean slate the vision you have for yourself, your baby, and your birth. What does it look like, and more importantly, what does it feel like? Take notes in a journal or draw anything that helps to hold this vision. Spend time with this vision every day, and hold a feeling of gratitude as if it has already been delivered.
- Share little with those who aren't in alignment with you–a mama may have her partner, her midwife, her doula, and/or a few real close friends in her circle. Be mindful about who you share your vision with because not everyone is able to connect with high energy like this … and that's okay … It's important to recognize that everyone is on their own journey, but you don't have to lower your standards to make others feel more comfortable about your life choices. And you must avoid conversations or sometimes people who lead you to feel inner tension and fear, which does not serve you at all during this most sensitive time.

- Get comfortable setting boundaries–you may simply need to tell those stressful family members and friends that you love them, you appreciate their concern, but you are pregnant and sensitive, trying to keep positive, relaxed, and upbeat, and you'd rather not talk about it or get into any disagreement. Many women, myself included, have spent time in life accommodating others. This is not one of those times, and pregnancy can help women shed their fears, limiting beliefs, and negative habits. Pregnancy is a time for a woman to focus on herself and her baby, and for some women, this may be the first time in her life when she experiences this. I give you permission to pleasantly exit the conversation, hang up the phone, or leave the room if they do not honor your request. Most will eventually learn and stop harassing you.
- Focus on surrounding yourself with positivity–this includes positive affirmations, inspirational birth stories, books, movies, radio shows, podcasts, and people. It's important for you and your baby to keep stress low and spirits high. Pregnancy provides an opportunity to release unconscious beliefs and emotions, so although it's rarely a completely smooth ride, it's one where you can always get back on board your wave of high vibes. Keep negative news media to a minimum and be mindful of toxic people and drama that just don't need your attention at this time.

Where and how a woman births her baby is her business. Feel confident in listening to your body, your baby, and your intuition when it comes to this very special time. It's not your job to convince anyone of anything, but only to show up for your own assignment, strengthen your faith muscles, and know that you come from a long line of birthing women. I have helped many women over the years face the critic in their own minds and in the minds of others, and once they start listening to the voice of their inner truth, they let go and enjoy the journey.

Your Support Team for Pregnancy, Birth & Postpartum

THE HOMEBIRTH MIDWIFERY
MODEL OF CARE

As a certified nurse-midwife with a full-scope group homebirth midwifery practice of over two decades who also provides similar care in wonderfully supportive hospital settings, I am often asked what the homebirth midwifery model of care actually is. I can speak for my philosophies, which are shared in general by many of my colleagues: we provide prenatal, labor, delivery, postpartum, and newborn care, as well as breastfeeding support for healthy, low-risk families planning to give birth at home. We provide gynecological and some primary care services to well women. We also support women with having a homebirth-like experience at a birthing center or in the hospital.

We offer a unique comprehensive model of maternity care that provides an exceptional level of holistic support and services to achieve optimum health. We believe there are several ingredients that contribute to a deeply positive and healthful pregnancy, birth, and postpartum experience, in addition to our midwifery care. These include wholesome nutrition, whole-food supplements, and regular exercise, as well as an ongoing practice of yoga and meditation, and other such methods to reduce inner stress, increase inner calm and healthy, joyful living (as discussed already). Relevant health education with books, movies, and childbirth classes, as well as connection with a supportive community are also crucial. We often draw on the expertise of additional professionals, such as doulas, childbirth educators, lactation consultants, acupuncturists, massage therapists, chiropractors or osteopaths, and mind/body medicine practitioners, to name just a few.

We encourage each woman and partner to take advantage of the many classes and support groups we recommend–from prenatal yoga, yoga-for-labor workshops, and postpartum mommy-and-me yoga classes, positive birth story pregnancy circles, community new-mother blessing ceremonies, annual family reunions, postpartum mom circles, pregnancy retreats, and a variety of other educational, supportive, and fun events, classes, and ways to connect with other likeminded people to build meaningful community. This is largely an effort to bring back the needed village it takes to raise a new baby and new parents.

While we continue to expand our academic, clinical, and intuitive knowledge and wisdom, we are also growing in understanding, appreciation, and awe of the sanctity of life and its many facets, transitions, and phases. Most women are candidates for midwifery care and home or birth center (out-of-hospital) birth. Over 92% of pregnant women in our home-birth practice will have a home birth, and we maintain a cesarean section birth rate of 5%.

Ongoing individualized care determines the needs of each childbearing family. We have developed practice guidelines in conjunction with other out-of-hospital midwives, evidence-based research, and the current midwifery literature. They reflect our philosophies and professional standards for practice, and they are reviewed and evaluated periodically as needed. We follow these practice guidelines to protect the health and safety of each individual in our care; and we try our absolute best, within our human capacity, to give our utmost attention and care with integrity, honesty, and heartfelt commitment and dedication.

We firmly believe that pregnancy and childbirth are normal, natural bodily functions, profoundly spiritual, truly inspiring, and an empowering rite of passage for women and their families.

We also believe that childbearing families are best served by caregivers who promote and encourage a loving, respectful, supportive, family-centered environment, and who maintain trust and calm confidence in the normalcy of the process until proven otherwise.

We have taken and will continue to take every reasonable precaution to ensure safety, comfort, and deep satisfaction, which are our top priorities. A safe and wonderfully positive birth experience requires the joint cooperative efforts of both the expectant family and healthcare providers, with a relationship based upon open communication, mutual respect, and shared responsibility.

Education of women and their families is an integral part of our services so that women are able to assume this responsibility for health maintenance and effective utilization of healthcare. Opportunity is offered to our clients to participate in the planning and implementation of their care, as the emphasis is placed on an outcome that satisfies emotional, educational, family, and spiritual concerns beyond the obvious physical needs.

We feel that every individual has the right to safe and satisfying healthcare by the provider of their choice, given with respect for personal preferences and cultural variations. We believe that normal, healthy women have the right to birth at home if they choose to do so. As licensed practitioners, we feel an obligation to make birth as safe and satisfying as possible for them. For the overwhelming majority of families, the childbearing experience is one of health rather than illness, and there is a need for preventative and loving supportive care that is not only safe, but also sensitive, compassionate, and empowering. We believe in enhancing the normal processes of the female reproductive cycle, pregnancy, and birth through education, physical and emotional support, and involvement of significant others according to the choices of each expectant mom and those she chooses and wants to be involved.

Our responsibilities include the review of each woman's complete health history, physical examination findings, and lab results to determine her eligibility for continued midwifery care and a home/free-standing birth center or hospital birth, as well as ongoing evaluation and guidance throughout pregnancy, labor, birth, and postpartum with attention to signs of normalcy and/or complications.

All findings are discussed openly, and there will be no routine procedures or interventions unless medically necessary and mutually agreed upon. While childbearing is a healthy, normal, and natural process for the vast majority of women and babies, problems can infrequently occur and need to be recognized and attended to.

Although many complications can be prevented or handled simply within our practice, some do require consultation with a collaborative physician or transfer to medical and hospital care to increase the likelihood of a safe outcome. It is our philosophy that decisions regarding each woman's care are informed and collaborative, and ultimately hers to make; however, rare emergent situations may arise in which the professional judgment of the midwife and/or consulting physician must be relied on exclusively for the safety of mother and baby. We are grateful for life-saving hospital, medical, and surgical care when there are serious complications and illness; and it is my hope that the homebirth midwifery model of care can be applied as much as possible in all birth settings, including the operating room if surgical birth is needed.

Home, Hospitals, and US Culture

There is an overwhelming cultural belief in the United States that hospitals are the safest place to give birth, regardless of the extensive scientific data that planned homebirths with skilled midwives suggest otherwise. Numerous studies around the world have documented the safety of planned homebirths by trained professional midwives, with outcomes at least as good, if not better than those occurring in hospitals.

This is especially true of women who have delivered vaginally before. The total slight increase in newborn mortality risk of homebirths is estimated to be 10 per 10,000 babies born at home, and that 1 in 1,000 babies born at home may be adversely affected by the extra transport time in reaching advanced care in the hospital. The absolute risk is small, however.

Despite spending the most money on obstetric care, the United States ranks among the highest of industrialized countries around the world in maternal mortality and morbidity and ranks among the highest in neonatal mortality and morbidity as well.

Countries that consistently demonstrate the best maternal and newborn outcomes have a large percentage of midwife-led maternity care for healthy women experiencing normal pregnancies—which constitutes the vast majority; they also have a greater percentage of out-of-hospital midwifery care with supportive hospital/medical transfer arrangements when needed, while the obstetricians attend to the women with high-risk complications and serious illnesses - which is how they are educated as surgeons and medical doctors.

When midwives and obstetricians work together as a team, both using their unique skills, knowledge, expertise, and training, the outcomes for moms and babies are far superior. Midwives are trained in guarding the normalcy of pregnancy, birth, and postpartum, not disturbing it when all is well, knowing when to compassionately observe with loving support, and when and how to use holistic remedies, or medical intervention only when necessary, as a last resort. We are also educated in the prevention, assessment, and treatment of complications, which most times can be managed simply and naturally, but sometimes involve consultation or referral to an obstetrician.

Although unforeseen events and emergencies can occur in any birth setting, some of which can be best handled in a high-risk hospital, a low-risk healthy woman entering the typical US hospital expecting a normal vaginal birth is subjected to a routine barrage of interventions. She also risks exposure to infectious pathogens and procedures that dramatically increase the risk of complications and problems with potentially longstanding physical and emotional ramifications for both mother and baby.

There are many other benefits of homebirth and out-of-hospital midwifery care, in addition to safety, which provides an alternative to the impersonal, fear-based, lawsuit-prevention-oriented medical and hospital care that has become prevalent in our society. These benefits include, but are not limited to-the power of human touch and presence;

the power of being surrounded by supportive people of a family's own choosing; and a feeling of security in birthing in the familiar and comfortable environment of one's home or another homey environment; feeling less inhibited...., eating and drinking as needed and desired; expressing or practicing individual cultural, value, and faith-based rituals that enhance coping—all of which can lead to easier labors and births.

In terms of homebirth, women express that not having to make a decision about when to go to the hospital during labor (going too early can slow progress and increase the likelihood of the cascade potentially harmful interventions, while going too late can be intensely uncomfortable or even lead to a risky, unplanned birth en route), being able to choose how and when to include children (who are making their own adjustments and are less challenged by a lengthy absence of their parents and excessive interruptions of family routines), enabling uninterrupted family bonding and breastfeeding, huge cost savings for insurance companies and those without insurance, and increasing the likelihood of having a deeply empowering and profoundly positive, life-changing pregnancy and birth experience.

Getting holistic prenatal-through-postpartum care and birthing in their own home or a homey free-standing birth center attended by a skilled midwife is a refuge for those who want to protect the normalcy and sanctity of pregnancy and birth. But focusing on the normal does not mean that problems go unrecognized or unattended; rather, they are viewed as issues that need to be dealt with, imbalances that need to be corrected, not expected or feared.

That being said, certain hazards do exist, however, in all settings, whether childbirth occurs in or out of the hospital; and there are risks unique to each setting. Some of these risks will never be eradicated no matter our state of technology or medical advancement. The safety of homebirths and free-standing birth center births is well documented, but childbirth by its nature is a threshold passage for the mom and the baby.

Some babies are born with defects and injuries despite all the technology, tests, and skills of the attendants. Birth defects may or may not be detectable by prenatal testing. In spite of the fact that births in hospital settings have failed to eliminate fetal or neonatal death, there is a cultural expectation that doctors and hospitals can guarantee a "perfect baby" every time. This is a pervasive myth. It is impossible for any provider to guarantee much of anything.

The practice of midwifery, nursing, and medicine are not exact sciences, and no assurances can be made regarding the results of examinations, diagnostic tests, treatments, procedures, or interventions. It is impossible for any provider to guarantee a normal, healthy birth for mother or baby. Part of the wonder of the miracle of birth is the inherent lack of guarantees in life and birth and the surrender to a power far bigger than ourselves. Part of life is death, and we often do not know why a person lives or dies.

We do have a spiritual perspective and believe that while we can do our best to do what is humanly possible, most of life, birth, and death are ultimately not in our control. We do believe that everything that happens is meant to happen because it did and that it happened for our benefit, even if it is beyond our comprehension, as we are souls temporarily residing in bodies and know that the G-d/Spirit of our own understanding is only good. Conception is the beginning of life, yet every life must end at some time.

Part of pregnancy is the excitement of new life and the fear of its loss. This is a normal human reality and is in part why pregnancy deepens and matures a woman and man spiritually and emotionally.

Types of Midwives

There are several options for midwifery care in the United States, during preconception, pregnancy, birth, and postpartum. There a variety of routes to becoming a midwife, with different types of education, licensing, and abbreviated titles that seem confusing to the public.

Each midwife has their own personality, philosophy, standards, level of experience, and practice guidelines–even within the field of midwifery. Some are more medically slanted or bound by the protocols of their collaborative obstetricians and hospitals, while others are more holistically minded and practice the midwifery model of care regardless of local medical standards of care, and there is a wide range in between. As you look at and begin to search for your midwife or group midwifery practice, here is a list of midwife titles, training, and what they can do to help you. I recommend you interview a few in your area if you have the option, so you can find one with whom you are most comfortable.

Certified Nurse-Midwife (CNM): a CNM is an individual who is trained and skilled in the disciplines of midwifery and nursing as a registered nurse (RN). The certificate in midwifery is a postgraduate training that requires a bachelor's degree prior to admission. In some states like New York, a master's degree is required for midwifery licensure. Occasionally you might see the term "registered or licensed nurse-midwife" used interchangeably.

A CNM's education and training are standardized across the country according to the requirements of the American Midwifery Certification Board (AMCB) and the professional organization that sets educational and practice standards, which is called the American College of Nurse Midwives (ACNM). A CNM provides care to all women from puberty throughout the childbearing and menopausal years, including newborn care, well-woman gynecology and primary care. A CNM can be legal and licensed in all 50 states, and their services are covered by most insurance companies. A CNM can work in all settings such as private practices, clinics, hospitals, freestanding birthing centers, and your home.

Of all the midwives, CNMs tend to be the most respected and accepted among physicians and hospitals, and the American College of Obstetricians and Gynecologists fully supports them.

Most CNMs' education touches on alternative healing modalities, and a midwife who is interested in these can learn more about them through continuing education required to maintain certification and licensure.

While CNM education includes out-of-hospital birthing, not all CNMs can get clinical training sites for homebirths or freestanding birthing centers, depending on the availability of those options in each locality. Many CNMs have worked previously as obstetric nurses, which provides additional skills and experience needed to deal with complications and emergencies, but also can impact how they practice.

Certified Midwife (CM): a CM is a relatively new credential in the US but is actually more similar to the independent midwifery profession in many other modern countries. A CM is an individual with a postgraduate education in midwifery without the required degree in nursing–although the training incorporates the knowledge and skills of nursing that are relevant to midwifery. A CM has to take the same certification exam as a CNM, and the ACNM considers the midwifery education and certification to be identical to that of a CNM, thus recognizing these degrees and scopes of practice as equivalent. Unfortunately, CMs are currently only recognized in a few states, including New York and New Jersey, but the ACNM's lobbying for change remains ongoing.

Certified Professional Midwife (CPM): a CPM is a national credential developed by the North American Registry of Midwives (NARM) in an effort to maintain rigorous and standardized education skills and experience for individuals to learn how to provide the midwifery model of care through other means.

Multiple routes of education are recognized–so both those who graduate from a midwifery education program accredited by the Midwifery Education Accreditation Council (MEAC) and certified nurse midwives can qualify for this credential, as can certified midwives without a requirement to be a nurse–although a high school degree is required. Learning by apprenticeship, self, and group study is highly valued.

The CPM is the only midwifery credential that requires knowledge about and experience in out-of-hospital settings. They generally train and practice only in homes and freestanding birth center settings, although this can affect their experience managing complications and emergencies seen more commonly in hospitals.

Many do not have gynecology or primary care education, although they tend to have some training in a variety of holistic alternative modalities. CPMs are legal in some states, neither legal nor not legal in others, and illegal and subject to a jail sentence in other states for practicing midwifery without a license. Their ability to carry medical supplies and administer medications if needed varies according to state laws. Midwives Alliance of North America (MANA) is their main professional organization, which is open to midwives of all educational backgrounds and practice styles. While only a CM or CNM can belong to the ACNM, quite a number of CNMs and CMs are MANA members, especially those who practice midwifery in out-of-hospital settings. Unfortunately, there has been some conflict between the ACNM and MANA, with strong opinions on either side, but ultimately these are the organizations that advocate for midwives and the families they serve and promote practice excellence in the midwifery model of care.

Direct-Entry Midwife (DEM): a DEM is a midwife who is trained in midwifery without having to be a nurse, via multiple routes of education. Her education and experience can vary widely. She may be educated in the discipline of midwifery through self-study and apprenticeship without a college degree, or she may have attended a MEAC-accredited midwifery school or graduated from a university-based program accredited by the AMCB. This includes CMs, CPMs, and any independent practitioner who decides to call themselves a midwife.

They may be highly skilled, experienced, and competent … or not. Their legal status varies according to the state where they practice. In the states where CMs are licensed, the scope of practice and settings are similar to a CPM. All other DEMs mostly practice midwifery in homes and some freestanding birth centers. A DEM who is not a CPM or CM/CNM tends to prefer to remain independent and autonomous of any institution or organization for personal, philosophical, or religious reasons.

Some choose not to be licensed or legally regulated at all, and as such, most insurance companies will not reimburse their services. These midwives are sometimes referred to as lay, community-based, granny, or traditional midwives. Such DEMs tend to feel that women have a right to choose qualified care providers regardless of their legal status and feel they are accountable to the particular communities they serve, not the state laws, formal educational requirements, or organizational standards of care.

Licensed Midwife (LM): an LM refers to any above practitioner who meets the requirements for legally practicing midwifery in a specific state. CNMs can qualify for their midwifery license in all 50 states while only some states provide licensure for other forms of midwifery education and degrees. So while you may be able to have a legal homebirth in states where only a CNM can be licensed, an unlicensed midwife could risk arrest by attending your home birth for practicing midwifery without a license–no matter their level of training and expertise. This can get complicated if a medical referral, hospital transfer, or emergency service is needed–as they will need to protect themselves by leaving or not being truthful about their role, and your medical provider will have difficulty obtaining needed medical records and reports of events to provide you with appropriate care.

Registered Midwife (RM): an RM is a midwife with a state-recognized legal licensure status to practice homebirths and for direct-entry midwives who have trained through a program approved by the Midwifery Education Accreditation Council (MEAC) or proof of equivalent apprenticeship and academic study. It is especially useful for midwives who do not qualify for the midwifery licensure of a CNM/CM but practice in a state where direct-entry midwifery is legal, like Colorado.

Now that you know some of the differences between the various types of midwives and their titles, you hopefully have some information to help you find a midwife with whom you are most comfortable. To further help you, the next chapter addresses questions to pose to midwives whom you are considering working with.

For more information on what to expect from care by an out-of-hospital midwife, watch my video : *https://homesweethomebirth.com/ nbsbookbonus*

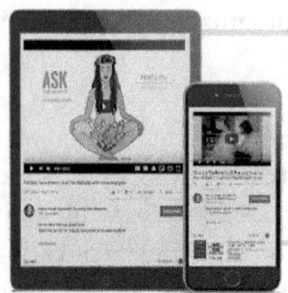

**Want to learn more or
have more questions?**

Grab your free Book Bonuses below:
https://homesweethomebirth.com/nbsbookbonus

QUESTIONS TO ASK WHEN INTERVIEWING A MIDWIFE

When it comes to both our own care and that of our babies, we want to leave no stone unturned in finding our best-suited midwife. And we all probably know the basic questions to ask when interviewing a midwife. But it takes a little more reconnaissance to uncover personality traits or practice philosophy that might not be immediately apparent when you are trying to decide which midwife will be best-suited to your needs and preferences.

The following is a list of queries you may want to consider bringing with you when interviewing a care provider for the first time. Don't worry that you are being too particular–we LOVE it when a potential client has done her research! So bring your list and inquire away!

Question: Who will be allowed to support me during labor and birth?

Ask if the midwife/practice allows other family members or friends to be present in addition to partners. And most definitely ask about doulas. Though most midwives welcome the presence of professional labor support, the staff culture where they have privileges might not be as open, accepting, or welcoming and supportive of doulas.

Question: Can you describe what happens during labor and birth?

This question really gets to the heart of the differences between having your baby at home, a free-standing birth center, or a hospital that is mother/baby-friendly vs. those that are, well, not so much.

According the Coalition for Improving Maternity Services, you'll want the answer to resemble these statistics:

- They should not try to start labor for more than one in ten women (10%).
- Cesarean birth rates should be 10% for community hospitals and 15% for hospitals that have a large high-risk patient population.
- They should allow full freedom to eat and drink.
- They should allow immediate and uninterrupted skin-to-skin contact between mama and baby, and all exams of the baby should be performed at the mom's bedside.
- They should offer the choice of intermittent fetal heart rate monitoring using a doppler or fetoscope periodically, which allows for complete freedom of movement, as you are not attached to continuous monitoring, which restricts mobility and often confines you to a bed.

Question: Do you support women with a wide variety of cultural beliefs and traditions around birth?

If so, is there anything you would like to bring, say, or do that they would not allow?

Question: What kind of mobility will I be allowed?

Laboring women should have the liberty to move around (and deliver their babies) according to what their bodies need at any given time. Mobility helps a mother's body open and her baby to journey down and out much more efficiently, and is one of the best comfort techniques a woman can rely on in her labor.

Question: What kind of collaboration do you have with other staff members, places to which I might be transferred, or organizations from which I may need assistance before and after the baby is born?

On the slim chance that a transfer from your home or a free-standing birth center is necessary, or your baby is born prematurely, does the midwife have a solid reputation with hospital partners who will respect her guidance and her clients?

Does the midwife have direct links to lactation consultants, breastmilk banks, postpartum therapists, and other practitioners who support prenatal and postpartum women? Will this be a seamless process, or might there be any potential issues?

Question: Do you support undisturbed birth?

In Childbirth Connection's ground-breaking report, *Hormonal Physiology of Childbearing and its Implications for Women, Babies and Maternity Care*, "Birth hormones are chemical messengers that your body makes. Your baby makes birth hormones, too. These hormones work together to guide important changes in your bodies—changes that help make labor and birth go smoothly and safely for both of you."

So, does your midwife and the place where they attend birth allow the natural, physiological process of birth to happen in its own way, in its own time, without disturbance when all is well? If not, what intervention is standard protocol, and what is only used when absolutely necessary?

Question: What coping techniques could you offer me if I'm planning a non-interventional birth?

If you would prefer not to use medication for pain relief, what can the midwife offer you so that you can best cope with the challenges of labor? They should be able to answer this with a fairly exhaustive list, as there are many, many ways in which women can access adequate comfort measures during labor and birth.

Question: Will you help me breastfeed?

Statistics show that women who are well-informed and buoyed by support and encouragement will fare much better regarding breastfeeding than those who aren't. Your midwife should be very knowledgeable in this area and have a relationship with at least one excellent International Board-Certified Lactation Consultant, should you need specialized help postpartum. Also inquire about what to expect from other staff, no matter where you are birthing your baby.

Question: What restrictions might be placed on me because of protocol where you attend births?

This refers to things like mother/baby separation, postdates, vaginal birth after cesarean (VBAC), twin and breech births. Find out whether you have choices regarding delayed cord clamping, circumcision, newborn procedures, LaBoyer baths (where your baby is washed right on or near you in quiet and dim lighting) or no bath at all, if that is your wish.

To learn more about this topic, watch my video: *https://homesweethomebirth.com/nbsbookbonus*

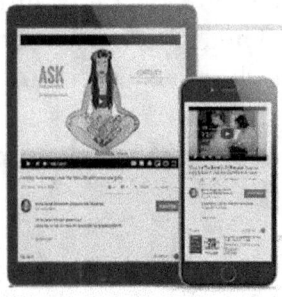

Want to learn more or have more questions?

Grab your free Book Bonuses below:
https://homesweethomebirth.com/nbsbookbonus

THINGS YOU MAY FIND AT YOUR MIDWIFE'S OFFICE

The list below shares 15 wonderful things you may find during prenatal care visits with midwives, especially those who practice in a relatively small group, private practices, out of the hospital, in free-standing birthing centers, and home settings across the United States. Other countries may have slightly different models, but authentic midwifery practices share many common core philosophies of care, so I suspect there would not be much difference. They are:

1. *Time*-as in actual time for connecting and developing a relationship with your midwife so that you can ask your questions and speak about your concerns. Time for the midwife to ask you the questions she needs to make assessments about your health and wellbeing, so she can best guide and support you.

2. *Continuity of care*-the midwife (or one of the few partners if in a small group practice) you see during your prenatal visits will most likely be the midwife who attends your birth.

3. *A big heart*-your midwife will give every ounce of her heartfelt knowledge, expertise, and care for you and your baby. You may feel very close to your midwife after a while. She is like your best big sister or wise friend, and her office is a safe space for you to share, laugh, or cry about anything.

4. *Education*-your midwife will teach you and your loved ones about your body, what's happening, what to expect along your childbearing journey, and what you can do to make it easier, healthier, and more positive. This includes diagrams and models of pregnant moms and babies, placentas, umbilical cords, membranes, and pelvises. Your midwife might just have a mirror for anatomy lessons of your own body if you are interested ... like seeing your cervix.

5. *Tea and healthy snacks*–for everyone.
6. *Inspiration*–inspirational quotes, affirmations, and art about pregnancy, giving birth, breastfeeding, babywearing, and parenting.
7. *Pictures*–photos of graduates on the wall and/or in photo albums.
8. *A collection of thank-you notes and birth stories*–I call these "love letters," and you could find them arranged in collages and/or scrapbooks.
9. *Midwifery and holistic health text/reference books*–these books as well as a lending library of books and movies on pregnancy, natural childbirth, breastfeeding, babywearing, and newborn care.
10. *Seating*–enough seating arrangements for the whole family and even some friends, as well as toys and books for the little ones.
11. *Hands*–your midwife's hands are skillful both in their assessment AND the supportive touch they offer.
12. *Tools*–all the supplies and knowledge of how to use them that could possibly be needed for your journey. These include equipment, such as a blood pressure cuff, stethoscope, fetoscope, Doppler and gel for checking the baby's heart rate, scale, measuring tape for assessing the height and growth of your uterus, and lab supplies for checking your blood, urine, screening for infection and pap smear, AND so much more! If she uses an exam table, the stirrups will be covered with oven mitts, and it will probably have a nice comfortable and decorative sheet and pillow on it, with a stool for climbing up and down and for the little ones to be involved.
13. *A boutique*–where you can buy needed items like supplements and natural remedies, books, affirmation cards, birth balls, birth kits, birth tubs for rental, pregnancy and postpartum support garments, postpartum mama and baby care supplies and baby carriers.
14. *Office and birth assistants*–your midwife may also have students, apprentices, and even a doula or two to choose from. She may have space to host childbirth classes, pregnancy and postpartum support groups, prenatal and postpartum yoga, parenting groups, and all sorts of relevant workshops and community events.

15. *Necessary medical and midwifery knowledge and clinical skills*–she will also be familiar with and use a variety of holistic, alternative, and natural modalities that can help you with pregnancy, birth, and beyond.

As you go about choosing your midwife and planning for your birth, you might want to ask yourself what is important for you from the above list. Does your midwife or obstetrician offer some of these things? What do you want and need? Start writing down your questions and preferences in a journal now, so that when you meet them, you have these handy.

Why a Doula Is a Must

World Doula Week is a week initiated by a doula in Israel to empower and support doulas around the world to improve the emotional and social health of birthing, postpartum women, and their families. This is so needed in modern times, with the breakdown of community and resulting lack of sisterhood in mothering, along with the medicalization, prevalent fear and lack of exposure to childbirth. Dr. John H. Kennel says, "If a doula were a drug, it would be unethical not to use it."

When I think of the many doulas I have been blessed to work with, I am reminded of strong, beautiful, kind, passionate, dedicated, fun-loving women who have found their calling supporting other women. These women rise by lifting others. Research the many proven benefits of having a doula, especially if you are giving birth vaginally for the first time.

What Is a Doula and Why Have One?

A doula or a labor support person like a doula is a must–someone calm and nurturing to mother you, who knows how to help mamas in labor, birth, and postpartum, and who trusts the process. Throughout history and even currently in large segments of the globe, women gave/give birth at home and were/are surrounded by and supported by other women in their communities. In the US and many parts of the modern world, more commonly, mamas don't have this, and it negatively impacts their birth and postpartum. My 7% transfer rate from home to hospital is mostly first-time moms with prolonged arrested labors, exhaustion, and with a common theme–they did not set themselves up with a doula or doula-like labor support, despite what I advised. I want mamas to optimize their chances of having an empowered, deeply positive, and healthy birth experience. See if your midwife knows great doulas, and if needed, with a sliding scale. An awesome one is worth every penny.

I could talk for hours about this, but here are the main reasons I believe pregnant moms, especially first-timers, those planning to VBAC, and those who are in a large group practice or have an obstetrician as their provider, should hire a doula. Most obstetricians do not learn about or actually provide labor support, and aside from periodic exams, diagnostic or treatment interventions, they will not be attending to you until your actual delivery. Midwives are more likely to be with a woman when needed, especially in the later part of labor, to provide supportive care, although their main job is lifeguarding the safety of mom and baby. In busy large group practices, a provider may have several laboring women at the same time, and need to rely on nurses if available, and doulas to fill in the gaps. Doulas and midwives complement one another even in out-of-hospital birth settings and preserve, rather than interfere with, partner and family support and privacy. Often partners are grateful they do not have to learn to be a labor coach.

In many cultures today, and throughout history–until relatively more recently when birth was moved into the hospitals and people live isolated from community–women supported women through childbirth and postpartum. Doulas fill this void. They are trained to provide emotional support, comfort measures, reassurance, encouragement, empowerment, advocacy, and basically to act as a mother to the laboring and postpartum mother.

Most doulas go through a short training and certification process, although many take continuing education and serve childbearing families in other ways, such as facilitating pregnancy and postpartum support circles, doing birth photography, creating mother blessing ceremonies, encapsulating placentas, and becoming childbirth educators to teach childbirth classes.

Doulas are not medical providers like midwives and obstetricians, responsible for the actual maternity and newborn care. Although midwives are more likely to provide doula-like care, which is integral to authentic midwifery, that is not their leading role.

There is an impressive body of research on the many risk-free benefits of the continuous support of an experienced doula during labor. For the mother-to-be, these benefits include improved coping, self-confidence, esteem, and empowerment, enhanced satisfaction and positive feelings about their childbirth, shorter and easier labors, an easier time adapting to motherhood with enhanced skills, longer breastfeeding, more positive feelings towards their baby, and even improved relationship with their partner!

Scientific evidence from gold standard medical studies also reveals less pain and fear, fewer childbirth interventions including cesarean, vacuum, and forceps deliveries, fewer episiotomies, less medication for pain and stimulating labor, fewer babies in poor condition needing intensive care and longer hospital stays, less of all the associated risks to the above interventions, and less postpartum depression. This is HUGE!

Having a doula is like having a personal coach so that you have the healthiest, most successful and wonderful experience possible. All successful professional athletes, performers, and most leading business people have coaches of some sort. "The wisdom and compassion a woman intuitively experiences in childbirth can make her a source of healing and understanding for other women," said the beloved Steve Gaskin. I honor all doulas and all superhero mamas who have given birth anyhow, anywhere.

Watch my video to learn more about doulas: *https://homesweethomebirth. com/nbsbookbonus*

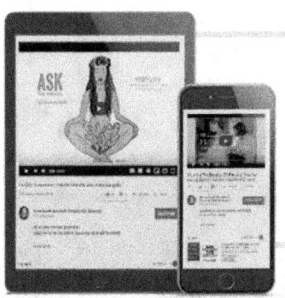

Want to learn more or have more questions?

Grab your free Book Bonuses below:
https://homesweethomebirth.com/nbsbookbonus

CHILDBIRTH CLASSES: WHAT'S THE SCOOP?

Since you have purchased this book you are clearly interested in learning about childbirth education. And there is a lot to learn! Let me break down a few burning questions you may have, like the many reasons why taking a childbirth class is so important today.

FULL DISCLOSURE: I am a midwife, labor support doula, and childbirth educator. But I'm writing this book also because I was once a pregnant mom faced with an overwhelming number of choices regarding how to prepare. It's tough out there in pregnancy-land! How are you supposed to know what you are supposed to know?

I have seen the difference on countless occasions that childbirth education classes make for women and their partners during labor and birth. Knowledge is power, my friends. Women and their partners who prepare in advance tend to have much easier labors, give birth vaginally, and cope better with the challenges they may face along the way. And they feel more positive about their experience.

The Basics: Why Take a Childbirth Education Class?

The anatomy and physiology of childbirth remain unchanged. So, if none of the actual process has evolved, don't we just know enough about birth by now? Well, we would, if this were the 1800s. Although we have made major technological advances that allow us to achieve truly magnificent and amazing things beyond our wildest dreams, our culture no longer provides us the opportunity to witness birth as a normal, everyday event.

In many places around the world, people still approach birth in the same ways that their ancestors have for generations. A woman is surrounded by her mother, sisters, cousins, aunts, grandmothers, and friends, creating a rock-solid foundation that cradles her through pregnancy, labor, birth, and postpartum. This means that these lucky people are around birth all the time. It was like this in developed countries as well until a few key events took place.

These key events: people began to move away from their communities, putting distance between new mothers and close relations. When childbirth moved out of the home and into the hospital in the early 1900s, it came to be viewed as a medical condition. As a result, clinical staff and hospital protocol created an even greater chasm between a woman and the support she would have received in the past from her circle of family and friends.

Therefore, a childbirth education class helps moms and their partners learn about and believe in the process, about how their bodies and babies really instinctively know what to do, about normalcy in labor and birth, about the importance of relaxation, and about how to gain confidence and find their inner strength.

If Your Body and Baby Know What to Do, Why Do You Need a Class?

Great question! It all goes back to our not being around birth. For most women in our country today, birth is something foreign that takes place in a medical institution. Many fear the great unknown. Childbirth is also viewed as something really scary. Why? Because most women in our society don't witness what birth really looks like until they have their own babies. Instead, they hear lots of negative stories that frighten the heck out of them. Or they watch birth scenes of hysteria and horror in movies and on TV. Although you may understand that a woman's body is designed to give birth as much as she is designed to breathe, taking a class to describe how it all goes down is really critical these days.

Perhaps you are now asking yourself, "Can't I just do my own reading or catch a webinar online or talk to my best friend's sister's co-worker?" For starters, you will have lots of questions. And you deserve answers to those questions. Not just standard, general, statistically-average, run-of-the-mill answers, but answers that answer YOU specifically by someone trained. And in real-time.

In addition, you'll learn comfort techniques for pregnancy and labor–things you can rely on yourself–and those that actively involve your partner. Trying to get a sense for these positions is a lot easier when a excellent instructor is right there with you, offering guidance along the way.

Next, you will be creating a community with your classmates. There is terrific value in going through such a profound, life-changing experience with others:

- You will understand each other on a level no one else really can.
- It's priceless when someone asks a question that you hadn't thought of, and it becomes one that you must have the answer to!
- You can learn a lot from one another and connect in the community for now and for post-birth. This is needed today to remedy the prevalent isolation. Remember, it takes a village to raise a baby and new parents.
- You might just meet your new best friend. This happens more frequently than you'd think!

How Do You Find a Class That Suits Your Needs and Preferences?

My first piece of advice is to do your research. Don't just check out an instructor's website. Get her on the phone and actually interview her. Read testimonials and online reviews, and contact former students. Get a sense of her philosophy and approach.

Secondly, ask to see a syllabus. Make sure a class offers the specific topics in which you are interested. **NOT ALL CHILDBIRTH CLASSES ARE CREATED EQUALLY.** Some spend a lot of time addressing common fears and exploring relaxation techniques. Some focus on medical intervention without going into much detail about natural coping modalities. Some include newborn care and breastfeeding; some do not.

My advice is to look for a comprehensive, non-judgmental class where discussion is encouraged and a safe forum is created so that you feel free to ask questions and share honestly.

A few of the things I hear all the time are: "I'm so busy. I don't have a traditional work schedule. I can't possibly dedicate all those hours. I just want to sleep in." It's easy to feel this way. I hear you. I really do. And a one-day intensive sounds like a perfect solution to this battle cry. However, I don't recommend it. First of all, there is far too much information to cover in one day, so you won't be receiving all that you need. Also, day intensives are exhausting for everyone. I taught them early on in my career and, trust me, instructors can't give their all when they are on hour six. Nor can a pregnant woman fatigued from hormones, her growing belly, and a full work-week possibly process all there is to learn. And when you are in a group, there is simply no way the instructor will have time to answer all of your queries.

What If You Really, Truly Can't Get to a Class?

If you are on bedrest; if there aren't any classes conveniently located near you; if transportation is a problem; if your schedule simply doesn't permit–seek out an instructor who offers in-home, private sessions, or take an excellent comprehensive online course–like mine!–ideally with an online consultation for your personal questions. You won't have the benefit of being with others in person, but you won't have to travel, you can schedule it according to your calendar, the class can be customized just for you and your partner, and you can join my online community. These tailored classes can address your own unique concerns from adoption, surrogacy, and gay parenting to sibling preparation, vaginal birth after cesarean (VBAC), and other health issues, etc.

If cost is an issue, ask about payment plans, barter deals, discounts, or promos. Scholarships are available in some locations too.

My motto is: "Don't wing it! Take a solid class. It doesn't have to be my class. Just take a class." Think of it as your marathon to run or mountain to climb. It takes lots of preparation, as any successful athlete will tell you. So, go for it. If you can only take a one-day intensive, at least do that, as it is indeed better than not taking anything at all. Just know that you will likely have to fill in some gaps with other resources, perhaps ones recommended by your care provider or my favorite and recommended books and movies–a comprehensive list is included in my online course.

Doing your research, taking a class, asking your questions–these are all tremendously worthwhile activities. They will serve you quite well as you continue this incredible journey. Don't shortchange yourself. Remember, there are no stupid questions. This is uncharted territory for most of you–let information be like hands that hold you up so that you can be and feel your best, and be as confident and prepared as possible!

For more information, watch my video on childbirth classes : *https:// homesweethomebirth.com/nbsbookbonus*

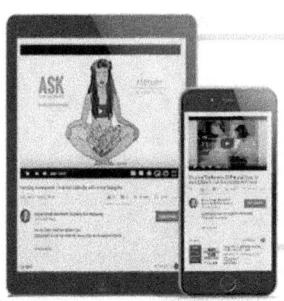

Want to learn more or have more questions?

Grab your free Book Bonuses below:
https://homesweethomebirth.com/nbsbookbonus

Pregnancy Troubleshooting:
Preventative, Natural & Gentle

CONSIDERING AN ULTRASOUND?

If you're worried about ultrasound safety, good for you! You should be. The use of ultrasound in pregnancy has become almost a given. Most women in the US and Canada experience at least one ultrasound during pregnancy. Some experience several. There are certainly appropriate situations for the use of ultrasound, but a healthy pregnancy isn't one of them.

If, after weighing the pros and cons of an ultrasound, you decide to have one, that's entirely within your right. What's important here is to make an informed decision rather than just exposing yourself and your baby to high-frequency sound waves as a matter of routine practice.

Is an Ultrasound Necessary?

The answer to this question really differs from person to person and even situation to situation. When a healthcare provider recommends an ultrasound to a pregnant woman, the FDA recommends that the mom speaks with their provider to understand exactly why the ultrasound is needed, what information will be obtained, how the information will be used, and any potential risks.

Medicine is big business. There is significant financial incentive for obstetricians to recommend ultrasounds to their patients, as they can bill many hundreds of dollars to insurance companies for each use. According to the Center for Disease Control (CDC), the overuse of technology is one of the major reasons for the rise in healthcare costs.

More and more modern obstetricians have been trained to use ultrasound in place of hands-on skills to evaluate the health of the pregnancy. They use it to evaluate fetal growth and position in the third trimester, which can often be assessed by a hands-on examination. They also use it to date pregnancies, which can typically be done with a little detective work.

Ultrasound is often used to determine whether a baby will be too large to be birthed naturally via the birth canal. However, ultrasound has been shown to be an inaccurate measure of birth weight. Further, our pelvic bones are joined together with ligaments that allow the pelvis to widen enough for birth to safely take place, especially when supported in upright and asymmetrical mobile positioning. This is true in almost every case, even when the mother is especially small or the baby is especially large.

There are some situations in which an ultrasound is warranted. For example, bleeding in pregnancy or a serious abnormality that requires immediate or high-risk hospital care. Or if mom has very irregular or absent cycles during breastfeeding, or she is unable to provide any real guideline for calculating gestational age and estimated due date. Sometimes, if mom has a lot of anxiety about the health of her pregnancy and baby, a normal ultrasound mid-pregnancy can provide some reassurance while still not being a guarantee.

The American Institute of Ultrasound in Medicine advocates for use of ultrasound solely for medical purposes, and never for things like keepsake images. And the American College of Nurse-Midwives' position is that "Ultrasound should only be used when medically indicated."

What Do We Know About Ultrasound Safety?

Ultrasound waves have the potential to produce biological effects on the body. They can heat bodily tissue, as well as produce small pockets of gas in bodily fluids or tissues (known as cavitation). The long-term consequences of these effects are still unknown.

Sarah Buckley, MD provides an extensive article in which she weighs ultrasound safety. In it she says:

"If there is bleeding in early pregnancy, for example, ultrasound may predict whether miscarriage is inevitable. Later in pregnancy, ultrasound can be used when a baby is not growing, or when a breech baby or twins are suspected. In these cases, the information gained from ultrasound may be very useful in decision-making for the woman and her carers. However the use of routine prenatal ultrasound (RPU) is more controversial, as this involves scanning all pregnant women in the hope of improving the outcome for some mothers and babies.

Studies on humans exposed to ultrasound have shown that possible adverse effects include premature ovulation, preterm labour or miscarriage, low birth weight, poorer condition at birth, perinatal death, dyslexia, delayed speech development, and less right-handedness."

Despite its rampant use, there has not been sufficient testing for ultrasound safety, especially concerning its routine use in healthy pregnancies. In fact, there has been very little testing at all since the 1980s even though the FDA allowed exposure limits to increase by eight-fold in 1992.

It's important to acknowledge here that technology is often assumed safe until proven otherwise. Just a couple of generations back, it was general practice to X-ray pregnant mothers. It sounds crazy now that we know more about the dangers of X-rays to the developing fetus, but back then it made perfect sense.

As Kelly Brogan, MD states:

"Multiple Cochrane reviews have demonstrated a lack of perinatal mortality benefit for routine ultrasound in a normal pregnancy, and an increased risk of cesarean section with third trimester screening. A review of outcomes literature condemns ultrasound when used for dating, second trimester organ scan, biophysical profile, amniotic fluid assessment, and Doppler velocity in high and low risk pregnancies."

While our reasons for using ultrasound are typically focused on healthy pregnancies and healthy babies, there has been virtually no proof that more ultrasounds in a population equate with better health. What's worse is there are concerns about their possible causative link to the alarming increase in autism. In addition, false positives of congenital malformations are not unusual. Sadly, this has led to more invasive testing and abortions misunderstood to be medically necessary when there is nothing actually wrong. At the very least, this puts undue stress on the mama, partner, and baby.

In my opinion, technology has put distance between mamas and care providers. In situations where a midwife historically would take a literal hands-on approach to a mom and baby's health, technology now allows for a disconnect where mom is sometimes never touched by her pregnancy and birthing support team. My belief is that this impersonal approach can do just as much harm as the technology can.

The overuse of ultrasound also undermines a woman's trust in her healthy body's ability to grow and birth her healthy baby, as modern-day families are putting more and more trust in technology over themselves.

Alternatives to Ultrasound

We do not fully understand the effect of directing loud sound waves at a baby, but it does alter DNA in the test tube and there is strong evidence to show that any damage done is cumulative. So, if you must have an ultrasound, keep it as brief as possible and limited to as few as possible. If all is well and you know your cycles or date of conception, but you really want an ultrasound, do it mid-pregnancy. And, of course, make sure to request a keepsake picture of your baby.

A Doppler is an ultrasound device that can detect fetal heartbeat as early as 10 to 12 weeks, depending on the device, the location of baby, and the position of the mom's uterus. It is used for each prenatal visit in many obstetrical care offices and clinics. If you want to minimize ultrasound exposure, ask for a fetoscope.

A fetoscope, which is similar to a stethoscope and works to amplify the baby's heartbeat, can be used in place of an ultrasound or Doppler after around 20 weeks gestational age to listen to the fetal heartbeat. It can also help assess the baby's position in later pregnancy.

When a baby starts to move regularly, especially in the third trimester, I teach fetal movement awareness and kick counts. Basically, babies sleep a lot, especially when you are busy running around; but they tend to get up and become active after you eat and when you're resting. Become aware of when and how often your baby is most active and take notice of your baby's typical daily patterns of movement. An active baby, moving as much as usual, is a sign of fetal health and wellbeing. If you did not feel your baby move as much usual on a given day, eat food that has previously stimulated lots of fetal activity—usually carbohydrates like a peanut butter and jelly whole-grain sandwich or cereal and nut milk—plus have two glasses of orange juice and a cup of coffee; recline and 30 to 40 minutes later aim to count at least ten separate kicks, body shifts, and punches in the hour. Most babies will produce more than that in a few minutes, but if you are not feeling ten separate moves in that hour, call your provider.

For most of history we did not know if we were having a boy or a girl until the birth of our baby. There is something special about the surprise. But for those wanting to know the sex of their baby, blood tests are now available and are actually more accurate than ultrasound for this purpose.

Your Choice

Medical interventions like ultrasounds often play into our fears and turn us away from our intuition. We have come to have less trust in the process and believe that we need to rely on technology to assure us that our babies are safe. As mamas, we have thousands of years of the birthing wisdom of our elders that we carry in our DNA. Is that less reliable than a relatively new, under-tested technology?

Midwives typically use touch and hand skills in place of technology like ultrasounds. As a holistic and integrative midwife that specializes in healthy pregnancies, I always give the option for an ultrasound and discuss the pros and cons with each family in my care. Some opt out unless there is an issue or complication when the benefits outweigh the potential risks. Some do want one to confirm they have a baby in the uterus with a heartbeat before it is too early to tell in the office, along with a basic scan between 18 to 22 weeks. For those birthing at home, some want a mid-pregnancy ultrasound to check the baby's anatomy and that the placenta is in the right place, so they are reassured there is nothing detected that warrants birth in the higher-risk hospital setting.

As midwives, we do not fix what is not broken. We instill trust in the pregnancy and birth process, and have confidence in a mom's ability to do it.

RhoGam Shot in Pregnancy

Risks and Benefits of RhoGAM

Many expecting parents have questions about whether or not to get the Rh immune globulin (RhoGAM) shot if the mama-to-be is Rh-negative. This applies to a small number of women, but it is extremely important for them to be armed with all the information prior to making a decision.

If you are among the roughly 10% to 15% of people who are Rh-negative, your pregnancy could be affected if your baby is Rh-positive. In this situation, obstetric providers often recommend RhoGAM.

However, it's not always that simple. If you're not sure you have all the information for an informed decision, you're in the right place. Below are some frequently asked questions and points to consider.

What Is the Rh Factor?

The Rh factor is a protein that can be found on the surface of red blood cells. If your blood cells have this protein, you are Rh-positive. If they do not have this protein, you are Rh-negative. This is the negative or positive after your blood type: A, B, O, or AB. It is simply about different normal variations in red blood cells. For example, you can be A positive or O negative. The negative or positive is your Rh factor. A pregnant woman will get a blood type, Rh, and antibody screen as part of the routine prenatal blood tests. If she is Rh-negative, her antibody response will get tested several times as indicated throughout the pregnancy to check for Rh sensitization.

What Is Rh Incompatibility and Sensitization?

Rh incompatibility is when the blood of a fetus is Rh-positive but the mama's is Rh-negative. In this situation, if the baby's blood gets into the mother's bloodstream, the mother creates a defense system against the different types of blood because her body perceives it as foreign even though it belongs to her baby. She will react against it by making anti-Rh antibodies. When a pregnant mother makes antibodies against the Rh factor on her baby's red blood cells, it is called sensitization. Once a mom is sensitized, it stays with her forever.

This rarely causes complications in a first pregnancy, as the primary immune response takes time to develop and initially produces IgM antibodies that are too large to cross the placenta. However, it could be dangerous in future pregnancies for the fetus or newborn baby because the secondary immune response is more rapid and the body has made smaller IgG antibodies that easily cross the placenta. Once these antibodies can cross the placenta, they try to destroy the fetus's red blood cells.

How Can Rh Problems Affect the Fetus During Subsequent Pregnancies?

Rh sensitization can lead to a wide variety of mild to serious health issues in a fetus or newborn of the next pregnancy. The main concern is a severe type of anemia in the fetus, in which red blood cells are destroyed faster than the baby can replace them. Red blood cells carry oxygen to all parts of the body. Without sufficient red blood cells, the fetus will not get enough oxygen, and this can result in hemolytic disease of the fetus and newborn, causing jaundice, brain damage, heart failure, and death.

How Can the Fetus' Blood Get into the Mother's Bloodstream?

During a healthy pregnancy, a mom and her fetus usually do not share blood, thanks to the placenta that keeps the fetal and maternal blood circulation separate. But sometimes a small amount of blood from the fetus can mix with the mother's blood. Typically, there is no mixing sufficient enough to risk sensitization unless there is are complications like miscarriage, placental abruption or previa, abdominal trauma, or an invasive medical/surgical procedure like chorionic villus sampling or amniocentesis, abdominal surgery, and even ultrasound.

Sensitization is usually associated with a rapid and large volume of fetal-maternal blood mixing. The most common time for Rh-positive fetal red blood cells to enter the mother's bloodstream is during childbirth, though it can occur at other points during pregnancy, mainly in the third trimester.

Traumatic and difficult births with a high level of invasive procedures increase the likelihood for the baby's blood to mix with the mom's. So can certain routine interventions including the use of the synthetic drug Pitocin to induce or augment labor, local or regional anesthesia, forced directed pushing, clamping the umbilical cord too early, pulling on the cord and putting pressure on the fundus to hasten the delivery of the placenta.

A gentle birth process with minimal intervention and time allowance for the placenta to separate provides a reduced risk of significant mixing of blood between the mother and baby. While not a guarantee, planning for a natural, undisturbed physiologic pregnancy and birth may certainly help prevent the mixing of fetal and maternal blood that leads to sensitization and hemolytic disease.

Can You Determine If the Baby is Rh-Positive?

There is a new non-invasive blood test which can detect fetal blood type using a blood sample of the pregnant mom. It is said to be highly accurate and almost as reliable as the conventional test that uses a blood sample of the newborn after birth. It is almost, but not 100% accurate, and it is not available everywhere or covered by all insurances.

If a pregnant mama is Rh-positive, there is no need for further testing or RhoGam. If she is Rh-negative, I recommend the father getting his blood type and Rh factor tested. If the father is Rh-positive and the mother is

Rh-negative, there is about a 75% chance the baby is Rh-positive, and providers will probably recommend RhoGAM. But if both parents are Rh negative, the baby will also be Rh-negative. In that case, there is no risk of Rh sensitization and no necessity for RhoGM.

What Is RhoGAM and What Are Its Benefits?

RhoGAM is a drug made from human blood plasma that prevents the mother from making antibodies against the positive Rh factor in her baby's blood. It is given via intramuscular injection to prevent the immune response of sensitization against the baby's Rh-positive blood and subsequent hemolytic disease of the fetus or newborn in future pregnancies.

RhoGAM's effectiveness has been demonstrated in multiple studies around the globe. According to Dr. Murray Enkin, one of the widely respected and authoritative founders of evidence-based care, and his team that wrote *A Guide to Effective Care in Pregnancy and Childbirth*, RhoGAM given after birth reduces the rate of hemolytic disease from 15% down to 1.6%. RhoGAM administration prenatally in the third trimester has been shown in studies to further decrease the incidence to 0.06%.

The administration of RhoGAM medication to Rh-negative mothers is thought to be a major achievement of modern obstetrics by many in the medical profession. Before RhoGam's introduction into routine practice in the 1970s, hemolytic disease of the newborn was a major cause of serious illness, death, and long-term disability in babies.

RhoGAM does not typically benefit firstborn babies unless the mom who is Rh-negative has previously experienced a reaction to a mismatched blood transfusion, abortion, miscarriage, or ectopic pregnancy untreated with RhoGam.

When Is RhoGAM Recommended and Why?

For women who are Rh-negative, healthcare providers routinely recommend a shot of RhoGAM around 28 weeks of pregnancy and then again within 72 hours after birth in order to protect the baby of a subsequent pregnancy.

Providers must decide about the RhoGAM shot and its dose based on how likely it is for the baby to have Rh-positive blood, as well as how likely it is for the baby and mother's blood to significantly mix during pregnancy and birth.

Is There Controversy around RhoGAM?

This standard approach is not without its critics, especially regarding its routine use during pregnancy, in which only about 1.5% of Rh-negative moms with Rh-positive fetuses develop antibodies and become sensitized against the baby's positive Rh factor. The risk of sensitization is significantly higher after birth. Administration of RhoGAM postpartum is much less controversial, where the benefits of the medication more clearly outweigh potential risks. As explained by celebrated midwife Ina May Gaskin, "The problem with routine prescription of prenatal RhoGAM is that many babies who are Rh-negative like their mothers will be exposed to the drug, and there has been no systematic study of the long-term effects of this product in babies."

Holistic midwife and author of several comprehensive midwifery textbooks, Anne Frye has the following take on it, "RhIG is not given for the direct benefit of the recipient or even her current fetus. The only beneficiary will be an RhD positive fetus during a subsequent pregnancy (although the woman would also benefit in the event of a wrongly-typed transfusion during the time of birth). Furthermore, prenatal prophylaxis unnecessarily exposes 35% of fetuses who are RhD negative to RhIG. These babies are at no risk of RhD sensitization. RhIG is completely unnecessary when a baby is the last child in the family. In the absence of clear answers to these pressing questions, the routine use of RhIG assumes that the birth process for RhD negative women is inherently flawed."

Reliable research and meta-analysis of the studies on benefit and harm of routine use of RhoGam in pregnancy are still limited, especially as it relates to whom, when, and which dose is needed, as well as its cost-effectiveness.

Some argue that there may be other factors that contributed to the marked decline in severity and prevalence of perinatal morbidity and mortality associated with Rh incompatibility and sensitization, and medicating healthy pregnant women undermines those who trust the inherent wisdom in the natural process of childbearing. That being said, the issue remains an issue that, still today, impacts babies of pregnant women who are Rh-negative.

What Are the Risks of RhoGAM?

Despite excellent results, the medication retains an FDA Pregnancy Category C: "Animal reproduction studies have shown an adverse effect on the fetus and there are no adequate and well-controlled studies in humans, but potential benefits may warrant the use of the drug in pregnant women despite potential risks."

The known possible side effects to RhoGAM include local swelling inflammation at the site, skin rash, body aches, and sometimes hives. Infection from the blood product of modern preparation is rare, but still a possibility.

Expecting mamas should also keep in mind that standard RhoGAM preparation in many countries contains the mercury compound known as thimerosal, which has a litany of health risks. However, pregnant mamas can request the use of the mercury-free RhoGAM if it is available where they live. In the United States, RhoGam is said to be mercury-free although it may still contain traces.

Is the RhoGAM Shot Absolutely Necessary During Pregnancy?

This is a hard question to answer for each individual. Although much of the research is compelling, it is dated, was largely funded by the pharmaceutical companies, and is not without bias, flaws, and some conflicting conclusions. For an eye-opening text analysis of the data through 2001 and guidance from a traditional midwifery perspective, check out Anti-D in Midwifery: Panacea or Paradox? Second Edition by Sara Wickham.

I encourage my clients to take great care of themselves, to be well-educated on their health-related issues, and to be in tune with their bodies. While I aspire to provide evidence-based information about medications and recommended treatments, I also know that there is much we do not know, and I am wary of routine medical and surgical interventions in a healthy, natural process. Too often they are widely used before sufficient evaluation of them or before their potential for harm has been identified. I feel informed and empowered moms are best able to make decisions for themselves.

Understanding that the vast majority of women who are Rh-negative will not become sensitized during pregnancy, as it is rare that mixing happens until birth, is an important consideration when balancing the risks and benefits of using a pharmaceutical therapy while pregnant.

If you are Rh-negative and the baby's dad is Rh-negative, no, you do not need the shot. If the baby's dad is Rh-positive, and you choose to refuse the shot in pregnancy, you may still need it later if you suspect bleeding or another reason for sensitization, or if you change your mind. If you have done your research, you believe you are low-risk, and you do not feel comfortable with the shot while pregnant, do not let a provider pressure you.

According to those who advocate a gentle birth process with minimal intervention and time allowance for the placenta to separate, there is usually less risk of significant mixing of blood between mother and baby. But mixing and sensitization can certainly still occur during healthy, natural birthing. Traumatic, highly-interventive, and difficult births increase the likelihood for fetomaternal hemorrhage and sensitization. So can certain routine interventions that possibly disrupt the delicate physiology of placental separation or cause tiny fetal blood vessels to rupture and bleed. Planning for a natural, undisturbed, physiologic birth may certainly help prevent the mixing of fetal and maternal blood that leads to sensitization and hemolytic disease.

As always, pregnant mamas should empower themselves with knowledge and talk with their provider to fully understand the benefits and risks of all medications unique to their situation.

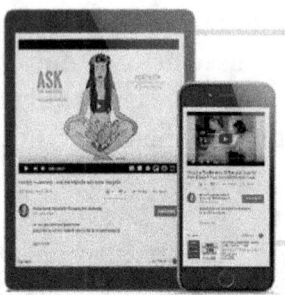

Want to learn more or have more questions?

Grab your free Book Bonuses below:
https://homesweethomebirth.com/nbsbookbonus

Screening for Gestational Diabetes

Gestational diabetes is rare in the healthy population. Occurring in about 6% of pregnancies, its incidence is increasing largely due to growing incidences of obesity, insulin resistance, adult-onset diabetes, and poor diet and lifestyle habits in the United States. There is much controversy around gestational diabetes, how it is screened for and diagnosed, and whether universal screening improves outcomes as opposed to testing when there are risk factors. If you do have it, however, treatment that includes appropriate actions like maintaining ideal weight and enhancing nutrition and exercise habits make a significant difference in reducing the serious health consequences for both you and your baby.

In the US, it is standard care that all women are screened for gestational diabetes at 24 to 28 weeks of pregnancy, although, in some other European countries, only women with risk factors are screened. Screening that is most common involves giving pregnant women a "Glucola" drink that has 50 grams of sugar in it in the form of dextrose and then testing blood sugar an hour later. Many holistic providers and the families they serve are concerned about this potentially toxic drink laden with chemicals that may make them feel sick, harm them and their babies, and can be associated with false positives that label them unnecessarily as "high risk." This increases stress and angst and leads to more testing, monitoring, and potentially other risky interventions. They want alternatives.

While it is within your right to refuse the test, you may want to consider screening for gestational diabetes in another way and discuss your concerns and options with your provider. If your provider is unwilling to work with you on this, consider switching providers to one who will.

Although we do not have enough evidence that alternative screens are as accurate as using the more extensively-studied Glucola drink to screen for diabetes of pregnancy, alternatives are not to be easily discounted and may be a viable option in the low-risk healthy population.

There is an option for screening for gestational diabetes by home testing. This involves checking your fasting blood sugar at home when you wake up in the morning and then again an hour after eating your usual breakfast, lunch, and dinner. While approved for monitoring blood sugar once diagnosed with diabetes, this method of screening is less studied and without clear standards. It is also more cumbersome and costly, as you need to get the supplies to do it, then take the time to get it right, and keep records to discuss with your provider at your next prenatal visit.

Alternative Gestational Diabetes Screening Options

Do note that not all sugars are the same, and they each have various effects on blood sugar. The Glucola drink is the most studied to screen for diabetes of pregnancy, and the blood test results are based on its ingestion. We are aiming to get as close to it as possible. Follow the instructions below to properly prepare for the test, increase accuracy, and avoid false positives and negatives, as well as improve your tolerance of it. Starting three days before your appointment, increase complex carbohydrates, such as whole grains, sweet potatoes, and winter squash.

The meal before the test should only contain protein and vegetables. A mixed veggie omelet is a great choice. Avoid sweetened foods, fruit, and carbs. If this last meal before the test is lunch or dinner, you can eat a normal breakfast but avoid carbs or sweets for the rest of the day.

To make a drink that is most equivalent to Glucola without the chemical additives, dissolve 50 grams of organic dextrose in eight ounces of filtered or spring water. It is ideal to be organic, produced from corn that has not been chemically sprayed or genetically modified. You will need to do some math. If there are 20 grams of dextrose in two tablespoons, for example, then you need five tablespoons of the powder. You ideally want dextrose, as it is the sugar made from corn that makes up the

Glucola drink, and it is most bioidentical to the sugar in your blood called glucose.

Therefore, it is the best alternative to screen for gestational diabetes as the standard Glucola drink does, according to the laboratory parameters designed and tested for this purpose.

Another alternative is to drink an equivalent amount of pure corn syrup dissolved in tea, as the sugar in corn syrup is dextrose. You can find organic non-GMO varieties of corn syrup in health food stores, but you still need to do some math to get 50 grams of sugar total.

Reputable research indicates that you can, instead, eat 28 all-natural organic jelly beans or enough that equals 50 grams of sugar, which has been studied to be a reliable alternative to the 50-gram glucose beverage. It is not standardized as is the Glucola drink, and amounts and types of sugars vary with each product, so you need to do the calculations and make sure you are eating 50 grams of sugar. The study was relatively small, but its results can certainly be considered.

Other less-ideal options are iced tea, organic Gatorade, or a cola drink that has 50 grams of sugar added in the form of added table sugar or dehydrated cane juice (sucrose), which is similar to the kind of sugar in jelly beans. These are not a first choice because they are not as extensively researched and the form of sugar is different than dextrose; thus, they may have a different effect on your blood sugar levels and test results, tests that were designed to screen for diabetes based on a person's response to dextrose.

As stated, the blood test to screen for gestational diabetes was studied and formulated to test your reaction to ingesting 50 grams of dextrose. Sucrose is made up of 50% glucose and 50% fructose. You will need to read ingredients and nutrition labels to use an alternative, an important skill to develop anyway. And you still need to do some math, as the nutrition label might say something like 23 grams of sugar per eight-ounce serving.

When going for sugars that are not dextrose extracted from corn, you can choose any sugar-sweetened drink without added fruit juice. Fruit contains a different type of sugar called fructose that makes the test less accurate as it has a different effect on your blood glucose levels than does dextrose and sucrose. If you cannot find or have no time to figure it out and have a low risk of gestational diabetes, a Snapple 16-ounce raspberry peach drink is an option. Although it is mainly sweetened with sugar (sucrose), it does have a little fruit juice, which again is mostly fructose.

Coconut water is another, but less than ideal, option, as it contains sugar in the form of mostly sucrose and glucose, and it does have some fructose. ZICO coconut water at 16.9 ounces has 20 grams of sugar in it, so you would need to drink 2.5 bottles. Honey is another alternative, but it is also not made up of an equivalent sugar; it is sucrose and fructose. Again, you need to read the label. Different honeys have different amounts of sugar per serving size too.

Hopefully, there will be more studies on these alternatives, but for now, those listed in this chapter are some to consider with your provider if for some reason you cannot take the dextrose or corn syrup equivalent and you are healthy, with a healthy weight and lifestyle, and with a low risk for diabetes.

Forty-five minutes before your appointment, eat the jelly beans or drink an amount that equals 50 grams of total sugar, ideally in the form of dextrose. Then consume nothing else until the blood test, which will be drawn one hour after you consumed the drink or candy. If you have time, do some form of exercise, like taking a brisk walk for 20 to 30 minutes after drinking or consuming the sugar, but before the test.

Bring a high-protein, whole-carbohydrate, and healthy fat snack (like a nut and seed bar, fruit and nut butter, hard-boiled eggs, meat, poultry or avocado on sprouted multi-whole grain bread) to eat after the test if needed to keep your blood sugar stable. This will help you avoid unpleasant symptoms once your blood sugar drops, like shakiness, lightheadedness, fatigue, anxiety, and irritability.

Rest assured, most healthy pregnant women (about 94%) do not have gestational diabetes. A positive screen simply means you need more testing to confirm it or rule it out. And if you do have it, you can learn how to keep your blood sugar normal throughout the rest of your pregnancy and life.

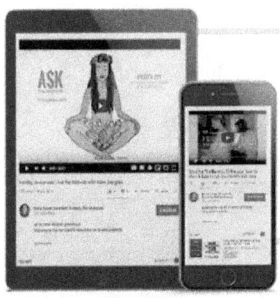

Want to learn more or have more questions?

Grab your free Book Bonuses below:
https://homesweethomebirth.com/nbsbookbonus

GROUP B STREP

Group B Streptococcus, otherwise known as GBS or Group B Strep, is a normally-occurring bacteria that lives in the lower intestines of human beings from babies to the elderly. It's a hot topic in the world of having babies, and there are no easy answers. I encourage you to educate yourself, weighing the risks and benefits of each option regarding testing, prevention, and treatment, and deciding what is best for you and your baby.

Around 10-30% of pregnant women are colonized with the bacteria depending on the population studied, but about 25% are reported to have vaginal GBS in the US. When there is a large amount of GBS in the colon and rectal areas, it can come forward to the vaginal and urinary tracts.

If detected vaginally in a non-pregnant woman, there is nothing wrong and no need for treatment. The main concern is if a pregnant woman has it in labor, and her baby is exposed to the vaginal bacteria after the "bag of water" breaks (during pregnancy, the baby is encased and protected in a double-layered membranous sac of amniotic fluid, in lay terms referred to as the "bag of water").

Although the vast majority of pregnant women with vaginal GBS have healthy babies, half are simply colonized and test positive for it but stay healthy. About one in 200 babies in the US who are exposed to it during childbirth can get this infectious illness. GBS infection can become very severe or life-threatening for about 1-2% of these babies, which is thankfully rare, but potentially devastating for those who are affected. Because every human life matters, I take those one or two babies per thousand very seriously, as would any parent of a very gravely ill newborn.

After a positive GBS test, don't let anyone pressure or scare you out of having a homebirth or free-standing birth center birth if that's what you want. GBS can easily be managed in the out-of-hospital setting. And know that you do have options and can speak up on how the issue is dealt with. Even though there is a standard of care that is strictly upheld in the US, there are different standards in other Westernized countries, like the UK, that might just make more sense for you. Let's look into it.

Risks During Pregnancy

Serious complications in pregnant women due to GBS are rare. Complications of GBS can lead to urinary tract infections in women, but often the positive test results are actually from vaginal discharge, even if a "clean-catch" culture was obtained. In my practice, I found that out early on, after sending women with persistent GBS on clean-catch urine culture tests to a wonderful local urologist. She found them all to be negative for GBS in the urine using a sterile straight catheter specimen and said there was no urinary infection to treat.

In the United States, GBS is routinely managed according to the Center for Disease Control (CDC) guidelines. It is tested for between the 35th and 37th weeks of pregnancy by taking a cotton swab from the vagina and rectal area and sending it to a lab. This is currently the best time for obtaining results closest to the onset of labor. It takes several days to get results, which are allegedly valid for five weeks.

Current testing is not completely predictive, as tests can yield different results at different times because GBS can come and go intermittently. A mom can test negative in late pregnancy but actually be positive for GBS if tested in labor. Likewise, but less commonly, a mom can test positive in late pregnancy and test negative for GBS in labor. There is a new home GBS test in the UK called Strepelle that gives accurate results three days from receipt of the sample, but it is not without controversy.

Unfortunately, at this time, there are no reliable, widely-available, cost-effective, rapid tests for GBS during labor, which would at least address this issue.

In other countries like the United Kingdom, women are not routinely tested in pregnancy for group B strep, according to recommendations by the National Institute of Health and Care Excellence. This is because they have determined that evidence of the effectiveness of routine GBS testing in all pregnant women remains uncertain. Per the guidelines of the Royal College of Obstetricians and Gynecologists, pregnant women are treated with antibiotics in labor only if there are risk factors, such as signs of infection like fever in labor, a prolonged time between "water breaking" and birth, or if a preterm baby is expected.

Until 2002, in the United States, GBS in pregnancy was managed this way as well. The change in American obstetrical practice guidelines was based on an analysis of some large studies around that time even though there are limitations to the quality of those clinical trials, as is common with research. One major bias that concerns integrative, holistically-minded practitioners, which most of the mainstream medical world discounts, is that this research is largely funded by for-profit pharmaceutical companies that manufacture the antibiotics. Dr. Kelly Brogan digs deeper into the research and points out what the Cochrane Database, considered the gold standard in objective evaluation of available research, found as follows:

> *"This review finds that giving antibiotics is not supported by conclusive evidence. The review identified four trials involving 852 GBS positive women. Very few of the women in labor who are GBS positive give birth to babies who are infected with GBS and antibiotics can have harmful effects such as severe maternal allergic reactions, increase in drug-resistant organisms and exposure of newborn infants to resistant bacteria, and postnatal maternal and neonatal yeast infections."*

Additionally, a retrospective study in Pediatrics found that all of the infants with GBS infection, were, in fact, administered intrapartum antibiotics. Of potentially greater concern is the increased risk of late-onset serious and drug-resistant bacterial infection conferred by intrapartum antibiotic exposure and the 40% increase in neonatal mortality (despite 68% decrease in GBS colonization) when infants are given antibiotic prophylaxis postpartum ... antibiotics for group B Strep positivity in pregnancy does not improve outcomes and is likely to negatively influence mom and baby flora. Similarly, liberal antibiotic use in neonates in the ICU has no effect on incidence of sepsis or on mortality as demonstrated in this trial.

Today, in the US, all women who test positive for GBS during the late third trimester screen are given IV antibiotics in labor. That is a lot of healthy women and babies exposed to antibiotics when the risk of serious infection in newborn babies is rare. Additionally, most cases of group B strep in term newborns occur after screened pregnant women tested negative.

Care Recommendations, Alternatives, and Issues

The current standard of practice in the US is based on the guidelines published by the Center for Disease Control and Prevention (CDC), which dictates that antibiotics are to be given during labor to all women who tested positive for GBS in current pregnancy. This is hospital routine and is based on the interpretation of the available research, indicating that IV antibiotics in labor significantly lowers the chance of infection in babies from one in 200 to one in 4,000. But antibiotics can have serious side effects.

Many healthy moms in my practice don't want routine IV antibiotics even though they can be given both in the home and freestanding birth center settings. It feels too medical for them. They are worried about it interfering with their ability to have a beautiful natural birth, and they have valid concerns about the consequences of the antibiotics and feel their risks do not outweigh potential benefits. Some pregnant moms do want the standard treatment, as they are more concerned with GBS than a few doses of intravenous antibiotics and do not feel the IV in labor will hinder them or their birth dreams.

If you do want the IV antibiotics, know you can still move around during the infusion and be in the tub or shower if the access site is covered properly. I was gifted with a home IV pole on wheels by a family in my practice. We had previously hung the IV on whatever we found in the house, a door hook, a hanger on a curtain rod, and once on the antlers on a wall-mounted moose head. When the mother needed to walk, someone would personally hold it up and follow her around with it. You also don't need to be attached to an IV the entire labor and birth but can have a saline lock, also known as a hep-lock. This is an IV catheter that's inserted into your vein, used only for the 15 to 30 minutes it takes for the medication to infuse. It is then disconnected from the access portal, so you are not attached to the IV tubing, pole, and solution bag in between doses for the majority of your labor.

Side Effects Associated with the IV Antibiotics

One reported side effect of IV antibiotics in women is a harmless rash. Another potentially annoying but treatable consequence is a vaginal yeast infection, which can lead to thrush in the baby's mouth and on your nipples and make breastfeeding painful for you until it resolves. A far more serious but fortunately very rare side-effect is anaphylaxis, an allergic reaction which can be life-threatening, but most often managed effectively with medication. What concerns us most are the short and long term effects antibiotics can have on us and our little ones.

Microbiome disruption is the disturbance of the intestinal tract balance of normal flora in babies (and mothers). More research is needed, but a recent Harvard magazine article tells us that this can cause life-long complications in infants. It also ups the antibiotic resistance in adults and infants, another life-long consequence, and can lead to other serious infections and health conditions for them both. The award-winning chilling documentary Microbirth delves deeply into the microbiome, the trillions of bacteria that live on and in us that is critical for human health.

If you opt for antibiotics, do what you can to help restore your and your baby's microbiome by drinking kombucha, eating lacto-fermented natural probiotic foods and the prebiotics that they feed on (like simple vegetable starches such as white rice and potatoes, and beans), as well as supplementing with probiotics that contain Saccharomyces boulardii, breastfeeding, and frequent skin-to-skin contact between you and your baby. You can heal your own gut by following a program for six to eight weeks that includes eliminating inflammatory foods like gluten, sugar, cow dairy, and those that are genetically modified, and feeding yourself organic fruits and vegetables, pastured meat, poultry, and eggs, fish free from pollutants, gluten-free grains, legumes, healthy fats from coconut oil, avocado, and clarified goat butter (ghee), and drinking half your body weight in ounces of pure clean water. Others require additional dietary changes and supplements like aloe, beta glucan, curcumin, licorice in the form of DGL and L-glutamine. Avoid exposure to common toxins in body care products and household cleaning products, as well as certain medications such as non-steroidal anti-inflammatories (like ibuprofen), hormonal contraceptives, stomach acid-blocking drugs (like Prilosec) and additional antibiotics, unless in cases of life-threatening infections.

Possible Alternatives

Chlorhexidine gluconate vaginal wash is commonly used in Europe for pregnant women who have been diagnosed with Group B Strep. Some studies have shown that the treatment of GBS using chlorhexidine is safe, cheap, and as effective as antibiotics, without negative side effects. Other studies suggest chlorhexidine reduces GBS colonization, but not GBS infection in newborns. It is known in the US as Hibiclens and is available over the counter without a prescription. It needs to be diluted, and there are several effective protocols in pregnancy or during labor. It is not natural. It's a potent antiseptic and does disrupt the vaginal flora, which can hopefully be restored with vaginal probiotics; but it doesn't travel through the body and cross over to the baby like IV antibiotics do. While it prevents the baby from exposure to GBS, it also does not allow exposure to the healthy vaginal bacteria during birth. But many moms in my practice prefer this to IV antibiotics in labor. I have tested its efficacy in my practice. After its use, I get back a culture swab negative for GBS and have had no cases of newborn infection after its use. Chlorhexidine for GBS is increasing in the US, mostly in out-of-hospital settings.

Another treatment in late pregnancy that has been used especially among out-of-hospital midwives is a vaginal antibiotic. Research is sparse but suggests possible effectiveness. There is currently only one vaginal medication that apparently works, if the strain of GBS is not resistant to it, called Clindamycin. Its IV use in labor is an alternative within the CDC guidelines, if the mom is allergic to the drug of choice. When testing for GBS, its sensitivity to the various antibiotics can and should also be tested, as antibiotic resistance is increasing.

There is a small study done by a colleague of mine on Clindamycin's effectiveness to reduce GBS infection in newborns of moms who had tested positive for GBS in pregnancy. My relatively large homebirth practice was included in her research, as for years I had been offering this option to pregnant women who tested positive for the bacteria but refused IV antibiotics in labor. The option includes a Hibiclens daily wash protocol, other recommendations for prevention of recurrence, and weekly GBS follow-up testing. The study demonstrated that this treatment was effective in the vast majority of women without any known complications, but it is only one small retrospective study, not a large, gold standard, randomized clinical trial. I am still impressed by the negative follow-up testing in my practice and that no baby in my care after this treatment had GBS infection or other problems. It is also not natural. It is an antibiotic medication, but with more of a local vaginal effect.

Moms who have follow-up cultures negative for GBS feel better about declining the IV antibiotics in labor, especially if there are no risk factors. But this protocol also disrupts the healthy balance of bacteria in the vagina, can similarly cause yeast and thrush, and can contribute to the issue of disease-causing bacteria developing resistance to the antibiotic.

Both of these treatments are easily accessible and thus convenient for homebirths, as well as birth center and hospital births. You can be empowered and learn to administer them yourself once you have the supplies. It is important to know that Hibiclens or vaginal Clindamycin is NOT the standard of care in the US, and they are not recognized to date by the medical world as a valid treatment to prevent GBS infection in babies. Women who choose either option are educated on the symptoms to watch for, advised to inform their pediatrician, and have the baby evaluated in one to two days. I also tell women who opt for either Hibiclens or vaginal Clindamycin that they would be considered untreated for GBS and given antibiotics if transferred to the hospital unless they refuse.

Although you have the option to decline IV antibiotics in the hospital, disturbingly, it can get nasty if they are not supportive. They could involve social services or report you to the child protection agency to be investigated for child abuse and negligence. Do discuss your plans with your provider and care setting in advance to avoid problems.

Although I prefer natural remedies when they are effective, unfortunately in over two decades of midwifery practice, I have yet to find one that works once GBS is detected. I have had numerous moms who have used just about all of them and then have a positive GBS test on follow-up. There is forever a place in my heart for a naturopathic mom who declined antibiotics and Hibiclens and her severely ill newborn with GBS infection. The outcome was tragic. She tested positive for GBS repeatedly despite using the best of the best of protocols of natural remedies. What baffled all of us was there were no risk factors; it was a relatively short, beautiful healthy birth with no interventions. Her water broke on its own during pushing. Yes, countless babies of moms treated naturally did not get sick even though follow-up cultures were still positive for GBS. But the one case was enough for me.

There is currently insufficient evidence of the effectiveness of any natural treatment remedy for preventing GBS infection in newborns. Holistic care includes all modalities, and sometimes there is a role for medication. When a pregnant mom tests positive for GBS, I discuss the issue, give her literature to read, present her with the pros and cons of all the options, from doing nothing to the alternative modalities, to IV antibiotics in labor, and I honor her informed decision. Some want to use the UK's risk factor protocol and decline GBS testing during pregnancy, and I respect their informed choice.

It must be said, however, that no treatment is 100%. Cases are still reported in medical literature where babies were infected with GBS after any treatment, including IV antibiotics, even though IV antibiotics have significantly reduced the incidence and severity of GBS illness in babies according to the research to date. I, therefore, recommend keeping a close eye on your newborn if you carry GBS, regardless of treatment. If any symptoms present themselves, consult your pediatrician immediately.

Symptoms to Look Out For (Scary But Rare)

Early-onset GBS occurs within the first week of life, most commonly within hours after birth. Signs and symptoms include lethargy; irritability; poor feeding; very slow or fast heart rate; abnormally high or low temperature; difficulty breathing such as flaring of the nostrils or grunting noises; too fast or slow breathing rate; and blueness of the skin of the baby's trunk and/or a pale or grey appearance.

Late-onset GBS occurs in one-third of babies with GBS infectious illness but is uncommon, affecting about 0.3 per 1,000 babies, mostly who are premature. It can happen anywhere between the first week and three months postpartum, but it is rare after one month of life. Unfortunately, there is no known prevention (IV antibiotic treatment given to women in labor who tested positive for GBS in pregnancy is only effective to help prevent early-onset infectious disease), and like early-onset GBS infection, it can occur even when mom tested negative in pregnancy.

An otherwise healthy baby can become critically ill within hours. Symptoms of late-onset GBS are the same as early-onset infection, but can also include having a high-pitched, inconsolable cry, whimpering or moaning sounds; blank staring or a trance-like expression; appearing floppy and listless; having an involuntary stiff body or jerking movements; not moving an arm or leg; excess sleeping and difficulty arousing; tense or bulging fontanelle (soft spot on baby's head); turning away from bright light; blotchy, tender skin; projectile vomiting; or pus and red skin at base of umbilical cord or at any puncture site (from internal monitor).

Let's Talk Prevention!

Probiotic supplements during pregnancy can't completely prevent GBS, but I highly advise taking them regardless, as I have had tremendous success with lowering the vaginal GBS rates in pregnant women who take the specific daily probiotic I recommend (like Klaire Labs Ther-biotic Women's Formula or Greens First Female Probiotic for Women). Many of my colleagues report similar success with these probiotics. There is finally a small but growing amount of actual research documenting the effectiveness of certain strains of probiotics to reduce the incidence of GBS. Probiotics are also safe and have many other health benefits. The other prenatal vitamins and minerals I recommend supplement a healthy diet with nutrients that enhance health and immunity. Please consult the chapter "Nutritional Best Practices for Mom" for my supplement recommendations.

You can lower the risk of infection also by minimizing exposure. You can try to lower the amount of GBS in your vagina with natural remedies, such as those given in Dr. Aviva Romm's protocol, even though there is no guarantee. If you have GBS in a healthy pregnancy and labor, you certainly can decline or limit vaginal exams, invasive procedures like internal fetal monitoring, and having your bag of water broken artificially. If your bag of water has definitely broken before or early in labor, you can use natural remedies to gently stimulate labor and lessen the time it takes to birth. Some studies suggest that a water birth can possibly help prevent GBS infection because it entails less interventions and invasive procedures, as well as the bacteria being diluted or washed away, so the baby is exposed to less of it.

Research is on the horizon regarding a vaccine for both early and late-onset GBS infectious illness, which sparks an entirely different debate, as well as more accurate and available rapid testing in labor. There is much to be done to decrease the risk and rates of preterm birth. But, my hope is for more research demonstrating prevention with probiotics in pregnancy, holistic modalities to improve immunity against infection, and the benefits of out-of-hospital midwifery care in terms of reducing newborn GBS infections.

My dream is that there is a widespread cessation of routine medical interventions in normal childbirth, one of the main pillars of authentic midwifery care. If there were more midwife-led birthing centers and out-of-hospital and homebirthing for the low-risk healthy population, according to evidence-based NICES recommendations, this would decrease the rates of invasive procedures and hospital exposure to pathogens, especially resistant ones, that all increase risk of infection. And hopefully, this would result in a major reduction of serious GBS illness in babies.

Can You Still Give Birth in a Birthing Center or Have a Homebirth?

Of course! And you might be better off doing so specifically in terms of GBS, by having a provider who honors your choices, possibly lessening infection risk by having a water birth, avoiding routine invasive procedures as well as avoiding exposure to bacteria and infectious illnesses that are common in hospitals. Again, testing positive for GBS in pregnancy does not risk you out of either. Even the usual protocol in the US to administer antibiotics by means of an IV can be done at home or a birth center with licensed midwives, which is good news, if that is your choice!

If you are a carrier of GBS and experiencing a healthy pregnancy, I hope that you now feel confident that a homebirth or birth center birth is still possible and actually a wonderful idea. I hope you have a better perspective on the issue and feel more educated and empowered to make an informed decision about how you want to deal with it. Know you have alternative options to consider, and most importantly, do what you can in terms of prevention. Definitely take top-quality prenatal supplements and probiotics!

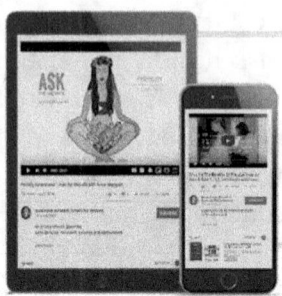

**Want to learn more or
have more questions?**

Grab your free Book Bonuses below:
https://homesweethomebirth.com/nbsbookbonus

IMMUNIZATIONS AND VACCINES

If you keep conscious and up-to-date with the goings-on of the health industry, you will know that the immunization of babies and young children through vaccination is not as simple as mainstream medicine makes it seem. It is indeed a controversial topic, especially among those that take their wellbeing into their own hands and prefer natural, more holistic approaches.

I encourage you to educate yourself, weighing the risks and benefits of each option regarding testing, prevention, and treatment, and deciding what is best for you and your baby. In the case where you're dealing with an illness that's potentially very serious, it may make sense to administer the associated vaccination whose known risks have so far appeared relatively innocuous. But often enough, it is not clear what is worse: the risk of infections or the risk of the vaccines, some of which are far from harmless.

What I'd like to do with this chapter is to give you a broad idea of what's being sold to us as consumers and what's truly out there in terms of factual information and sound research.

The Advisory Committee on Immunization Practices (ACIP) is "a group of 'thought leaders,'" writes Dr. Kelly Brogan, who goes on to say:

> "[The ACIP 'thought leaders' are] charged with the task of determining what vaccines will be pushed upon you during your doctor's check-ups and wellness visits. It consists of heads of pharmaceutical companies such as Novartis and Sanofi Pasteur and is a prime example of the enmeshment between the Center for Disease Control (CDC) and [the] industry. The surprising news

is that vaccines, the pharmaceutical product in question, have never been studied in a truly placebo-controlled manner, in single, or multiple deliveries, and not for long-term outcomes, even in a general population."

For example, in the US, all major health regulators including the CDC advise all pregnant women to get the flu vaccine to decrease the risk of flu-related complications. It is said to be safe in all trimesters as based on short-term studies by various pharmaceutical companies. The complications in question, however, are rarely severe enough to cause preterm labor and even death. Furthermore, the studies did not take into account healthy lifestyle and holistic modalities to strengthen immunity against the flu virus, commonly seen and used in out-of-hospital midwifery practices. The flu vaccine has been administered to millions of pregnant women in recent years, exposing millions of unborn fetuses.

Dr. Kelly Brogan in her thought-provoking scholarly analysis of the flu vaccine in pregnancy calls into question the validity and flaws of these studies, and discusses risks families are not told about. What is striking to me is that long-term effects on the unborn babies have not been studied and are, therefore, unknown. Fetal loss (miscarriage or stillbirth) has been excluded from the studies when a huge increase in fetal deaths after the flu vaccine has been reported. Risks to the healthy mother have been downplayed. Plus, the vaccine's benefits have been falsely exaggerated.

This hits home as I had two moms in my practice who had healthy pregnancies miscarry in the second trimester the day after they were given the flu vaccine by their primary physician. As is commonly the case, the flu vaccine was not reported as the causative factor. After the second tragedy, I did some research. Not only did I hear similar incidences among my colleagues around the country, but the Vaccine Adverse Events Reporting System (VAERS) found over a 4,000-fold increase in fetal deaths after the flu vaccine in 2009 and 2010.

In an eye-opening blog article on her website, Aviva Romm, physician, herbalist, and midwife, speaks to the way the medical industry portrays our health as a whole, writing, "There is a lot of fear-mongering in medicine. As a public, we have a skewed, media-driven, fear-based view of our health and of disease prevalence. And it is impossible to ignore the fact that there are massive profits to be made by the very limited number of pharmaceutical companies producing the influenza vaccine." Dr. Romm continues, in this article regarding the flu vaccine, to state that the very reasons why we are told to have the flu vaccine are actually not as severe as the media makes them out to be.

In fact, a mother with a PhD in immunology, Tetyana Obukhanych, even wrote to legislators with hopes to debunk some of the consequences the media forcefully and fearfully propagates. It is important to note here that she did not write to them in order to push her own right not to vaccinate her children, but simply because she feared the discrimination against non-vaccinated children in school. Dr. Obukhanych pointed out, "In summary, a person who is not vaccinated with IPV, DTaP, HepB, and Hib vaccines due to reasons of conscience poses no extra danger to the public than a person who is. No discrimination is warranted." If you can take the time to read her letter, please do so. In it, she shows that the school environment is not affected any more or less by either a child who is vaccinated or not.

While an illness can lead to certain potentially serious complications in a pregnant mama and/or her baby, those complications are actually more exceptional and more uncommon than the pharmaceutical industry and modern medical authorities make them out to be. Although medical doctors take the Hippocratic Oath upon graduation from training, with the essential component included, "First, do no harm," I am concerned the risks of each injection into a healthy mom, impacting her baby are downplayed and may be doing more harm than realized.

Dr. Kelly Brogan does not mince words in her brave research-based statements not only, writing about:

> *"... a known 4,250% increase in fetal demise during the 2009/10 flu season, but also about evidence-based inefficacy and risks of the pertussis vaccine pushed on pregnant women, about Gardasil killing healthy girls across the globe, fear-mongering about SIDS*

that is actually caused by a visit to the pediatrician, corruption of an infant's birthday by the hepatitis B vaccine ... As parents around the world have known for seven decades, and basic science has supported, vaccines do cause autism."

The Truth about Disease and Vaccines

While the intentions and the aim of the pharmaceutical industry can be seemingly profit-driven, and concerns about the various infectious illnesses seem valid, this does not address the facts about the vaccines themselves. Can vaccines truly help to prevent today's diseases in our children? What are the facts about disease-prevention and vaccines?

Fortunately, or unfortunately, there is no clear or direct answer. In tackling this issue of navigating immunizations for your baby, the only sure thing to do is to personally conduct your own research and to then come to your own conclusion. Each vaccine and the infectious illness it is directed against needs to be looked at individually.

Interview several pediatricians who share your philosophies and choose one that you trust. There are pediatricians who do not accept a baby into their practice if parents do not follow the standard vaccination schedule. Fortunately, there are more and more holistic or integrative family and pediatric physicians out there who can teach you about disease prevention as a whole, address each vaccine separately, as well as appropriately plan a wide variety of alternative healing modalities.

A wonderful example is pediatrician Dr. Elisa Song of Whole Family Wellness in California, who believes the following:

> *"The decision to get the flu vaccine for your child, just like any other vaccine, is your choice as a parent, and it's a very personal choice with many factors that have to be weighed. This decision must be made on an individual basis, taking into account the unique healthcare needs and concerns of your child. There is no right or wrong decision. By informing yourself, you are doing the best thing for your child and for your whole family. Trust your mama or*

*your papa 'gut,' and you will always do what is best for your child.
Whatever you decide, using your natural medicines toolkit will get
your whole family through the winter cold and flu season healthier
and stronger." She empowers the families in her practice to treat
your child's flu - naturally!"*

Dr. Song, like other more progressive pediatricians, she accommodates
a variety of approaches from administering all immunizations according
to the CDC recommendations, to giving them one at a time over a period
of time instead of giving several of them at once, to only giving those you
decide upon, to not giving any at all. She integrates conventional and
holistic pediatrics to help children thrive to their fullest potentials of
wellness, prevention, and healing from illness.

Dr. Sears, famed American and midwifery-friendly pediatrician, wrote
The Vaccine Book solely to address this convoluted subject. He wrote it
in order to answer parents' questions and address their deepest concerns
about vaccinating their children. He tackles the pros and cons as well
as information about the diseases themselves in a relatively unbiased
fashion. He adamantly suggests that you take the time to learn how the
vaccine you're considering is made and what ingredients are contained
within it. If you decide to vaccinate, this will help you to get clear on
which particular quality brands to ask for, in what order the vaccines
should be taken in succession with others, etc.

The aim of Dr. Sears' book is to give parents enough information and
clarity so that they feel confident enough to make their own decision
whether they decide to vaccinate their children or not. Despite his being
pro-vaccine, he does not take a stance in this book and simply provides
facts.

For a powerful award-winning documentary and science-based website
regarding vaccines, visit greatergoodmovie.org/learn-more/science/, as
well as the non-profit National Vaccine Information Center www.nvic.
org/, an independent clearinghouse for information on vaccine science,
policy, and laws, dedicated to preventing vaccine-related injuries and
helping people make informed decisions about them.

How Your Immune System Works

Research is increasingly showing that there may not be as big of a disease threat as we've been taught to believe. Vaccines do not always work or confer long-lasting immunity, as would be the case after creating your own antibodies from the actual infection. For example, chicken pox (varicella) is usually a harmless infectious illness in children but results in life-long immunity. The vaccine is now given to babies but does not often produce immunity lasting into adulthood, the time when the illness is potentially more serious.

The recent resurgence of adult pertussis (whooping cough) is largely occurring in vaccinated individuals whose immunity after the childhood vaccine waned, risking non-immune newborns who can get dangerously ill if exposed. The German measles (rubella) vaccine is given to babies, but their immunity commonly does not last into adult childbearing years, risking serious complications for fetuses of non-immune pregnant women. People still get the flu after the flu vaccine.

In reference to the flu shot, Dr. Romm and Dr. Brogan share with us that in a Cochrane analysis of 50 studies, there was a 2% incidence of presumed influenza in the unvaccinated population as opposed to a 1% incidence in the vaccinated, thus a difference of 1%.

What this means, then, is the fear we've been taught to harbor isn't actually necessary. There are risks to each vaccination injection given that need to be weighed against the risks of each infection. There is way more to the story than most parents are told, and it is not a topic to be taken lightly.

While it is not much within in our human control who gets sick, we can do what we can to prevent exposure to someone with a known infection. We can maintain good hand-washing and hygiene habits, avoid sharing personal items, observe safe eating and traveling practices, as well as preventing illnesses unique to each infection.

Something as simple as a regular practice of yoga, visualization, and meditation—prenatal yoga in pregnancy—can help boost your own immune system, which can be passed on to your baby, against many types of infections. Yoga and simple meditation reduce the incidence and severity of many of the modern world's most recent and common ailments: infection, cancer, various inflammatory and autoimmune diseases, and allergies. Regularly visualizing yourself as already being healthy and vibrant, with a strong resilient immune system, and feeling the strong positive emotions that reality brings with the passion and excitement of a child, is a powerful and effective practice, that can literally improve how your body functions, may not only prevent infection, but also can hasten healing if you do get sick. As Dr. Joe Dispenza advises, speaks and writes extensively about, using the latest cutting-edge research and science, "Be Your Own Placebo."

Eating healthfully has a huge impact on preventing illness, as does reducing inner stress, getting enough sleep, plenty of fresh clean air and sunshine. Eating a wide variety of plant-based whole foods and with sufficient protein and healthy fat are major steps to robust wellbeing. You'd be surprised at how well your body can actually defend and heal itself against disease when given the proper nutrients and care.

In terms of nutrients, Dr. Sears has a concise and simple article on how our body's immune system works. If you understand how your body heals itself from within, you may be more able to decide which vaccines are worth investing your time in. In this article, Dr. Sears addresses the army that is your immune system and how it works to defend your body from sickness. He also shares why some more serious diseases can attack your body. What he does point out at the top of the article is something foundational to our and our children's health and wellbeing: "Because of poor diets, many school children and adults have immune systems that don't operate at peak efficiency. They get sick more often." Breastfeeding, without question, results in healthy immunity, and breastfed babies have significantly reduced rates and severity of infection as compared with formula-fed babies.

Something as simple as including probiotics and whole-food supplements into your diet can boost your immune system and improve your overall health and wellbeing, and treating common infections naturally can be very effective. And these are nutrients that pass into the breastmilk you give to your baby, boosting your baby's health and immunity.

Factors for Making Your Decision

I think what Drs. Brogan, Romm, Song, and Sears have in common is their mission to provide facts to their readership in order to improve health and wellbeing. They want to help us to make better decisions that empower and help us to grow healthfully and live to the fullest potential. As I've mentioned previously, Dr. Sears always refers back to how crucial it is that you learn about the product you're using so that you can make a conscious decision. Dr. Brogan strongly advises that when doing research, you take into account a few things:

- Who funded the study?
- Was a proper placebo used?
- What did the results show?

I would also add these:

- How large was the study?
- Were long-term consequences properly researched, as well as the short-term effects?
- What were the study's limitations and biases?
- Is there a meta-analysis of multiple, large, random, double-blind, placebo control trials that provides compelling results, or are there only a few small and limited studies on the subject?
- What were the results of studies chosen not to be published?

Even the doctors conducting the study might have to use "strategic tactics to paper over the truth," as Dr. Brogan puts it in an article she wrote addressing the overlooking of certain medical data pertaining to premature babies. Our tendency is to think that because we're reading a clinical study, it must be accurate; because our doctor says so, it must be true. Making conclusions based on a meta-analysis of multiple, properly conducted, random control trials carries much more weight than one clinical study, the opinion of a healthcare provider, or a medical "expert."

In the same article I mentioned earlier from Dr. Romm, she finds that the data given to us on the prevalence of the flu as well as its severity among pregnant women is highly inflated. And, in doing her own research, she has found that the "CDC does not know exactly how many people die from seasonal flu each year."

This is the same organization that was spreading fear-ridden media about how catastrophic the H1N1 disease was going to be. And Romm is directly quoting from the CDC's website. On top of this, she has learned that they also state, "About 90% of influenza-associated deaths occur among adults 65 years and older." Sometimes, inaccuracies are staring us right in the face. It's worth taking the time to root them out.

While there is an extensive amount of information online and in libraries about the pros and cons of vaccinations—from isolated tragic cases to conflicting opinions to reputable research—that can be daunting, I hope that this chapter provides you with the first building blocks to guide your personal journey to decide what is best for you and your young ones.

To summarize the answer to the question, "How do you navigate immunizations for yourself and your baby?" take the time to learn not only about immunizations as they pertain to preventing infectious illnesses, but also consider the short- and long-term risks of each vaccine, and learn more about how the body can minimize common ailments, avoid sickness, heal itself, and what you can do to aid the process.

Do your research and be mindful of the difference between fear-based news and actual facts. Consider all of the evidence and sound investigation, as well as your options and your own principles. Seek professional guidance from those you trust, but then trust your intuitive wisdom to make the decision that is right for you and your family.

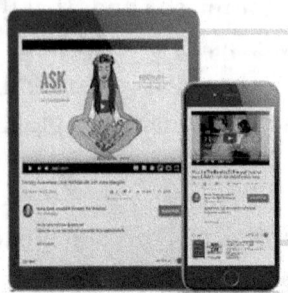

**Want to learn more or
have more questions?**

Grab your free Book Bonuses below:
https://homesweethomebirth.com/nbsbookbonus

GENERAL RECOMMENDATIONS FOR COMMON DISCOMFORTS AND HEALTH ISSUES

What follows are my general recommendations based on a long career of research from trusted sources and over two decades of experience helping the thousands who seek my guidance. Although part of holistic care is embracing all safe and effective modalities, obviously reserving the use of allopathic medicine only when absolutely necessary, there are risks to medications. What follows are lots of suggestions and natural remedies for issues most people struggle with on this journey. There are pros and cons to everything; from doing nothing when something needs to be addressed, like unhealthy diet and stress to taking herbs alone or in combination. Even though the herbs I suggest are widely used, they work well, and are considered relatively safe, they are less studied than the pharmaceuticals, many of which have known toxicities. So I encourage you to do your research and take charge of your health. There is no one-size-fits-all. Listen to your body and see what works best for you.

I recommend starting with addressing root causes in habits of eating, drinking, sleeping, exercise, stress management, toxic exposures, etc., supplementing with necessary vitamins and minerals, food-based and lifestyle medicine, and safe, topical, or external applications. The body reacts super intelligently when supported appropriately, and often the best course of action is doing nothing but watching and marveling in awe at its brilliance.

My preference in pregnancy is to try, in addition to modalities like acupuncture, osteopathic or chiropractic care, massage and physical therapy, is to try homeopathic remedies first when possible, before ingesting herbs, as they have no risk other than taking the wrong remedy, which is simply not working, and switching to another one that is better indicated. Homeopathy honors the wisdom of the body's symptoms as indications the body is doing what it needs to do to heal itself. Symptoms are positive adaptive responses to some sort of imbalance and stress, messages that need our attention and support. Suppressing symptoms interferes with the body's brilliant defense mechanisms, masks the real issue, and increases its complexity. When you get the correct remedy to your particular symptoms, it stimulates the body's defenses and can support your body to heal quickly and naturally on its own. Homeopathic remedies are totally safe and remarkably effective for treating common ailments. You can consult with a classical homeopath or refer to excellent reference books like Homeopathy for Pregnancy, Birth and Your Baby's First Year by Miranda Castro, A Homeopathic Handbook of Natural Remedies by Laura Josephson and Everybody's Guide to Homeopathic Medicine by Stephen Cummings, MD and Dana Ullman, MPH.

If you need to take herbs, rest assured, there are wonderful well-tolerated options, that are usually much safer than medications with benefits that far outweigh potential risks. While gold-standard research on the safety of herbs, as well as medications in pregnancy, is limited, there are a number of herbs that have been used historically and that have been scientifically investigated as safe for expecting mamas, with an excellent track record, some dating back to ancient times. Conversely, many previously-thought benign drugs and over-the-counter medications recommended by allopathic medical providers have later been found to be harmful.

While there are many herbalists, like Susun Weed, and holistic midwives whose books line my shelves, Dr. Aviva Romm remains one of my favorite resources for the safe and effective use of herbs in childbearing. She is an integrative physician, midwife, and herbalist who has done extensive research and compiled the most comprehensive, scientific, evidence-based reference guide I have come across called Botanical Guide for Women's Health.

Stick to herbs well-known to be safe for use in pregnancy and avoid those known to be potentially toxic. Herbs in the form of spices, teas, and infusions tend to be considered most gentle and nutritional tonics when used in moderation. As an extra precaution, avoid using herbal tinctures and capsules in the first trimester, unless absolutely necessary. For any natural herbal remedies or supplements you use in acute situations, try one at a time or safe, formulated combinations for the shortest duration and in the lowest dosage possible.

For more long-standing issues, give an herb or a formulated herbal combination up to a two-month trial to see how it affects you. Some work right away, others take more time, or may not work for you and you can try another alternative. Go for high-quality sources like Pure Encapsulations, Gaia, Wish Garden, HerbPharm, Nature's Way, and Eclectic Institute, or professional-grade brands like those in my online holistic apothecary, which offers the natural, premium, hand-picked supplements and remedies that have gone through my thorough screening process and includes those that I personally use and recommend to my family and the women in my practice over the years with great success. Just because it is natural does not mean it is safe in any amount or combination for you to take. When in doubt about herb and supplement dosing unique to you, interactions, side effects, and concerns, or you simply need more personalized guidance, consult your holistic or integrative medical provider, seasoned naturopath, herbalist, or schedule a consultation with me, so you can be advised about the best supplements, remedies, and dosages specific to your situation.

If you experience any sort of chronic emotional and physical symptoms in which serious causes have been ruled out and none of the natural and conventional medical remedies help, read Dr. Kelly Brogan's *Own Your Self: The Surprising Path beyond Depression, Anxiety, and Fatigue to Reclaiming Your Authenticity, Vitality, and Freedom*, and follow her program which is covered in more detail in her first book Mind of Your Own. Read the book The Mindbody Prescription by John Sarno, MD. He is an amazing pioneering physician whose brilliant approach has helped hundreds of thousands of people without drugs, physical measures, or surgery. Even though he started out curing chronic pain with his approach, people were ridding themselves of many chronic ailments, and it illustrates how intimately the mind and body are connected.

Check out Brandon Bays' book The Journey for extremely effective cutting-edge mind-body methods that have also led to transformational healing for thousands of people worldwide. In adjunct, a must-read is You are the Placebo by Dr. Joe Dispenza; he, backed by powerful science and the latest research, has helped thousands globally completely cure serious mental and physical illness and positively transform their lives using the power of the mind and imagery, in cooperation with the innate brilliant intelligence within each of us and its capacity to heal, regenerate and fully recover. Consider going for deeper, powerfully effective healing with Clarity Breathwork, another practice that has helped countless people around the globe release trapped energy of stress, painful emotions and trauma causing all sorts of dis-ease, reset their system and restore their health and wellbeing.

ANEMIA IN PREGNANCY— PREVENTION AND TREATMENT

Physiologic "anemia" in pregnancy is healthy and natural. Increased amounts of iron are needed to make additional red blood cells for your developing baby and for your body's preparation for blood loss at delivery. Anemia also results from the dilution of red blood cells as the fluid volume expands to nearly double the amount normally present before you were pregnant. It is evidenced by a gradual two-gram drop in hemoglobin by the seventh month, followed by a gradual return to pre-pregnancy levels by three to four weeks postpartum. Iron stores (ferritin levels) also tend to drop.

While iron deficiency anemia is the most common type, it's important to note that anemia can be caused by a number of factors. Also, vitality is a great gauge of wellbeing. If your hemoglobin is a little below normal but your iron stores are fine and you feel fit and healthy, you need not worry. Just make sure your diet is rich in foods high in iron and vitamin C.

If you are truly anemic, you may experience the following symptoms:

- Extreme exhaustion and weakness
- Shortness of breath
- Heart palpitations
- Dizziness or faintness
- Headaches
- Irritability
- Poor concentration and confusion
- Feeling weary and run down with a lowered resistance to infection
- Poor appetite and unusual cravings for non-food items.

Whether or not you have the above symptoms, you are smart to be paying attention. As already mentioned, the formation of additional red blood cells for both mama and baby, coupled with their dilution by increased fluid in the circulation, can often lead to iron deficiency anemia during pregnancy. It can be especially aggravated by:

- A diet low in iron, both before and/or during pregnancy
- Severe nausea and vomiting
- Being pregnant with multiple fetuses
- Closely spaced pregnancies
- Alcohol or drug addiction
- Severe or chronic infection
- Significant blood loss
- More serious medical conditions.

Treatment Options for Anemia in Pregnancy

Untreated anemia in pregnancy that becomes severe may increase the risk of harm to your baby and to you. You may be more susceptible to infection, less likely to handle the stress of labor, the normal blood loss at delivery, and the needed healing during the postpartum period.

Treating iron deficiency anemia can be tricky because many sources of iron are not easily absorbed into your system and some products, like coffee, soda, black tea, dairy foods, bran, antacids, calcium and magnesium supplements, and certain medications, actually inhibit iron absorption. However, careful attention to diet and the use of natural, easily-assimilated forms of iron have produced excellent results without the detrimental side effects of the commonly prescribed ferrous sulfate.

Ferrous sulfate is not only poorly absorbed, but also very constipating, can cause indigestion, black tarry stools, skin rashes, and is said to be hard on the digestive tract, liver, and kidneys. Too much ferrous sulfate has been associated with serious complications and can produce the same deficiency state that it was prescribed to correct. There are a number of ways anemia in pregnancy can be addressed without ferrous sulfate. I recommend combining several of the suggestions below to boost your chances of successfully increasing your iron stores (ferritin), hemoglobin, and hematocrit, and for keeping them at healthy levels.

Get as much iron as you can from your daily diet. Good food sources for iron (as well as other needed nutrients) include:

- Organ meats like beef or chicken liver
- Red meat and poultry
- Shrimp, oysters, and clams
- Egg yolks
- Dark green vegetables like spinach (ideally boiled briefly to increase absorption), watercress, alfalfa, parsley, seaweed, collards, kale, turnip greens, and dandelion greens
- Seaweeds (kelp and dulse/kombu)
- Beets and fresh, raw beet juice
- Jerusalem artichokes
- Legumes like red beans, chickpeas, lentils, and split peas
- Whole grains
- Blackstrap molasses
- Seeds and nuts
- Dried, unsulphured fruits like raisins, apricots, cherries, black mission figs, and prunes
- Black cherries and pomegranates
- Prune juice
- Carob powder
- Brewers yeast.

To further enhance iron absorption, eat iron-rich foods in combination with foods high in vitamin C. For example, fresh, organic uncooked grapefruit, oranges, vegetable or tomato juice, strawberries, blackberries, raspberries, mangos, cantaloupes, papayas, tomatoes, red or green peppers, cabbages, broccoli, cauliflower, and leafy greens. Regular exercise will also help with absorption, as will cooking in cast iron.

Herbs and Tonics

Choose one or two of the following natural sources of iron to prevent iron deficiency or alternate between a few.

Vegetarian iron tonic—mix one tablespoon of blackstrap molasses, one tablespoon of brewers yeast, one tablespoon of wheat germ, one tablespoon of coconut oil, and four ounces of orange, grapefruit, or pomegranate juice. If you like warm drinks, try two tablespoons of blackstrap molasses in one cup of hot water with fresh lemon juice. Drink one to three times daily.

Fresh juice—fresh beets and apples make a yummy, absorbable, iron-rich juice. Drink two cups, twice daily. You can add a half to one ounce of wheatgrass juice, a half-cup of fresh parsley, and/or other green leafy veggies (except raw spinach) to boost the iron content.

Wheatgrass—take no more than one ounce per day. If it causes stomach upset, half the dose or add it to beet, carrot, or another vegetable juice for the first week. Then take the full ounce by itself or in the vegetable juice.

Herbal infusion—steep up to one large handful of dried nettle leaf and/or red raspberry leaf in a quart of boiling water for at least four hours. For increased iron, you can add a pinch of dandelion root and/or a pinch of yellow dock root. Strain and drink several times throughout the day. You can add a splash of lemon or lime juice, fresh mint, one to two tablespoons of blackstrap molasses, or a dash of honey to taste.

Capsules—take three to four capsules of freeze-dried nettles or eight capsules of seaweed daily.

Tinctures—for prevention, take a dropperful of yellow dock root or dandelion root tincture in orange juice. For treatment, take up to three dropperfuls, one to three times daily.

Liquid chlorophyll—take one to three tablespoons per day, depending on your individual requirements.

If You Decide to Take an Iron Supplement

If an iron supplement is needed, I recommend taking a non-sulfate, whole-food variety like ferrous gluconate or fumarate combined with vitamin C and bioflavonoids. 30-60 mg of elemental iron daily should suffice for those with normal iron stores, while higher doses may be needed if your iron stores are depleted. Your dose should be adjusted according to your lab results and individual needs. Take your supplemental iron daily until two to four months postpartum.

For optimal absorption, it is best to spread supplemental iron intake out over the course of the day to avoid stressing your system with the unabsorbed portions. Do not take it with dairy foods, caffeine, or soda with phosphates. Be sure to take it between meals on an empty stomach with 500 mg of vitamin C and bioflavonoids.

Although it can take a few months to correct iron deficiency anemia, you should start to see an improvement in the lab values within two weeks of treatment. If not, try a different combination of natural iron sources. If there is still no improvement after another two to four weeks, your anemia may not be related to low iron and a more thorough medical evaluation is needed.

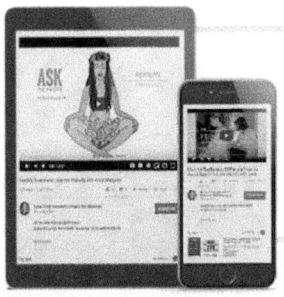

Want to learn more or have more questions?

Grab your free Book Bonuses below:
https://homesweethomebirth.com/nbsbookbonus

BLEEDING IN PREGNANCY: WHY IT HAPPENS AND WHAT TO DO

Vaginal bleeding during pregnancy can often cause us to freak out and start thinking the worst. However, there is a multitude of less serious and more common reasons for light bleeding at this time, such as:

- A burst of a tiny blood vessel in the vagina or cervix engorged from pregnancy hormones, especially with minor local infections, during the friction of sexual intercourse, internal exams or Pap smears, and when there are vaginal varicosities
- Cervical polyps, which are often benign growths on the cervix that usually increase in size during pregnancy.
- Hormonal fluctuations, especially around the time of usual monthly periods
- The normal implantation of the fertilized egg within the uterus, which occurs one to two weeks after conception, around the time of your expected period, and lasts just a few days.
- Bloody show at the beginning of labor, a welcome event only if your baby is at least 37 weeks, but more concerning if preterm.

Vaginal bleeding in the first trimester of pregnancy affects approximately 25% of all pregnant women. Less than half of these bleeding women actually miscarry, and even more rarely experience an ectopic pregnancy. Once the fetal heartbeat is detected at the prenatal visit or on a sonogram, miscarriage is rare and unlikely, especially in a healthy pregnancy where there is no prior history of problems like recurrent pregnancy loss. About one in ten pregnant moms will have some bleeding in the third trimester. More often, the cause of bleeding is never found, the bleeding stops, and the pregnancy continues to a happy conclusion.

Vaginal bleeding during the second half of pregnancy can infrequently indicate potentially serious complications, such as:

- The placenta partially to completely separating from the uterine wall before birth (placental abruption).
- A placenta that is located close to or over the cervix (placenta previa), instead of higher in the uterus. A note of reassurance is that while approximately 45% of placentas are classified as "low lying" during the second trimester, the majority "migrate" upwards far enough away from the cervix by the third trimester and are not a cause for worry.
- The umbilical cord first inserts into the fetal membranes, then the exposed blood vessels without the protection of the cord travel to the placenta (velamentous insertion).
- Preterm labor.

When to Call the Midwife or Doctor

You should be evaluated by your midwife or physician anytime there is bleeding during pregnancy in order to rule out anything concerning or deal with something that is treatable. Call your practitioner if bleeding is light but lasts more than three days or is getting worse, is heavy like a period or a continuous flow (you completely soak through a regular sanitary pad in an hour or less), or accompanied by any of the following:

- Pain in your pelvic area, abdomen, back, or shoulder
- Rhythmic uterine cramping
- The passage of tissue or clots bigger than a 50-cent piece
- Foul-smelling discharge
- A gush of fluid from the vagina
- Symptoms of a urinary tract infection, like feeling you have to urinate frequently, but only little amounts come out, burning or foul-smelling urine, low mid-pelvic pain when you pee
- Fever or chills
- Decreased fetal movements
- Weight loss, premature resolution of early pregnancy symptoms

like nausea, vomiting, fatigue, and breast tenderness, or the return of your normal breast size
- You have a history of ectopic pregnancy, miscarriage, molar pregnancy, placenta previa or abruption, or another significant health problem
- You simply feel that something isn't right.

Once you have been evaluated and the more serious causes of the bleeding have been ruled out or dealt with, you should do the following:

- Make sure any issues that can be treated, like infections, MTHFR mutations, or low progesterone, have been addressed.
- Do what you love, what brings you joy, and use your imagination to make routine tasks more enjoyable, even turning on the music while you work.
- Reduce stress and keep calm inside. Practice relaxation techniques with meditative breathwork, as given in the chapter "Meditation, Breathwork, and Visualization."
- Take it easy and avoid heavy lifting until a few days after the bleeding subsides, with frequent breaks in a comfortable lounge chair, bed, or couch.
- Limit non-essentials, delegate, and ask for extra help from family and friends.
- Stock up on some good books, inspirational podcasts, and movies.
- Put nothing in the vagina (this includes no sexual intercourse) until one to two weeks after the bleeding has stopped.
- Eat warm foods, drink fresh ginger tea (steep a piece of raw ginger in a quart mason jar of boiling water for several hours), and limit cold and frozen foods.

For a friable cervix that bleeds easily, small amounts of bleeding from a subchorionic hematoma or persistent spotting from placental implantation, eat foods high in vitamin C. Good choices are citrus fruits, berries, and dark leafy greens, as well as other fresh produce. You may need to supplement with 500-1,000 mg of vitamin C with bioflavonoids, and add vitamin E (the alpha-tocopherol form), 400-800 IU daily for a few weeks only, to support stronger placental adherence to the uterus in early pregnancy. Chasteberry (Vitex) can enhance pregnancy hormones, and natural progesterone can be prescribed if levels are low in the first trimester. There are natural supplements recommended like whole-food B complex with 2-3 mgs of l-methylfolate, and at least 400 mg of DHA/EPA omega-threes for those with the MTHFR mutation, as well as eating more herbs like ginger, turmeric, cinnamon, and cayenne pepper that can thin the blood enough to help it circulate through the tiny vessels of the early placenta without clotting and prevent miscarriage if that is the issue. Speak to your integrative provider about supplementing with ginger as a safer alternative than the commonly prescribed low-dose aspirin if additional blood thinning is advised.

Cramping But Not Bleeding

If all is otherwise well, and you are simply having a lot of cramping without bleeding, make sure you are drinking enough water and getting plenty of calcium and magnesium in your diet. Start by eating lots of green leafy and seaweed veggies, ground sesame seeds (tahini), wild-caught fish like salmon, almonds, whole grains, and pastured organic dairy (preferably goat and sheep). Minimize or avoid cow dairy intake, coffee, and soda, even spinach, which decreases calcium absorption. You may need additional supplementation, at least 400 mg of magnesium and 1,200 mg of calcium daily in 2-3 divided doses; or make your own infusion of nettles and red raspberry leaf tea, using the recipe in the chapter on nutrition.

Also, helpful herbs to reduce cramping are cramp bark, black haw, and wild yam. You can experiment with one of them at a time or use them all together in combination. Take 1-5ml of each tincture every 30 minutes to a few hours, depending on how often and intense the cramping is.

For a Threat of Miscarriage

Women can bleed and cramp and still have a healthy pregnancy. But not all miscarriages can be prevented. Miscarriage is actually pretty common, and its possibility rises with age and the more pregnancies a woman experiences. About 10% to 20% of women with known pregnancies miscarry before 20 weeks. Many miscarry around the time of the first missed period before they even realize they are pregnant.

Heavy bleeding with cramping, lower abdominal or back pains, and/or passage of tissue or fluid from the vagina during early pregnancy usually indicates that a miscarriage is in progress, and there is little that can be done to stop it. In most cases, a miscarriage is your body's natural way of rejecting an unhealthy or abnormally implanted fetus. Try your best to surrender, even embrace what is happening, and trust that all is for your ultimate benefit, even though you may not understand what that is right now.

Once you know you are pregnant, it is still often experienced as a huge loss and the grief can be intense. I am so sorry if that is what is happening, and I encourage you to mourn as you need to, tap into your strength, look for the silver lining, and notice how you grow as you heal.

Other less-common reasons for an isolated miscarriage include infection, dehydration, poor nutrition, severe trauma, and exposure to significant doses of hazardous substances (toxic industrial or environmental chemicals, drugs, alcohol, smoking, and radiation). It is still important to get evaluated, though, to be sure of what is going on, and get treatment if needed.

If you have been informed that a miscarriage is threatening, follow the suggestions above for treatment of bleeding, plus the following:

- Drink a small glass of wine or beer, or a shot of whiskey in juice to lessen the cramping at night if it is interfering with sleep and you do not have a history of alcohol addiction, but alcohol should be used in very limited amounts during pregnancy.
- Keep well hydrated with plenty of water.
- Light some candles and take relaxing warm baths in a clean tub, with your favorite essential oils.
- Take 200 IU of vitamin E, three to four times per day, for no more than three weeks to strengthen placental attachment and reduce spotting.

- Take 500 mg of vitamin C with bioflavonoids, twice a day, during the crisis period.
- Do a yoga nidra, mindfulness practice, or a progressive relaxation meditation to maintain your inner calm. Whenever worrisome thoughts occur, use them as an opportunity to practice being present in the now and doing breathwork. For example, for five to ten minutes twice a day, do slow, deep, extended exhalation breaths (inhale for a count of three, exhale for a count of six) while allowing yourself to feel whatever you feel.
- In a meditative state, tune into what is true for you and what you really want. If it is your heartfelt desire to continue the pregnancy, let that feeling expand, as that will enhance whatever else you are doing. You can send loving thoughts to your baby and visualize your womb surrounded by love, light, and spiritual protection. Affirm that your baby is welcome in your life, that you and your baby are healthy and vibrant, that your placenta is strongly attached to your uterus, and that you are providing safety, security, and nourishment to your baby. Visualize how it feels to hold your baby in your arms and let those expansive high vibrational feelings expand within you.
- You and your partner can place one hand on each other's hearts, the other hand on your womb, and imagine enhancing your family bond. Send love from your hearts to one another and to your baby. Focus on deepening and strengthening your love and connection, especially if there is tension between you. Never underestimate the close relationship of the mind and heart to the body, and the power of love and harmony to heal, transform, and even prevent a miscarriage if the pregnancy is healthy. This can be a wonderful opportunity for healing and transformation for all of you.
- It helps to love yourself unconditionally and with compassion, to have a clear intention to release all self judgement and blame. Visualize the blame leaving you with each exhalation or melting away from your body, sinking down into the earth beneath you.
- Connect to other wise women in sisterhood, those who uplift, inspire, and support you. Have a good cry, a good laugh, and a good hug several times a day.

- It also helps to pray, and as much as possible. Then let go, surrender to what is greater and wiser than us all, the benevolent infinite, and release trying to control what is not in your control. Can we dare to love what is, even when we do not understand the hows and whys?

If you are interested in herbal remedies to help prevent a threatened miscarriage, you can make your own infusion or tincture combination by mixing the following bulk dried herbs or the same herbs in tincture form:

Combine equal amounts of partridge berry, cramp bark, black haw, and wild yam, false unicorn root, and chasteberry (Vitex), with a dash of lobelia. Take 2.5-5 ml of the mixture every half to few hours until symptoms resolve. Then a few times per day for a week. This mixture can be taken prophylactically twice a day in the first trimester if you have a history of miscarriage in prior pregnancy. These herbs are said to aid the miscarriage if the fetus is not normally formed, but prevent it if it is strong and healthy.

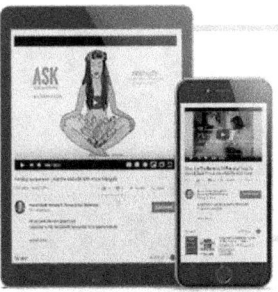

Want to learn more or have more questions?

Grab your free Book Bonuses below:
https://homesweethomebirth.com/nbsbookbonus

MISCARRIAGE: EVERYTHING YOU NEED TO KNOW FOR NATURAL HEALING

Early miscarriage is very common. Bleeding in pregnancy is even more common, but only about half of women who have first trimester bleeding will actually miscarry. It's believed that virtually every woman will have at least one miscarriage sometime in her reproductive years, occurring in as many as 40% of all conceptions. Many miscarriages fortunately go unnoticed as an unusually heavy, crampy, or late period. This explains the lower general statistic of 10% to 20% of pregnant women known to miscarry before 20 weeks.

Sometimes the initial symptom is spotting or premature resolution of early pregnancy symptoms. Sometimes, there is no sign that anything is wrong, but the early ultrasound and labs are diagnostic of a miscarriage, blighted ovum, or chemical or abnormal pregnancy. Heavy bleeding with cramping, lower abdominal or back pains, and/or passage of tissue or fluid from the vagina during early pregnancy usually indicates that a miscarriage is in progress, and there is little that can be done to stop it. In most cases, a miscarriage is your body's natural way of rejecting an unhealthy or abnormally implanted fetus.

However, once the pregnancy has been diagnosed, the grief and emotional pain that you feel with miscarriage can be very acute. It's often quite physically uncomfortable and can even be a little scary.

When a miscarriage is confirmed by your symptoms, blood tests for pregnancy hormone levels (quantitative beta HCG and progesterone), and ultrasound as indicated, consult with your practitioner regarding the risks and benefits of each option and a plan of action. You can choose whether to let nature take its course (expectant management) if deemed a safe option and/or use natural remedies, acupuncture, and traditional Chinese herbs to assist in the process. Alternately, you can take a medication to encourage its completion (medical management) or have your uterus cleaned out surgically with a procedure known as a D & C (dilation and curettage or surgical management). Whatever you choose, you may still benefit from many of the suggestions when watching and waiting and healing.

Watching and Waiting

If your condition has been evaluated as stable and you want to go home to await the inevitable, you can do so, and here is what you can do to help. Have a close, nurturing, and able family member or friend stay with you, so you are not alone until the miscarriage is complete and the intense cramping and bleeding significantly diminish. Remain in close contact with your practitioner. Usually, the bleeding, cramping, and possibly low back pain increase in amount and intensity over the next few days until the bleeding is heavy, and the cramping is severe. Women tend to be surprised by the intensity of cramping, how heavy the bleeding can become, the size of clots, and what else they pass in a normal, uncomplicated miscarriage. Most often, the severe symptoms should not last more than a few hours and end when all the products of conception have been passed (fetus, placenta, and membranes, which may not be discernible prior to eight weeks).

Sometimes the process may take longer, occurring over several days to weeks. In any case, once you have passed all products of conception, the cramping gradually subsides and the bleeding tapers down to occasional spotting for the next week or two. The earlier you are in the pregnancy, the more medically uncomplicated a miscarriage is. The main risks, especially later in the first trimester, are incomplete miscarriage from retained products of conception, hemorrhage, and infection.

Be sure to contact your practitioner and go to the emergency room if severe symptoms persist beyond a few hours or if you experience any of the following:

- You are steadily soaking through a regular pad in less than one hour (especially after you miscarry).
- You have a total blood loss of more than two cups.
- You pass large clots (congealed globs of blood larger than a tennis ball).
- You pass clusters of grape-like vesicles suggestive of a molar pregnancy.
- You feel drowsy, weak, spaced out, or oddly unwell.
- You feel dizzy, lightheaded, or faint.
- You are sleepy, incoherent, or unusually anxious.
- You look pale or feel cold and sweaty.
- You develop severe pain.
- You experience a foul-smelling discharge.
- You have a fever over 100.
- You experience a persistence or worsening of symptoms despite following these suggestions.

While you are miscarrying, go easy. Keep warm and comfortable, and listen to your body, but do not fall asleep while you are bleeding heavily. It is helpful to try to visualize your body letting your fetus and placenta go fully, your cramps emptying your uterus completely and minimizing bleeding, your placenta coming off easily from the wall of your uterus, and letting go of a pregnancy that was not meant to be.

Imagine your uterus surrounded by light and contracting in a rhythmic wave-like pattern, like ocean waves that come and go. Totally surrender to the pain and to a power greater power than yourself, and try to fully accept the miscarriage and that which you cannot control. Trust that your body knows just what to do and that this is for the best in the grand scheme of things, even when you do not comprehend.

Experiencing physical and emotional pain is humbling, and it can be a chance for personal growth. It can be an opportunity to practice techniques like breathwork, mindfulness, and befriending and relaxing into intense sensations that will help with life beyond. Pain provides a chance to learn how to prioritize, delegate, let go of routine activities, and allow others to help and support you. It can teach you compassion for yourself and others, patience, acceptance, surrendering to what is. It can enhance your connection to a higher intelligence or the spiritual realm. It can sensitize you to other people's pain and enable you to be of service to another who is suffering, especially from pregnancy loss. Is there something else that it can teach you? Is there a silver lining or gift in this experience? It may be too early for you to know these answers or even want to think about them in your grief, but this is your journey that you were given, and it is key to ending your suffering and healing fully.

Breathing and Coping Techniques

Breathwork exercises are simple to do and can be done any time and place, and can help you tremendously go through your experience with more ease.

Refer to the many different breathwork practices given in the chapter "Meditation, Breathwork, and Visualization," and choose the breathing technique that helps you the most now.

Conscious Relaxation

Notice habits of increased muscle tension, especially around your upper back, shoulders, neck, forehead, and jaw, and make an effort to release these tightened muscles while doing slow, deep abdominal breathing. Relax the muscles that are tensing up, as you are breathing. Breathe slowly and deeply while thinking about relaxing each muscle from your head down to your toes. Focus on releasing all of your muscles, more and more with each exhale. Visualize feeling heavy and limp like a rag doll or like your napping dog or cat.

As the cramping intensifies, assume any position for comfort like hands and knees, kneeling, or leaning forward on an exercise ball. Rhythmic movement is comforting, like gentle bouncing, rocking, swaying, or pacing. Moaning through your cramping helps as well as saying chakra syllables, mantras, or simple affirmative words or sounds like those mentioned in the chapter "Meditation, Breathwork, and Visualization."

Ask your support person to massage areas of persistent muscle tension with arnica oil mixed with a dropperful of St. John's wort topical oil and a few drops of lavender. Periodic firm massage or pressure to your feet, lower abdomen, upper back, and sacrum is soothing. Use a hot or cold pack, heating pad, hot water bottle, or a very warm wet towel with a few drops of lavender oil over your pelvic area or lower back. Tightly hold small combs so that the teeth are pressed into the mounds at the base of your fingers. This stimulates acupressure points to facilitate uterine contractions.

Make sure to stay well-hydrated by drinking plenty of clean water every day. Try to sip a cup of clear fluids like water, electrolyte-infused Smart Water, pure coconut water, herbal tea and honey, juice or frozen juice pops, Recharge or organic Gatorade, or miso, bone, or vegetable broth or chicken stock every hour. Urinate frequently, so your uterus can properly contract. You may need more fluids and electrolytes if bleeding is heavy or prolonged and you feel dehydrated. To make your own electrolyte concoction. Combine:

- 1/8 to 1/4 teaspoon of sea salt
- 1/4 teaspoon of baking soda
- One teaspoon calcium/magnesium powder
- One to two tablespoons of honey
- One quart of spring or pure coconut water
- Juice of a fresh lemon or lime to taste.

If a miscarriage has been confirmed with an ultrasound and you're interested in herbal support, try the following formulations. *These are only for a known miscarriage and are not safe or recommended to induce abortion in a healthy pregnancy.*

For Herbal Miscarriage Support

In The Natural Pregnancy Book Dr. Aviva Romm advises the following wonderfully effective remedies:

1. Combine a one-ounce bottle each of cotton root bark and black cohosh tinctures with a half an ounce of blue cohosh tincture.
2. Take one teaspoon of the combination every four hours on the first day and every hour for four hours on the second day.
3. Then half a teaspoon every 30 minutes for 4 hours the rest of the second day.
4. Skip a day and repeat the second day dosing one more day if you have not started cramping. Consult your provider if you still do not experience results after doing this.

To prevent mild to moderate bleeding from becoming heavy, combine equal parts shepherd's purse, witch hazel, and bayberry bark tinctures, and take half a teaspoon every hour. You can add 1/4 to a half of a teaspoon of beth root tincture every 15 minutes during the acute stage, then every 2 hours until the bleeding has tapered down.

You can also brew a teaspoon of basil or cinnamon in a cup of boiling water and sip the tea throughout the period of miscarriage to support contractions and minimize bleeding.

If you are feeling anxious or feeling emotionally off-balance after a complete and normal miscarriage, drink strong lavendar, lemon balm, skullcap, motherwort, passionflower, hops, and/or chamomille tea as often as needed using two bags and steep them for 10-15 minutes. You can take any of the calming herbs in capsule or tincture form that work best for relieving your internal stress and steadying your emotions. The healing herbs of Dr. Bach's Rescue Remedy used as directed can have a calming influence during this stressful time (take a few drops of it as often as required). Avoid alcohol, mood-altering drugs, and medications like sedatives, as they can cloud your thinking, suppress your body's natural responses, and, thus, interfere with healthy grieving.

To prevent retained products of conception and ensure the uterus clears out completely, take a dropperful of angelica tincture, three to four times per day that first week, or up to every few hours until the heavier bleeding lessens. Add one to two dropperfuls of ground ivy tincture every few hours if the bleeding and cramping are still persisting. Consult your provider if this does not help.

After the Miscarriage

After a complete miscarriage, it takes some time to heal physically and emotionally. The amount of time varies with each woman, but it is helpful in the first few weeks to get plenty of sleep, take it really easy, stay warm and cozy, drink lots of fluids, and eat hearty and wholesome real foods.

Remember to take your vitamin, mineral, and nutritional supplements to make sure you are fully nourished. I recommend taking an herbal iron in tablet or liquid form for two months. If you were anemic and/or lost a significant amount of blood, follow the suggestions in the "Anemia in Pregnancy" chapter, about diet and natural remedies to boost your iron stores.

To prevent infection, for the first week:

- Take 1,000 mg vitamin C with bioflavinoids, one to two times daily.
- Sweeten your teas with plenty of manuka honey.
- Eat a bulb of garlic daily (baked or sautéed cloves in olive oil, salt, and pepper) or take a capsule of supercritical garlic, a few times per day.
- Take oil of oregano, one to two times daily.
- Take one dropperful of Gaia's alcohol-free Echinacea Supreme, three to four times per day.
- You can also add a dropperful each of calendula and goldenseal herbal tinctures a few times daily to not only prevent infection, but to promote healing.
- Echinacea supreme, goldenseal, and calendula can also be taken in capsule form.
- To further support your immunity, take Host Defense Asian Mushrooms, two per day.

Refrain from a bath until the major bleeding subsides, but showering is fine. Once the bleeding stops, enjoy a daily warm bath in a cleansed tub, with a few drops of the essential oils of lavender, neroli, frankincense, cinnamon, and/or rose to help ease stress and promote healing after a miscarriage. You can also place a few drops of your favorite essential oil in a diffuser.

Periodically check your temperature to ensure you are not developing a fever. Do not put anything inside the vagina until your bleeding stops (it could be a few weeks for the bleeding to taper to light then spotting). Change your pads every few hours and wipe front to back after going to the bathroom.

You can ovulate as soon as two weeks after a miscarriage. Most women get their period in four to six weeks if not pregnant again. The first period or so after a miscarriage may be a little different, so give yourself time to get back to your usual cycling. It is advisable to use contraception and wait at least one to two regular periods in a row before trying to conceive again, more time if you had complications or simply need to get your iron levels back to normal. There are helpful online resources like on natural pregnancy sites such as mamanatural.com to guide you as well for general healing and getting pregnant after miscarriage.

For a wonderfully nourishing herbal infusion for four to six weeks after miscarriage:

1. Combine a handful each of red raspberry leaf, nettle leaf, dandelion root, and strawberry leaves.
2. Mix in a pinch of fresh or dried ginger root, a small piece of cinnamon stick, and a teaspoon of alfalfa.
3. Place a small handful of the mixture into a glass canning jar.
4. Add one cup of boiling water and brew for two to three hours.
5. Strain it, and drink a half to one cup, two to four times per day.
6. You can add juice of lemon or lime, fresh mint leaves, or a dash of honey to taste.

Many integrative holistic practitioners recommend additional herbs like vitex or chasteberry, don quai or angelica, red clover, wild yam, false unicorn, licorice, ginseng, ashwagandha, maca, rhodiola, and/or holy basil to support your hormones and reproductive organs, as well as your stress response and adrenals during this healing time, specific to the situation. Acupuncture and Chinese herbs can be very effective as well. Consult a professional regarding which ones and the dosing that is best for you.

You will need to be examined in a few weeks to make sure you are healing properly and to discuss future plans. It is ideal to check pregnancy hormones until they return to non-pregnant levels, and, if needed, to get an ultrasound to confirm the miscarriage is complete. If your blood type is Rh-negative and the father of the baby is Rh-positive, an injection of Rhogam is strongly recommended within 72 hours. This is to prevent you from developing antibodies against Rh-positive fetal blood cells that mixed with your circulation during the miscarriage. These could dangerously attack another Rh-positive baby's blood cells should you become pregnant again.

Ask your practitioner and hospital for reading material or handouts specific to miscarriage and pregnancy loss, as well as for a local support group, therapist, and member of the clergy with whom you and your spouse can speak. This will help you better cope with your grief, disappointment, and guilt, and enable you to go through the process of mourning in a healthy way.

Many find it very healing to hold a special memorial ceremony to name, grieve, provide closure, and remember the baby. You can also write something to your baby, like a poem or letter, plant a tree or perennial plant or flower, buy or create art - a small remembrance figurine, necklace, or bracelet to symbolize, honor and remember your loss.

Spiritual Support

On a mind/body/spiritual level, you can give the baby permission to go if they need to. Treat yourself with love and care, and try to love yourself and your body without toxic feelings of blame or guilt. This can be a wonderful and healing opportunity to stay in the present moment and practice mindfulness. Simply watch all the various sensations you experience, accepting and surrendering to what is true, and the often intense feelings you may experience without judgment. Instead, choose compassion and love for yourself and others close to you.

Slowly and deeply focus on your breath, meditate, and simply sit quietly, letting thoughts come and go without attaching to them. Breathe into the pain or visualize healing light or energy directed at the emotional pain you feel, dispersing it into the atmosphere or falling deep into the earth beneath you. Know that you are going through one of the deepest lessons of life's impermanence and our lack of control over it. You will find your inner strength, heal physically and emotionally in time, and one day be more able to help others who go through this common but painful experience. Many of the suggestions in the chapter for managing emotions in pregnancy still apply now. What really helps is to allow yourself to feel everything you feel and move it through your body with music. To help you process, release, and heal intense, stuck, painful emotional energy and trauma from the experience, schedule a Clarity Breathwork session with me. This is a great way to get the support and guidance you may need to get yourself back.

If You've Had Multiple Miscarriages

Women who have suffered from three or more consecutive pregnancy losses need expert medical care and counseling. A number of factors can contribute to repeated miscarriages, including:

- Increased maternal age
- Chromosomal or genetic abnormalities
- Hormonal imbalances
- Cervical incompetence (the cervix opens prematurely, especially if scarred after a traumatic procedure)
- Uterine abnormalities (as in structure, fibroids, or scar tissue)
- Immunologic problems, serious illness, or chronic health problems
- Blood elevation of a kind of lipid or certain clotting factors
- Poor lifestyle choices like dehydration, unhealthy diet and nutritional deficiencies, smoking, drinking too much alcohol, drugs, and other toxic exposure - including chronic inner stress.

Consider an experienced doctor of Chinese medicine and acupuncture in adjunct to any medically needed treatment, which can be very effective for preventing recurrent miscarriage and strengthening you for a healthy pregnancy next time around. It's also essential to decrease internal feelings of stress and promote inner peace as well as joy by doing more of what you love. Taking yoga classes and regularly practicing your breathwork and meditation are wonderful places to start.

Please be reassured that many of the causes of repeated pregnancy loss are medically or surgically treatable. Never give up hope. There are many success stories. Some are accomplished with simple attention to correct nutrition, hydration, and lifestyle habits (like quitting smoking, avoiding alcohol, drugs, and other noxious substances), taking supplements and herbs, reducing stress, and enhancing spiritual practice and prayer.

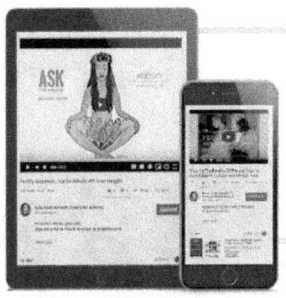

Want to learn more or have more questions?

Grab your free Book Bonuses below:
https://homesweethomebirth.com/nbsbookbonus

Managing Fatigue During Pregnancy

Fatigue during pregnancy is a very common experience. Growing a baby is an enormous task and requires a tremendous amount of physical and mental energy. There are a number of factors that can contribute to fatigue during pregnancy, for example:

- The increased demands on your body, mind, heart, and spirit
- Lack of quality sleep or rest periods
- Overworking yourself inside and/or outside of the house
- Excessive or chronic stress
- Short pregnancy spacing, breastfeeding, and caring for other children
- Too much time on a computer or cell phone
- Inadequate diet and hydration
- Nutritional deficiencies like low B12 and anemia
- Sedentary living
- Unexpressed or unresolved emotional difficulties
- Depression or anxiety
- Acute infection or illness
- Under-active thyroid function
- Toxic exposures (such as from pesticides, chemicals in your water, common household cleaning and body products)
- Other health problems
- And even boredom

Resolving Fatigue During Pregnancy

Look at the whole picture. Consider what in your life could be contributing to your fatigue, and take common-sense measures to take care of yourself. Go clean, green, and organic with food, body, and household products, and minimize time online. Connect more with others you love to be around, in person.

Lack of Rest and Inner Calm

Get more sleep by going to bed earlier, sleeping later in the morning, and/or taking a nap during the daytime. Getting enough sleep is especially essential during pregnancy.

Take frequent breaks or "healing intervals" throughout the day to simply rest, and center and calm yourself. You can do this by lying down or sitting quietly with your eyes closed, slowing down your thoughts by focusing on slow, deep breathing while gazing internally between your eyebrows or towards the tip of your nose.

Meditation, breathwork, visualization, and yoga nidra/progressive muscle relaxation are all great ways to relax the body. There are many books, audio CDs, and hypnobirthing MP3s for pregnancy to help you learn these important life skills. There are also wonderful phone apps like Breathe and Calm. Make it a regular part of your daily routine to practice them, even just for 15 to 20 minutes. Refer to the chapter on "Meditation, Breathwork and Visualization" for more details. Breathing in certain ways helps you to maintain internal peace no matter what is going on around you, and certain breathwork exercises create energy and give you an amazing sense of vitality.

Inadequate Diet

Paying close attention to your diet can go a long way in avoiding fatigue during pregnancy, as your nutritional needs soar during this time.

Make sure you're drinking and eating well, taking in lots of protein (at least 20 to 30 grams, three times daily) and healthy fats. For more details on diet and prenatal supplementation, refer to the chapter on "Nutritional Best Practices for Mom."

Avoid white flours, cane sugar, and high fructose corn syrup, as they make you feel more tired after an initial brief boost in energy. Use fruit, raw honey, and maple syrup instead, but in a meal with quality protein and fat to keep your blood sugar stable.

Most also feel best physically and emotionally off gluten and dairy products, for example, on a Paleo or ancestral diet. When eating whole grains, try gluten-free varieties like gluten-free oats, buckwheat, and quinoa, and combine it with a protein or fat like avocado, seeds, nuts, pure nut milks or nut butters, wild-caught fish from non-polluted waters, or pastured, organic poultry, meat, and eggs.

Eat small amounts several times throughout the day rather than heavy infrequent meals.

Vitamin and Mineral Deficiencies

If you are anemic (which is very common in pregnancy, especially during the second and third trimesters), eat iron-rich foods. Check out the chapter, "Anemia in Pregnancy: Prevention and Treatment" to learn more about iron supplementation.

If your vitamin B12 levels are low - under 600 (common in women today, especially those who have had several successive pregnancies or are breastfeeding, and with vegetarian/vegan diets), supplementing with 1,000 to 5,000 mcg of vitamin B12 (in the form of methyl, hydroxo, or adenosyl cobalamin) sublingual (under the tongue) or more will be needed, depending on your labs and can really make a huge difference in how you feel.

Have your thyroid function and antibodies checked, and address any imbalances with a functional medicine or integrative doctor.

Also, be sure to take a good, all-natural, whole-food-based prenatal vitamin and mineral supplement.

A daily nutrition-rich fresh juice made with a combination of veggies and superfoods like spirulina, kelp, or wheatgrass can help you feel more alert and energized. Start slowly with one to two tablespoons of the superfoods and build up to 1-2 ounces. Drink it first thing in the morning on an empty stomach. Superfoods also come in all-natural powdered mixes that can be added to your daily smoothie. Note: *if you have a lot of accumulated toxins in your body, wheatgrass may cause slight nausea at first as it cleanses your system. This is harmless and eventually passes.*

Nature and Movement

Get plenty of fresh air and adequate exposure to sunlight on a daily basis. Try to spend at least 30 minutes outside with nature in the early morning or late afternoon sun each day without sunscreen. If spending a lot of time indoors, at least open the windows–especially in the winter.

Engage in moderate exercise for 30 minutes at least 5 days per week. Good options during pregnancy include swimming, brisk walking, cycling, dancing, or low-impact aerobics. Even though you feel tired, this type of exercise creates energy and does wonders to minimize fatigue, depression, and anxiety. Incorporating yoga (especially prenatal, yin, gentle, and restorative) as a regular part of your daily routine can also be very powerful.

Try to maintain correct posture and body mechanics. Use your abdominal muscles to straighten your upper back and tuck your pelvis in to straighten your lower back. Engage your core by bringing your breast bone and lower ribs and belly toward your back, and bringing your front pelvic bone towards your breastbone. Use your arm and leg muscles instead of your weaker back muscles to lift, carry, pull, and push things.

Emotional Health

It is important to be open and honest about your feelings to yourself. Some women find it helpful to keep a journal or diary to increase self-awareness and understanding. Share your feelings with your spouse, close friend, or a family member. But talking about our feelings only goes so far. Periodically release pent up emotions with a good cry, followed by a hug, and a good dance.

Move strong emotions through your body. If you are angry or overstressed, play an angry song; if you feel grief, play a sad song; or simply play a track of African drumming and let your body move to the music while making the sounds you need. Our little ones have their temper tantrums to move and release their emotions, so they are not repressed and stuck in their bodies. Then they get back up and resume playing. Some indigenous cultures dance their grief, anger, joy, and celebration in community drum circles. We have much to learn from them. Invite friends and have your own drum circle to express and release emotions. You might just feel so exhilarated by it you will want to do this regularly.

Avoid overexertion and trying to be "super mom" by re-examining your priorities, limiting unessential activities, and learning how to say no. Delegate tasks to others and let friends and family help.

Try to allow yourself regular time each day without guilt to do something that you fully enjoy, that inspires and uplifts you. Make it easy and fun. Some ideas are:

- Watching a musical, romance, comedy, or uplifting drama
- Reading a good novel or inspirational biography
- Taking a stroll through the park or a gentle hike in the woods or a beautiful spot in nature
- Gardening
- Going on an outing with your partner or good friend
- Cultivating a hobby
- Learning something new that interests you

Add more laughter and play to your life. Many women are surprised to find how health-enhancing and energizing this can be.

Seek out a transformational life coach or, if needed, a professional, holistic therapist if the above ideas do not help and you are troubled by psychological distress or emotional discomfort. Suppressed feelings can worsen fatigue as well as cause all sorts of other problems if not properly dealt with.

Herbs and Oils

Take an invigorating bath with a few drops of essential oils of peppermint or eucalyptus, lemon, wild orange, grapefruit, and/or rosemary. You can add a few drops of these essential oils to a bowl or spray bottle of cool water and spray yourself with the uplifting scents throughout the day.

Nettle is a great herb to be taking in pregnancy as a nourishing tonic. It also has the added benefits of blood sugar regulation, adrenal support, improving nutrient intake, and building iron levels. Make a strong infusion by steeping a handful of this dried herb in one quart of boiling water for three to four hours, and strain it into a glass canning jar. Drink one to three cups daily (with fresh lemon or lime juice, mint leaf, or a dash of honey to taste). A fresh spearmint or peppermint tea can also provide a lift of spirit and energy.

If you're interested in other herbs to improve energy, combine equal amounts of herbal tinctures of schisandra, eleuthero, and American ginseng, and take 1/4 to 1/2 of a teaspoon, once or twice per day. Start with the lowest dose and work your way up as needed.

Minimize or avoid caffeine. It is addictive, too much is harmful, the energy boost is artificial, and it can be agitating and impair sleep. Many feel more tired when its effects wear off.

Avoid stimulant drugs (including diet pills) and sleeping medications, as most have side effects for you and your growing fetus, and can cause you to become dependent on them. Many substances, such as cocaine, are outright dangerous to you and your baby. You must seek professional help if you cannot stop using them, your symptoms don't improve or worsen despite implementing these suggestions or you need more professional guidance.

Other Resources

Homeopathy and acupuncture can both be great for soothing stress and increasing energy. Also, check out Clarity Breathwork for extremely effective, mind-body, cutting-edge methods that have led to transformational healing for thousands of people around the world.

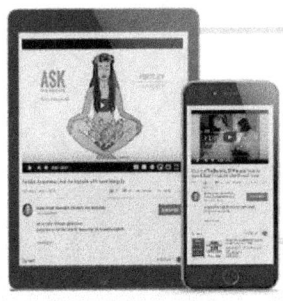

Want to learn more or have more questions?

Grab your free Book Bonuses below:
https://homesweethomebirth.com/nbsbookbonus

Natural Remedies for Nausea During Pregnancy

Nausea is one of the most common complaints of pregnancy. It seems to be related to the massive increase in hormones to support the pregnancy and an individual's unique sensitivity to the physical and emotional changes that result.

Nausea during pregnancy will resolve on its own by the third or fourth month for most people. In the meantime, there are several effective ways of dealing with it naturally.

Consider keeping a diary of what makes your symptoms better and worse to increase your awareness of what to avoid and how to help yourself. Nausea is often made worse by dehydration, fatigue, stress, unresolved emotional issues, sedentary indoor living, an inadequate diet, nutritional deficiencies, an empty stomach, and offensive odors. Plan accordingly!

Dietary Recommendations for Reducing Nausea During Pregnancy

A drop in blood sugar from the added work of making a baby can make nausea worse, so it is important to eat small amounts of whole food with complex carbohydrates, protein, and healthy fat, at least every 2-3 hours, and eat real, local, organic food products as much as possible. Include in your daily diet small, frequent meals of what is most healthy and wholesome of foods recommended in pregnancy, as discussed in more detail in the "Nutritional Best Practices for Mom" chapter.

Stay away from refined white flour foods, high fructose corn syrup, and cane sugar, as they lead to a rapid rise then fall in blood sugar, which actually worsens nausea and causes other symptoms like fatigue, dizziness, headaches, brain fog, anxiety, and depression. Avoid letting your stomach become empty or stuffed, and try to separate eating solids and drinking liquids by about 15 to 20 minutes. Try to eat a small portion of food that you can tolerate after vomiting. Eat what agrees with you for now from the advised healthy foods, as your baby will take nutrients from you. You can replenish when the nausea resolves.

Keep some healthy snacks by your bedside to eat before rising in the morning and going to bed at night–like a yummy raw crunch Paleo nut/seed bar. Always carry an assortment of the foods you tolerate best when out.

In general, plain foods are usually better tolerated than hot, spicy, rich, greasy, and overly sweetened, or processed junk foods. Avoid coffee, alcohol, and cigarettes, as they irritate the stomach, in addition to causing health problems for you and your baby.

Hydration Is Key

Keep well-hydrated by drinking lots of water daily (at least half your body weight in ounces). Pure filtered, spring or well water with a splash of lemon, lime, orange, or grapefruit juice, or seltzer or sparkling water (plain or naturally flavored) are great options.

Good choices in addition to water are:

- Herbal teas of ginger, peppermint, spearmint, chamomile, raspberry leaf, cinnamon, peach, catnip, lemon balm, anise or fennel seeds with honey, or fresh mint leaves to taste
- Warm pure almond milk with lemon juice or honey, as soon as you get up in the morning
- A small glass of grapefruit juice before meals
- Sipping natural ginger ale throughout the day
- Soup broth (vegetable, chicken, or bone).

If you are vomiting, try to drink a small amount of liquid each time you throw up. 1/4 of a cup of fluids every 15-30 minutes is crucial to keep hydrated. Place a pinch of Himalayan sea salt on your tongue to help replenish electrolytes.

Try to drink the health food alternative to the standard Gatorade or Pedialyte (which is full of chemicals) called Recharge to replenish lost fluids and electrolytes. Gatorade now makes an organic variety. Another option is electrolyte-infused water like Smart Water. Fresh or all-natural coconut water is nature's rehydration drink. Eating watermelon is also great for hydrating yourself and is well tolerated. You can also make your own concoction by combining:

- 1/8 to 1/4 teaspoon of Himalayan sea salt
- 1/4 teaspoon of baking soda
- One teaspoon of calcium/magnesium powder
- One to two tablespoons of honey
- Juice of one fresh lemon or lime to taste
- One quart of spring or coconut water
- Drink a cup slowly every 1-2 hours. Even if you vomit it up, you will still get some and it often reduces the number of vomiting episodes.

Take Time for Self-Care

This is a very sensitive period. You need to find extra time for your own much-needed pampering, and remind close friends and family that you need lots of additional love and understanding.

Soak in a warm bath with a few drops of essential oils of lavender, sandalwood, peppermint, citrus, or rose. You can also bathe in a few tablespoons of fresh ginger juice—made by juicing a piece of ginger a few inches long or a half-cup of grated ginger to the bath.

Get more sleep by going to bed earlier or sleeping later, and taking a nap or frequent rest periods during the day. Allow more time to get out of bed in the morning. Get plenty of fresh air and sunshine.

Open windows when inside, weather permitting. Every day, try to spend at least 30 minutes outside with nature in the early morning or late afternoon sun. This does wonders!

Engage in regular moderate exercise such as brisk walking, cycling, dancing or swimming for 30-60 minutes, 5 days per week. Even though you may not feel like doing this, it helps immensely and you will feel better afterwards.

Practice breathing exercises for 10-20 minutes, once or twice per day (like before rising in the morning and going to sleep at night) and whenever you feel very nauseous or stressed. Try to relax with yoga, meditation, progressive muscle relaxation techniques (yoga nidra), visualizations and imagery work (see the chapter, "Breathwork, Meditation, and Visualization").

Enjoy a light distraction like watching an engrossing drama, comedy, or musical, reading a good book, or listening to music that you love. Get a change of scenery by unplugging from your smartphone or computer and spending a day in the park or at the beach, hiking in a beautiful place, getting a spa treatment, exploring a museum or a local town, going to the theater, taking an art or music class, volunteering for those in need, getting together and connecting with those who support and encourage you, going on a mini-vacation with a family member or friend to a place you enjoy.

Natural Remedies for Nausea During Pregnancy

Herbs

If you are interested in herbs, there are several options to try alone or in combination.

- **Peppermint.** Make your own mint-smelling remedy. Place one or two drops of essential oil of peppermint in a spray bottle and spray it near your nose periodically. You can also put the drops on a piece of cloth or in an essential oil diffuser, or place fresh mint leaves in a covered container, crush the leaves each time you open it, and smell it throughout the day as often as you need.

- **Red raspberry leaf.** Take one to two capsules or one dropperful of tincture, one to two times per day.
- **Wild yam tincture.** Take 20-30 drops, 3-6 times a day, or one dropperful, up to every few hours depending on the severity of your symptoms.
- **Dandelion tincture.** Can be taken on its own, but is especially effective in combination with wild yam. Take 20 to 30 drops, 3-4 times daily.
- **Ginger root powder.** If you have no history of two or more miscarriages, take 250 mg capsules, up to 4 times a day.
- **Ginger Honey Tonic.** Can be taken in 1-2 teaspoon doses as often as needed, as can all-natural ginger lozenges, ginger sucking candies, and dried, crystallized ginger pieces.
- **Slippery Elm.** Can be taken in lozenge form or as a thin porridge by adding water to the powder and honey to taste.
- **Umeboshi (sour plum).** Can be taken as sucking or chewable candies, and are available in most health food stores.

CBD from hemp oil. This is the new rage, as it helps to relieve morning sickness without the potential risks of the THC component of cannabis on the developing fetus. Results from anecdotal evidence and preliminary research, although sparse (as is common with most natural remedies in pregnancy), are promising. Make sure it is absolutely pure and from a reputable source who can recommend proper dosing or from pharmacies licensed to dispense it, as it is largely unregulated. It is usually taken as several drops under the tongue.

Fresh homemade herbal teas can work wonders for nausea during pregnancy. Do some experimenting to find what is most helpful to you:

- Immerse a tiny piece of fresh ginger or one teaspoon of grated ginger in a cup of boiling water for 5-15 minutes. Strain into a glass, and sip up to two cups throughout the day.

- Dandelion root can be taken with or without the ginger. Add approximately five tablespoons of dried root or about ten tablespoons of fresh root to one quart boiling water. Let it brew for 3-4 hours, strain into a glass canning jar, and periodically sip, totaling up to two cups per day.
- Add one tablespoon of dried chamomile to one cup of boiling water, and steep covered for 10 minutes. Strain into a glass and sip periodically, up to two cups daily.
- In one cup of boiling water, add a teaspoon of dried or two tablespoons of fresh leaves of peppermint or spearmint. Immerse covered for 15 minutes, and drink as often as needed.
- You can add a dash of honey and/or lemon or lime juice to any of the above teas to taste.
- Try making ice cubes of strong ginger, peppermint, or red raspberry tea, and suck on them every few hours.

Supplements

Take a good whole-food, all-natural prenatal vitamin as explained in the Nutrition chapter. Add an additional supplement of 25-50 mg vitamin B complex, one to two times per day, depending on how much nausea, vomiting, and fatigue you are experiencing. A whole-food or herbal iron supplement can also be taken after meals as needed if you are anemic. It tends to be well-absorbed and better tolerated than the pharmaceutical formulations, especially ferrous sulfate that actually upsets the stomach. But if you cannot tolerate swallowing capsules or tablets at this time, add a powdered superfood combination to your smoothie that is loaded with nutrients.

If your symptoms are severe and you cannot tolerate taking supplements, just take 25 mg of vitamin B6, three times a day. If even that is too much and your nausea is accompanied by the great exhaustion of early pregnancy, consider vitamin B6 injections from a compounding natural pharmacy, with methylated B12 and folate.

Another option when dealing with severe symptoms is to combine vitamin B6 with a relatively safe over-the-counter antihistamine medication doxylamine, known as Unisom, which is available in most drugstores. Take half of a tablet or 25 mg before sleep with 25 mg of vitamin B6. You can take the other half in the morning with your first B6 dose, but it may make you drowsy. And do not forget the midday 25 mg dose of B6. The combination of vitamin B6 and Unisom or the prescriptive version called Bongesta can be phenomenally successful at reducing severe nausea during pregnancy, and is considered the best, most nontoxic pharmacological treatment around.

Additional Remedies

In Dr. Aviva Romm's *The Natural Pregnancy Book* she advises a wonderfully effective Japanese remedy if you feel like a bout of vomiting is coming on or if you have been vomiting multiple times:

- Heat a half-cup of sea salt in a skillet for three minutes.
- Put the salt in a pillowcase or other suitable sack.
- Fold into a rectangular pad or small square, and wrap it in another towel if too hot.
- Apply pack directly to your stomach on your upper right abdomen (not lower belly).

Wear acupressure wristbands, or Seabands, which place constant pressure on the acupressure points related to nausea. These can be purchased in most health food stores and some pharmacies, and have been very effective for some women. Or get regular acupuncture treatments.

Consult with a classical homeopath or an excellent reference book for a remedy most specific to your symptoms. Some women report much success with Weleeda's homeopathic combination Nausin (7-10 drops, four times per day).

Do not take over-the-counter medications without checking with your healthcare provider, as many are not safe during pregnancy, especially during the first trimester.

Final Consideration: Your Nausea May Have an Emotional Component

Mental conflict and emotional turmoil can greatly contribute to nausea and vomiting, as does ambivalence about your pregnancy. Make a conscious effort to work on increasing feelings of forgiveness, appreciation, love, joy, optimism, and healing. Likewise, try to let go of anger, resentment, fear, sadness, and other negative thought patterns that are not serving you. Conscious, connected breathing as in Clarity Breathwork is a highly effective way of doing this naturally, without much effort.

Try to avoid things, thoughts, and people that agitate your mind and raise your internal tension. Surround yourself as much as possible with calm, centered people, things, sounds, and places that inspire you, relax you, and cause you to feel at ease and restore you to inner peace and serenity.

Talk through ambivalent or troubling feelings with your partner, close friend, or therapist as needed. Don't be afraid to seek counseling if you need help with this, as it is not only helpful to express your feelings with a sympathetic ear, but also to develop skills of self-mastery and empowerment. Breathwork, however, will release issues that cannot be resolved through thinking and talking, and shave off years of therapy.

Please call your health care provider if your nausea is extreme or persists in spite of following the above guidelines, if you have severe persistent vomiting such that you cannot keep anything down for more than 24 hours, you are losing weight, dehydrated, and/or you feel faint, as you may need medication, or even intravenous hydration.

40 Ways to Manage Emotions in Pregnancy

Powerful, often conflicting emotions, can feel concerning. Hormonal and physical changes, as well as the associated stresses of pregnancy and having a baby may cause pronounced mood swings. Common and normal feelings include:

- Excitement, joy, elation
- Gratitude, enrichment, love
- Creativity, clarity
- Ambivalence, impatience, vulnerability
- Apathy, indifference
- Confusion, self-doubt, insecurity
- Guilt, shame, burden
- Fear, anxiety
- Sadness, grief, resentment
- You may feel beautiful, sensual, and voluptuous. Or you may feel fat, unattractive, and asexual. Pregnant women often have increased sensitivity, a heightened sense of perception and awareness, and notice stronger reactions than usual.

These emotions can be especially troublesome if you are not eating or sleeping well, have ongoing exposure to common toxicants in food, water, home cleaning, and body products, and/or have experienced psychological problems in the past, have other health problems or pregnancy complications, do not have sufficient support from family or friends, the pregnancy was not planned, or there are other major stresses in your life.

First and foremost, know that you are not your emotions. They usually come after thoughts; some call them "thoughts in motion." Look at emotions as sensations in the body without the story, that come and go like waves, or like the sun, clouds, and rain. They are never permanent but change like the weather. Emotions are a part of you, they all are a sacred part of being human, but see your true essence above and unaffected by it all. Just as there is the perfect warm sunny day with a cloudless blue sky, there are thunderstorms with great wind and rain, and blizzards with snow; there are periods of darkness and periods of light. You can absolutely be in charge of how you feel rather than at the mercy of your emotions. You can learn to embrace all of your sensations without attaching to any particular one and ride the waves of life with grace, ease, and a deep sense of joy. It takes regular practice, yet it is so doable.

40 Ways to Manage Emotions in Pregnancy and Beyond

1. Seek balance in your emotional life, instead of going for the highs and lows that follow.
2. Get extra needed sleep in pregnancy by going to bed earlier, sleeping later, and/or napping during the day, as well as allowing periodic rest from a hectic routine.
3. Limit or avoid highly processed foods, refined white flour, high fructose corn syrup and all forms of cane sugar, refined vegetable and partially hydrogenated oils, and artificial colorings and chemicals.
4. Make sure to eat a nourishing, wholesome organic diet. Many feel best completely off gluten, sugar, and dairy; instead, go organic Paleo and eat plenty of high-quality fats and protein (see the chapter on nutrition for details). Try it for a month. You will be amazed at how much better you feel physically and emotionally.
5. Stay hydrated by drinking lots of clean water.
6. Take a good all-natural, whole-food-based prenatal vitamin and mineral supplement (also covered in the nutrition chapter).
7. Avoid alcohol and caffeine.
8. Do regular moderate exercise that you enjoy and are accustomed to, 30 minutes daily, five times per week.

9. Get plenty of fresh air and time in nature.

10. Get adequate exposure to sunlight by spending at least 20 minutes each day outside in the early morning or late afternoon sun, ideally without sunscreen (or if sensitive or fair-skinned, use a very low dose, all-natural sunscreen).

11. During the early part of the day, if you cannot go outside, use 150- to 200-Watt incandescent bulbs or full-spectrum fluorescent lamps that supply 2,500 or more lux, and keep the light within three feet of where you are sitting.

12. Go green and all-natural with body and cleaning products, and maintain a toxic-free home and reduced exposure as much as possible at work (see resources in the chapter called "Preparing for a Healthy Pregnancy" for details).

13. Become intensely conscious of the present and acutely sensitive to your feelings and inner experiences, using all of your senses. Get curious. Observe, watch, and allow whatever comes up without judgment or thought.

14. Practice breathwork daily for 10-20 minutes, once or twice a day. See the chapter "Mindfulness, Breathwork, and Visualization" for details. Schedule a Breathwork session and allow yourself to experience its wonderful life-changing benefits!

15. Stay away from things (like certain books, movies, and news), situations, and people (like those who are angry, stressed out, negative, pessimistic, critical, fearful, or demanding) that agitate your mind, raise your internal tension, bring you down, and worsen your emotional state.

16. If someone who you are close with continually criticizes, belittles, demands, or negates your feelings, try to give positive, straightforward suggestions about approaches that would be more helpful to you, or consider having this person come with you to some professional counseling sessions.

17. Surround yourself as much as possible with calm, centered, and positive people, things, sounds, and places that inspire, uplift, relax, and restore you to inner peace and serenity.

18. Periodically rub the essential oil of rose into your pulse points and spray rose water on yourself throughout the day.

19. Treat yourself to a massage each month, or ask your partner or friend for one regularly. Include a few drops each of any

combination of the essential oils of lavender, orange, citrus blend, rose, St. John's wort, and/or chamomile. Make your own mixture in a bottle of almond oil.

20. Bring more art and music into your life.

21. Try to allow time each day to do something you enjoy and something that makes you laugh.

22. Collect at least eight deep, soul-nurturing hugs daily.

23. Keep a journal or diary as a way to be honest with yourself about your feelings and increase self-awareness and understanding. Try to write free-flow without editing; draw and write poems as you are inspired.

24. Share important feelings with your partner, a close friend or family member, a transformational life coach, or a professional therapist. Suppressed emotions are ultimately more damaging, and they can cause all sorts of physical, psychological, and relationship problems if not properly dealt with.

25. Periodically release pent-up emotions with a good cry, followed by a good hug. Do not hesitate to share with your friends and family, so they can be more sensitive to your needs.

26. Even more effective, get out of your head and into your body. Put on some music like African drumming and start dancing and moving to the music as if nobody is watching. Dancing will help you move through the tough emotions of grief and anger, tap into your inner joy, your playfulness, your aliveness, even your sensuality, and sassiness. Toddlers embody and move their strong emotions with temper tantrums, reset, and then get back to playing. Many indigenous cultures dance their emotions in community drum circles.

27. Make the practices of authentic yoga (especially gentle, prenatal, and/or restorative), meditation, breath awareness, breathwork, visualization, and yoga nidra/progressive muscle relaxation a regular part of your daily routine, even if just for 20-30 minutes each morning or evening (see the related chapters on yoga, breathwork and stress reduction for more details).

28. Check out the emWave personal stress reliever from the Institute of HeartMath for a wonderful hypnotherapy and biofeedback tool to lessen your body's reactions to stress.

29. Surrender to and embrace the cycles of life and its ups and downs and ups again, and know that day always follows night, and light always comes after darkness.

30. Take a soothing bath each night, or when stressed, enhanced with one cup of Epsom salts and a few drops of essential oil of lavender, orange or rose or a few fresh rose petals and lavender. Light a few of your favorite candles and enjoy some quiet, relaxing "me" time.

31. Sprinkle a few drops of the above essential oils on your pillow or put them in a diffuser next to your bed to promote more restful sleep and reduce irritability.

32. Make a commitment to unplug as much as possible, to reconnect with yourself, others, and the world around you … and feel so much better. For incredible insight and guidance about breaking the common modern addiction to the smartphone and computer, read *How to Break Up With Your Phone* by Catherine Price. Wear shungite or black tourmaline jewelry to mitigate EMR exposure.

33. Avoid overscheduling yourself.

34. Change work hours to avoid rush hour traffic and allow more time to get places.

35. Be clear about your priorities and rearrange your schedule to protect your own health and that of your growing baby.

36. Ask family and friends to help you with chores or childcare.

37. Treat yourself to hired help and healthy take-out meals.

38. Let go, and delegate work responsibilities that you can. You do not need to do everything.

39. Rescue an affectionate and playful dog or cat to snuggle and have fun with.

40. If you feel depressed, anxious, or are troubled by strong feelings and emotions that persist or worsen despite these suggestions, take renowned holistic, integrative psychiatrist Kelly Brogan's online course, and explore the books and courses of Dr. Joe Dispenza. They are lifesavers. There are many ways to heal emotional pain and trauma naturally and holistically, whether or not you need medication.

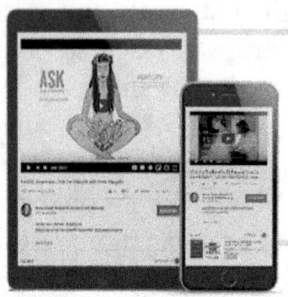

**Want to learn more or
have more questions?**

Grab your free Book Bonuses below:
https://homesweethomebirth.com/nbsbookbonus

Natural Stress Alleviation in Pregnancy and Beyond

Pregnancy can be an emotional rollercoaster, a time of increased sensitivity, and life circumstances often feel heightened. However, there are a wide variety of natural remedies and resources to help steady moods and enjoy the beautiful experience of pregnancy. The following recommendations will not only assist you with stress relief during pregnancy, but during many stages of life.

Diet and Supplements

For general health and physical and emotional wellbeing during pregnancy, make sure to eat healthy foods, stay well hydrated, and take supplements. For my specific recommendations in these areas, refer to the chapter "Nutritional Best Practices for Mom."

Vitamins and minerals that support the stress response and promote inner calm include vitamin D, calcium, and magnesium, as well as B-complex, with additional methylated B12 if your lab level is below 600. I also recommend you get screened for iron deficiency anemia, which is common in later pregnancy, as it can exacerbate your emotional symptoms and is easy to treat. Please refer to the chapter "Anemia in Pregnancy: Prevention and Treatment" for detailed information on this important topic.

Relaxation Through Mindfulness Practices

A wonderful life-changing approach to internal stress and uncomfortable or intense feelings and emotions is learning about present moment awareness, mindfulness, breathwork, and visualization, and incorporating them into your daily life. Please refer to the chapter "Meditation, Breathwork, and Visualization" to learn more about these stress-relieving practices and to find many options for practicing them.

I also encourage you to check out my yoga recommendations given in the chapter "Yoga During Pregnancy and Labor." There are many books, audio CDs, and hypnobirthing MP3s for pregnancy to help you learn these important life skills, as well as wonderful phone apps like Guided Mindfulness Meditation Series, The Mindfulness App, Headspace, Insight Timer, Breathe and Calm. Try practicing breathwork, meditation, progressive muscle relaxation, yoga nidra, or gentle prenatal or restorative yoga, Qi Gong, Tai Chi, visualization, and guided imagery on a regular basis. Locate your nearest Zen Center (Zen is NOT a religion and does not conflict with any religion) or read any book by Thich Nhat Hanh, Pema Chodron, or Shunryu Suzuki to learn the basics of meditation and Zen practice.

Conscious Relaxation

Notice habits of increased muscle tension, especially around your upper back, shoulders, neck, forehead, and jaw, and make an effort to release these tightened muscles while doing slow, deep abdominal breathing. It would be very beneficial to you if you could learn how to relax the muscles that are tensing up. It is an essential skill for labor and can be used in any stressful situation. Make a conscious effort to be aware of anxiety-provoking, tension-causing thought patterns that are not serving you, and to stop them or shift your attention to something more positive and ultimately change your mental state. You can always try to focus as much attention as possible on the present moment, literally without letting your thoughts wander into the past or imagined future (unless it's phenomenal!).

Modern life is getting more stressful. Eliminating all outside stress, especially that which we cannot control, is not an option. We can only work on changing our outlook about stressors we cannot change. This involves deep, profound, and rewarding transformation, cultivating spirituality, and an attitude of surrender and acceptance. Realize that very little in life outside of our own way of thinking, feeling, reacting and behaving is within our control, and know that everything happens for our ultimate benefit, even if it is beyond our ability to fathom. You can learn to activate your own relaxation response to stressors and quiet your nervous system with breath awareness and relaxation techniques, mastery over your thoughts and reactions to difficulties, and also by modifying what you can in your day to make it less stressful and more in alignment with your core values.

Minimize time online, especially addictive, stressful apps, social media, and computer games. Try to stay away from things and people that agitate your mind and raise your internal tension, and instead surround yourself as much as possible with calm, centered people, things, sounds, and places that inspire, relax, and restore you to inner peace and serenity. Make a conscious effort to work on increasing your own feelings of forgiveness, appreciation, love, joy, optimism, and healing while letting go of anger, resentment, envy, fear, sadness, and negativity.

Know that you are in charge of what thoughts and feelings you host, and how you react to stressful or painful situations. You have the ability to change your attitude and reaction to life experiences to more health-enhancing responses. For example, you can surrender to and totally accept unpleasant life events over which you have no power. You can also view them as potential gifts, powerful stimulus to change, a wake-up call, and an opportunity for personal growth, redirection, and spiritual practice.

We all need to be very careful about what we say to ourselves repeatedly, as thought is creative and can lead to manifesting our reality. What we say to ourselves—the good stuff and the not so good stuff—we can often make happen. Literally. Never underestimate the power of the spoken word and your inner self-talk. To learn more about rewiring your brain and reconditioning yourself to make lasting positive, transformational change in this arena, visit drjoedispenza.com.

If a thought supports, empowers, and inspires—and leads to good or uplifting feelings—let it flow. If your internal dialogue leads you to feel more stressed, anxious, unhappy, upset, not good enough, victimized, limited, or increases your suffering in any way, drop it like a hot potato.

Know you can avoid going down a slippery slope and that you have the power to turn off the spiraling record player of negativity. It takes great personal work to replace those lower vibration thoughts with higher ones that are actually more true and supportive, but regular practice will elevate your life immensely. You can turn those negative, often false, thoughts around to the opposite. Examples could be:

- I am good enough at … (instead of—I am not good enough).
- I have the strength to handle this (instead of—I have no more strength to handle this).
- I am a great mother (instead of—I am a bad mother).
- They should have done that, or that should have happened (instead of—they should not have done that, or that should not have happened because it did happen, they did do it, so it was actually meant to happen (without condoning harmful actions that were done by someone)).
- I am loved and cared about (instead of—no one loves or cares about me).
- That was just what I needed (instead of—that ruined my day).

Learning Materials

For more information about thought and emotional mastery, and other great ways to improve your overall wellbeing, read more from the variety of resources below. Make a commitment to practice and transform your life for the better. It is beyond worth it to feel your absolute best. There are amazing books about miraculous tools to remedy wounds from the past, relieve internal stress, tap into your inner power, and basically heal almost all stress-related problems of the heart, mind, and body to live a vibrant, joyful life.

Some great books include:

- *Just Breathe* by Dan Brule
- *Breathe: Strategizing Energy in the Age of Burnout* by Dr. Ela

Manga
- *Breath Love* by Lauren Chelec Cafritz
- *Breathe Deep Laugh Loudly* by Judith Kravitz
- *Conversations with the Goddesses* by Agapi Stassinopoulos
- *Pussy: A Reclamation by Regina Thomashauer*
- *You Can Heal Your Life* by Louise Hay
- *Practicing the Power of Now* by Eckhart Tolle
- *Breaking the Habit of Being Yourself: How to Lose Your Mind and Create a New One* by Dr. Joe Dispenza
- *You are the Placebo: Making Your Mind Matter* by Dr. Joe Dispenza
- *Awaken the Giant Within* by Anthony Robbins
- *From Panic to Power* by Lucinda Bassett
- *Prescriptions for Living* by Dr. Bernie Siegel
- Change Your Thoughts Change Your Life by Wayne Dyer
- *A Thousand Names for Joy* by Byron Katie
- *Question Your Thinking, Change the World* by Byron Katie
- *Loving What Is: Four Questions That Can Change Your Life* by Byron Katie
- *Lit from Within* by Victoria Moran
- *Creating a Charmed Life* by Victoria Moran
- *The Mindful Way Through Depression* by Mark Williams, John Teasdale, Zindel Segal, and Jon Kabat-Zinn
- *Full Catastrophe Living* by John Kabat-Zinn
- *Radical Acceptance* by Tara Brach
- *True Refuge* by Tara Brach
- *Accomplishing More by Doing Less* by Marc Lesser
- *The Journey: A Practical Guide to Healing Your Life and Setting Yourself Free* by Brandon Bays
- *The Healing Code* by Alex Loyd and Ben Johnson
- *The Mindbody Prescription* by Dr. John Sarno
- *Spontaneous Healing* by Dr. Andrew Weil
- *Natural Health, Natural Medicine by Dr. Andrew Weil*
- *A Mind of Your Own: The Truth About Depression and How Women Can Heal Their Bodies to Reclaim Their Lives* by Kelly Brogan MD

- *Own Your Self: The Surprising Path beyond Depression, Anxiety, and Fatigue to Reclaiming Your Authenticity, Vitality, and Freedom* by Dr.Kelly Brogan
- *The Mood Cure* by Julia Ross
- *The Chemistry of Calm* by Dr. Henry Emmons
- *The Chemistry of Joy* by Dr. Henry Emmons.

Websites

- *www.drwaynedyer.com*—for more resources from Wayne Dyer
- *www.thework.com*—for more from Byron Katie
- www.stresscenter.com—to learn about attacking anxiety and depression, a self-help, self-awareness program
- *www.behavioraltech.org*—to locate a cognitive behavioral therapist closest to you
- *www.mbct.com*—for resources and info on a proven mindfulness-based cognitive approach to feelings of chronic unhappiness and depression
- *mindfullivingprograms.com*—offers courses using the mindfulness-based stress reduction program (MBSR)
- *thejourney.com*—offers retreats and local practitioners teaching deeply awesome and extremely effective mindbody approaches to health
- *kellybroganmd.com*—for wonderful holistic and integrative psychiatric approaches to mental wellness without medication
- *mamagenas.com*—the official site for Mama Gena's School of the Womanly Arts, leader of a global movement to reclaim the feminine, helping countless women to reclaim their power, feel exquisitely comfortable within their bodies and souls, and live with radiant pleasure
- *Ibfbreathwork.org*—the international organization for conscious breathing and breathwork for optimal health and well-being; also lists local practitioners and retreat workshops that are extremely transformational and profoundly healing for thousands and thousands of people around the world.

Herbal Stress Relief

Herbs are mentioned last, as they can be used as supportive to your personal growth and self-mastery efforts; but for best results, they should not be used without those other efforts or relied upon alone. Inner peace and happiness is an inside job.

Drink red raspberry leaf, skullcap, motherwort, chamomile, lemon balm and/or lavender tea to relax yourself. Peppermint or spearmint tea will lift your spirits. You can make a lovely calming infusion, which is more effective than the ready-made teas, by mixing a pinch of each dried herb: chamomile, lavender, and lemon balm. Then add it to one cup of boiling water. Steep covered in a glass jar for 15-20 minutes, strain, add lemon, fresh mint or honey to taste, and drink.

Nettle and dandelion are common herbs recommended in pregnancy to take as a nourishing tonic, but they are also wonderful for regulating blood sugar, supporting the adrenals, improving nutrient intake, and building iron levels. In turn, this can balance your emotions and lessen mood swings and irritability.

To make an infusion:

1. Soak a handful of each dried herb in one quart of boiling water for three to four hours.
2. Strain in a glass canning jar.
3. Add lemon or lime juice, fresh mint, or honey to taste.
4. Drink one to three cups per day.

Nettle and *dandelion* can also be taken as a tincture: one dropperful each, three to four times daily.

Oatstraw works best to nourish and calm the nervous system when taken over time. You can add a generous pinch of the dried herb to the infusion above. Or, take one dropperful of the tincture of fresh creamy milky oat tops in its most potent form, one to two times daily.

Motherwort is great for occasional use after the first trimester to help restore emotional balance when feeling stressed, restless, irritable, or overwhelmed. Take 1/2-1 dropperful of the tincture; repeat if needed every 15-30 minutes for 3 hours or up to 2-3 times daily for 2-3 days.

Skullcap has a similar effect as motherwort, but more helpful to calm, and can be used regularly. Take 1/2-1 dropperful of tincture a few times per day. Both skullcap and motherwort are helpful to have on hand in labor as well as postpartum.

Passionflower is a great herb to take when feeling cranky, short-tempered, experiencing frequent changes of mood, or anxious, which is interfering with sleep. Try 1/2-1 dropperful of the tincture or two capsules of the standardized extract up to three times per day as needed.

Reishi mushrooms are a nice natural remedy for stress and anxiety. They are calming and also help with sleep. Take one to two capsules, up to three times daily.

Valerian can be taken on occasion, especially if you cannot fall asleep at night because of feeling stressed or anxious. Take two capsules of standardized extract or one dropperful of the tincture in juice to help with taste.

CBD from hemp oil—make sure it is absolutely pure, from a reputable source who can recommend proper dosing, or from pharmacies licensed to dispense it. It is usually taken as several drops under the tongue.

Bach Flower Rescue Remedy can be used in stressful situations, four to six drops, every 10-15 minutes for a few hours. Repeat as needed. There are many flower essences that are effective and safe for specific transient emotional symptoms on an energetic level, developed by Dr. Bach. If you are interested in exploring this modality, get yourself a wonderful reference like "The Encyclopedia of Bach Flower Therapy" by Mechthild Scheffer and a starter kit to use now and beyond for your growing family. *Homeopathic remedies*—you can consult with a classical homeopath or refer to an excellent homeopathy reference book for a remedy specific for your symptoms.

St. John's wort can help relieve mild to moderate depression. Take it if you are not pregnant (although if you are expecting, it may be a safer alternative than the common antidepressant prescription medications to take in consultation with your provider). Dr. Andrew Weil advises 300 mg, three times per day of an extract standardized to 0.3% hypericin. Allow at least two months for the full effect, and minimize sun exposure if you develop a photosensitivity reaction.

If you are not pregnant, take one to two 80 mg capsules of lavender oil for the occasional bout of anxiety, or try blue vervain, 1/2-1 dropperful, one to three times daily. Also take rhodiola as a tonic herb for mild depression, anxiety, and stress, 100-200 mg, twice daily. Choose an extract standardized to 2% to 3% rosavins and 0.8% to 1% salidrosides. This usually improves anxiety and sleep, but needs to be taken more regularly. Obviously stop it if it is too stimulating and worsens insomnia. You can also try ashwagandha if you feel overstressed and burned out. Dissolve one to two teaspoons of the powder in your smoothie, tea, or warm milk for 5-10 minutes, two to three times per day; or take two to three dropperfuls of the tincture twice daily and before sleep; or two to five grams of the capsules daily in divided doses. Gaia's kava kava 1-2 liquid capsules one to two times per day is excellent for calming anxiety, as long as you are not drinking alcohol or do not have any liver issues.

SAMe is another natural remedy for mild to moderate depression and/or anxiety. Dr. Andrew Weil recommends the butanedisulfonate form, in enteric-coated capsules or tablets, 400 to 1,600 mg per day on an empty stomach.

Dr. Aviva Romm is an excellent resource for herbs and natural remedies for depression and anxiety, and if you are struggling with psychological symptoms, integrative holistic psychiatrist Kelly Brogan's online course and associated resources mentioned in the previous chapter on emotions are a must.

Contact your provider if these suggestions do not help and your negative emotions are persistent and becoming too frequent or strong to cope with, especially if:

- You have a history of depression or anxiety needing prescriptive medication.
- You are having trouble functioning.
- You are eating or sleeping too much or too little.
- You have frightening thoughts.
- You experience severe oscillation of moods between wild elation and despair.
- You feel at risk for harming yourself or others.

Such severe symptoms require psychiatric evaluation and often medication to prevent or treat a more serious illness. However, try to avoid mind-altering drugs and medications (such as sedatives, tranquilizers, sleeping pills, antihistamines, and steroids) unless absolutely and medically necessary.

Do not take any herb especially long term, or medication before discussing it with your provider, as many are not approved or safe for use in pregnancy. Do not take any prescriptive anti-anxiety or anti-depressant drug unless you are really suffering and none of these suggestions help, and you are closely supervised by your psychiatrist, who is ideally an integrative holistic one who focuses on the whole you, the whole picture, and addresses root causes with more effective lifestyle medicine approaches.

Insomnia During Pregnancy: Natural Relief

Insomnia during pregnancy is often related to the other various symptoms, aches, pains, and worries commonly experienced in pregnancy. While insomnia is extremely frustrating at night, if you are managing well during the day, you are probably getting enough sleep and should not worry. Your negative moods, fatigue, poor energy, and overall absence of wellness will let you know when this lack of sleep is taking its toll. Stress reduction and maintaining internal calm are crucial for health and wellbeing—please see the chapter "Natural Stress Alleviation During Pregnancy and Beyond" for my recommendations in this area—as getting enough sleep is just as important, if not more so, than diet and exercise, so make them among your top priorities.

Please consult your integrative practitioner if this has been a chronic problem for you even before pregnancy, as you may need their support for a serious health condition that's contributing to the insomnia. Once more serious conditions have been ruled out, try the suggestions below. Also, consider seeking out a classical homeopath, acupuncturist, hypnotherapist, holistic counselor, or breathwork practitioner who can offer wonderfully effective alternatives to dealing with this problem.

Natural Insomnia Prevention

Many foods, drinks, and drugs contain stimulating substances that disturb sleep. For example, coffee, tea, chocolate, and some sodas contain caffeine, and certain cold, asthma, allergy, pain, and psychiatric medications can also keep you awake. Avoid these whenever possible, especially after 4 pm, and ask your provider about alternatives.

Avoid alcohol as well. Aside from its potentially harmful effect on your unborn baby, it may help you fall asleep initially, but can disrupt your sleep cycle, causing early or frequent waking during the night.

Four to five hours before bedtime, depending on the severity of your trouble falling or staying asleep, avoid the following:

- Large meals
- Unhealthy vegetable oils, processed, and refined foods, gluten, high fructose corn syrup, and cane sugar
- Drinking lots of fluids
- Vigorous exercise
- Stimulating or upsetting books, movies, or news reports
- Performing busy work or frustrating tasks
- Intense or stressful conversations or arguments in person, via email or text
- Electronic media.

These activities rev up your nervous system, cause inflammation and blood sugar imbalances, and make you feel tense, agitated, or excited, and, thus, interfere with sleep. You do need to stay well-hydrated by drinking plenty of pure water, but try to get most of your hydration during the daytime.

Do not go to bed hungry. Eat high-quality protein and fat at dinner, and a bedtime snack before bed like a bowl of gluten-free oatmeal with organic nut milk, avocado and an egg, apple and nut butter, or a yummy, nutrient-dense nut/seed crunch or bar.

Shorten your daytime nap to no more than 20 minutes, or awaken earlier if this is the culprit.

Engage in moderate exercise for 30 minutes, 5 days per week during the morning or afternoon. Regular aerobic activity has many health benefits, as well as helping you to feel more energized during the day and to sleep better at night.

Honor your body's circadian rhythms and maximize the time you are sleeping during the late evening hours - the most restorative part of sleep. Go to bed around the same time each day, but make sure to wind down around 8:30-9:00 pm, and fall asleep around 9:30-10:00 pm. Ideally, go to bed not much later than 10:00 or 11:00 pm and get up at a consistent time each day. Try not to sleep in more than an hour, even on weekends, to keep within your circadian rhythm. The later you go to bed, the more trouble you will have sleeping, even though you are exhausted.

Make sure you get plenty of fresh air and adequate exposure to sunlight. Weather permitting, try to spend at least 30 minutes outside with nature in the early morning or late afternoon sun each day. At night, keep lights dim. This is why people sleep better when camping, so if you need a reset, spend a week vacation camping way out in nature!

In the evening, avoid prolonged exposure to blue and artificial bright light. Block out blue light with special glasses, and if you must be online, download the free f.lux app to minimize blue light on your device. Ideally, your rooms should be lit by no more than a reading light with an amber light bulb, and amber-colored fire-like light like calming Himalayan salt lamps. During the day, get out in bright natural daytime light. If you cannot go outside, use 150- to 200-Watt incandescent bulbs or full-spectrum fluorescent lamps that supply 2,500 or more lux (equivalent to 150 to 200 Watts.) Keep the light within three feet of where you are sitting.

Minimize the time you are on the computer and smartphone, especially in the evening. Remove them from your bedroom to create an environment that is a calming haven for rest and sleep. For help breaking addiction to your smartphone, read How to Break Up With Your Phone: The 30-Day Plan to Take Back Your Life by Catherine Price. Put anti-electromagnetic radiation devices, crystals, including those made from genuine shungite or black tourmaline, in your bedroom to reduce EMF exposure. Sleep with an EMR protective blanket. Explore additional resources like on wellnessmama.com and kellybroganmd.com for more information and other practical suggestions to mitigate EMR exposure, especially in pregnancy.

If you like making lists of what you need to do or buy at the store, do your to-do lists during the day. The day is a better time to journal your feelings, or even better, move them through your body with music.

Preventing Insomnia Through Stress Reduction

Activate your own relaxation response and quiet your nervous system with breath awareness, breathwork, meditation, relaxation techniques, yoga, thought control, and cutting down on the added burdens in your life. Please visit the chapters in this book related to these practices to learn more and begin your own practice. While easier said than done, this is an important time to be clear about your priorities. If you feel overstressed, which is interfering with your ability to sleep at night and then function during the day, your body is sending you a warning signal to rearrange your schedule to protect your own health and that of your growing baby.

After you have visited the several chapters in this book related to stress reduction, breathwork, and visualization, you can incorporate some of those practices to make a regular bedtime relaxation routine. For example:

- Gentle stretching
- Yin, restorative or gentle yoga, like spending 10 minutes lying down with your legs resting up the wall
- Meditating
- Visualize yourself sleeping well and let yourself feel what that feels like
- Gentle breathing exercises
- Soaking in a very warm bath with Epsom salts and five to ten drops of your favorite essential oil for 20 minutes (you can do your meditation, visualization and breathwork in tub while staying awake but calm).
- Reading from a boring, soothing, or light drama book before bed
- Reciting a calming mantra if needed as you close your eyes
- Listening to effective audio programs that actually train your body to sleep, using sleep phones

- If noise or lights are keeping you awake, use noise-canceling headphones and an eye mask combined, and/or install blackout curtains.

You can create a regular winding down and soothing ritual at night before going to bed, combining a few calming and nurturing techniques like preparing a cup of the relaxing chamomile, lavender, or lemon balm tea, turning on some soft, tranquil music and lighting a candle while you take a warm Epsom salt bath with a few rose petals or lavender. Follow this by 5-15 minutes of various restorative yoga poses in silence, eyes covered with a lavender-infused eye pillow. Don't forget to pee just before bed. Read a little inspiration and settle into sleep. If you can't fall asleep after half an hour, read or do something relaxing and sedating until you feel sleepy. Try again in 30-60 minutes, and recite a calming mantra.

High calcium/magnesium and soothing herbs can help, which include nettle, red raspberry leaf, oat straw, and dandelion greens prepared as infusions. To make an infusion:

1. Combine a handful each of nettle, red raspberry leaf, and dandelion with a pinch of oatstraw.
2. Add mixture to one quart boiling water in a glass canning jar.
3. Cover and steep for four to eight hours.
4. Strain.
5. Add fresh lime or lemon juice, mint leaves, or a dash of honey to taste (optional).
6. Drink one to four cups daily.

Experiment with essential oils, either alone or in combination in your bath with Epsom salts, and see what will best help you sleep. Add five to ten drops of the essential oils of chamomile, vanilla, lavender, rose, geranium, frankincense, jasmine, marjoram, basil, citrus, sandalwood, and/or neroli to your evening bath, in your diffuser, and onto your pillow if needed. Soak for a while in the bath, and practice your mindfulness. Let the feel, sound, and smell of the water and essential oils ease your tension and consciously allow your muscles to release and relax.

Make sure your mattress is comfortable, you have enough pillows and blankets, the noise is at a minimum, and the light, temperature, and ventilation are adjusted to your comfort level. Use natural bedding to minimize toxic exposure that disrupts sleep. Try sleeping on earthing grounding sheets. Many have had much success with using a white noise machine, which creates soothing sounds that help promote sleep. Others like the Dream Pad Pillow or pillow speaker, or find that earplugs and an eye mask help to cut out noise and light they cannot control. Create a restful environment in your bedroom, and keep all of the things that cause you stress (like a computer, smartphone, to-do lists, unpaid bills, unfinished work or projects) in other rooms. Get a simple alarm clock without light instead of using your phone, and keep it out of your easy reach or vision while in bed. Or use a Sunrise alarm clock with sunset nightlight.

Many sleep better when the room temperature is cool (in the mid-60s degrees), and they are not hot by adjusting the thermostat, opening a window, using a cooling mattress pad topper or Chilipad. Be sure to make your bedroom as dark as possible.

Sleep Supplements

Take 500-1,000 mg of calcium and/or 500-1,000 mg of magnesium before sleep. Natural Calm is a wonderful powdered liquid magnesium as is Innate Response's or Pure Encapsulation's capsule form. It is important to understand that individual needs will vary. Some individuals will need more magnesium than others. To see what works best for you, start with 300-600 mg of the capsules or with one teaspoon daily of the Natural Calm, and increase your dose up to the point of soft stools. This will be the dose you will need to maintain for regular use. This could be taken all at once or split into two to three smaller doses throughout the day. If you get diarrhea, it is a sign that you used too high a dose, and you need to cut it back to the point where the diarrhea does not reappear, but you are relaxed and sleeping well. Also, some feel better using an equal ratio of calcium to magnesium, others do best taking double the amount of calcium than magnesium, or vice versa.

Try homeopathic Calms Forte if your symptoms are related to stress. Refer to books for a remedy specific to your unique symptoms, or consult with a classical homeopath for more personal guidance. Get a flower essence kit and look for a Bach Flower remedy that fits your particular situation, such as white chestnut if persistent unwanted thoughts or mental conflicts are preventing sleep.

Also, you can try fresh creamy milky oat tops. Take one dropperful of the tincture in its most potent form, one to two times daily. It is especially effective when taken over time.

Add a tablespoon of all-natural, organic, grass-fed gelatin collagen hydrolysate in a little applesauce or gluten-free oatmeal in the evening, or about an hour before bed.

Other herbs helpful for insomnia for occasional use only are listed below. Try each of the natural remedies for a few nights to see what is most effective. If it is going to help, its benefits should show up within a day or two (unless otherwise specified).

- If insomnia is related to feelings of internal stress and anxiety, try passionflower. You can take capsules with at least 0.8% flavonoids, as directed on the bottle, two to three times per day as needed, or one to two dropperfuls of tincture, one to two times before bed (after the first trimester).
- Motherwort—a half to one dropperful of the tincture in water or juice, no more than every two hours or up to three times per day in a period of more acute stress (after the first trimester).
- St. John's wort—one dropperful of tincture or 300-600 mg of capsules at bedtime (after the first trimester).
- Skullcap—a half of a dropperful, twice before bedtime at a 15-minute interval.
- Chamomile tincture, one to two dropperfuls before bed.
- Valerian—two capsules of standardized extract or one dropperful of the tincture in juice to help with taste, a half an hour before you go to bed.

- CBD from hemp oil—make sure it's pure and from a reputable source. It is usually taken as several drops under the tongue, every hour or so in the evening, a few hours before bed.
- Lemon Balm in doses of 300 mg early evening and before bed. This can be quite sedating, so take precautions, or try lower doses in effective combination formulas.

When not pregnant, you can try the following and see what works best for you:

- Encapsulated lavender oil—one to two 80 mg capsules, an hour before sleep, is as effective as benzodiazepine medications.
- Magnolia—200-500 mg an hour before sleep.
- Hops—if your sleeplessness is related to muscle tension or poor quality, broken, light sleep from feeling stressed, then take two capsules of freeze-dried extract of hops at bedtime or a dropperful of tincture, twice, a half an hour apart, starting an hour before bed, for a nice, deep sleep.
- Ashwagandha—if you feel burned out, overstressed, exhausted, but too wired to sleep, dissolve one to two teaspoons of the powder in your smoothie, tea, or warm milk for five to ten minutes, two to three times per day, or take two to three dropperfuls of the tincture, twice daily and before sleep, or two to five grams of the capsules daily in divided doses.
- Rhodiola—as a tonic herb, take 100-200 mg twice daily (an extract standardized to 2% to 3% rosavins and 0.8% to 1% salidrosides). This usually improves anxiety and sleep, but needs to be taken more regularly. Obviously stop it if it is too stimulating and worsens insomnia.
- Reishi mushrooms—take one gram (two capsules) an hour before bed.
- Kava kava—a few drops or up to a dropperful of the tincture or 150-450 mg of the capsules before bed can be taken for occasional short-term use only. Do not use if you are taking any substance including alcohol or medications that affect the liver or if you have any liver issues.

- California poppy—also for periodic use only, take one to two dropperfuls of the tincture before bed.
- Melatonin—best for jet lag and after working the nightshift. Take under the tongue before bedtime starting at 2.5 mg and increasing up to 6 mg if needed, lozenges or liquid.
-

Another helpful approach is using natural amino acid supplements:

- 5-HTP (hydroxytryptophan)—50-150 mg, before going to sleep, or up to 100-300 mg, two to three times daily if anxious.
- L-theanine—100-200 mg, twice daily, at lunch and bedtime is also very calming.
- GABA—up to 500-700 mg, depending on how much you need to get to sleep.
- Glycine (Glysom)—it comes in a nice three-gram powdered stick that dissolves in water and tastes good that is helpful for maintaining deep, restorative sleep.

Pure Encapsulations makes a nice, effective herbal-and-amino-acid combination sleep supplement called Best-Rest Formula, which you can take as directed.

For more information on using amino acids and increasing them naturally in your diet, read *The Mood Cure* by Julia Ross. Also read *The Chemistry of Calm* and *The Chemistry of Joy* by Dr. Henry Emmons for more detailed and thorough information on the supplements, as well as wonderful suggestions for what really is most effective in the long term: self-relaxation and visualization exercises to deal with stress and quieting the mind, and for finding a stronger sense of long-lasting, true happiness.

During Times of Insomnia

When sleeplessness strikes, don't worry or fight it. Instead, try forcing yourself to stay awake with your eyes open and simply lie there and rest. You may suddenly find yourself waking up in the morning. If you are still up after 30 minutes, turn the light on and read, do a crossword puzzle, listen to soothing music, a podcast, or a radio talk show, fold laundry, or do some other repetitive, sedating chore, and then try again only when you start to feel sleepy.

To break an insomnia pattern, set a time one to two hours after your usual bedtime and force yourself not to go to bed until then. You'll probably worry more about how to stay awake that long than about your inability to fall asleep, and you'll be tired the next day, which should help you fall asleep easier the following night. Each night, move your "later bedtime" 15 minutes earlier until you've forgotten about your insomnia altogether.

If you are having difficulty stopping all the worrisome and anxiety-provoking thoughts, write them down with an action plan to deal with them in the morning. Now is the time to get out of your mind and focus on your breathing, practice your muscle relaxation techniques, visualization exercises, or meditation, and use your skills of self-mastery.

Ideally, it is best to avoid sleeping pills on a regular basis, as some can have negative side effects for you and your baby, and they can lead to addiction. Please let your practitioner know if none of the suggestions mentioned above helps and you are suffering and at your wit's end.

DIZZINESS DURING PREGNANCY

O ccasional feelings of lightheadedness or being about to faint without actually fainting is most often related to the pooling of blood in the lower body from circulatory changes but can also be caused by:

- Pressure of the enlarging uterus on maternal blood vessels
- Warm or overcrowded environments, especially if you are overdressed
- Exposure to toxic agents, including some medications
- Poor diet and eating habits
- Low blood sugar
- Not enough water
- Anemia
- Hyperventilation
- Sunstroke
- Eye strain
- Anxiety.

How to Avoid Dizziness During Pregnancy

Some amount of dizziness during pregnancy may be unavoidable, but following the suggestions below will likely reduce the frequency and intensity. Try to note any patterns that provoke your dizziness so that you can implement preventative measures.

Positional Dizziness

Avoid sudden positional changes by making gradual adjustments. Avoid prolonged periods of standing by taking periodic rest breaks. Prolonged periods of sitting (for example, at work or during travel) should be interrupted by getting up every few hours to stretch and do some moderate form of exercise like marching in place or taking a brisk walk wherever possible.

In later pregnancy, if you feel lightheaded while flat on your back, stick to side-lying positions.

Nutritional Dizziness

Going too long without quality food or drink can cause a person to feel lightheaded, but it's best not to overstuff yourself either. Eat smaller, more frequent meals and light snacks with quality protein and healthy fat. Drink lots of clean water. Follow my suggestions on what to eat and drink in pregnancy as given in the chapter "Nutritional Best Practices for Mom."

Make sure you are taking whole-food prenatal vitamin and mineral supplements, and herbal iron as advised if your iron levels are low. Both of these important topics are addressed in the chapters "Nutritional Best Practices for Mom" and "Anemia in Pregnancy: Prevention and Treatment."

Avoid caffeine, sweetened drinks, and heavily-processed foods, especially those with lots of sugar and/or refined white flours. Although they can give you a quick "fix," a quick drop in blood sugar usually follows, resulting in more dizziness. Processed foods that contain certain additives and chemicals, like MSG, also cause dizziness in sensitive individuals.

Medications

Avoid medicating yourself without first consulting your healthcare provider. Many medications–even those sold over the counter–have a side effect of dizziness.

When Dizziness Occurs

Dizziness during pregnancy most commonly occurs:

- After eating a large meal
- After a long interval without food, drink, or rest
- When eating white flour, refined sugar foods, or fruit without a protein and/or fat
- When feeling overheated
- Upon quickly rising from a sitting or lying position.

Warm, stuffy, or crowded places can cause the sensation of dizziness in pregnancy. If you find yourself in such situations, loosen or remove a layer of clothing and/or get some fresh air and sun by going outside or sitting near an open window. Wearing support stockings may also help.

Try to increase circulation to your head by lying down with your feet elevated. Do this by assuming the yoga position *viparita karani* or "legs up the wall," a wide child's pose, or do any yoga inversion with your head lower than your heart. Modify your exercise or yoga practice as needed, and get out of poses slowly and with care.

If you are at work, try sitting or kneeling down with your head between your knees until the dizziness passes. Splash some cold water on your face and, if available, rub some oil of peppermint, orange, citrus blend, or lavender under your nose, so you can breathe in the strong, refreshing smell. Cup your hands over your nose and mouth for a few minutes as you take some slow deep breaths.

Practice breathwork regularly. Please consult the chapter "Meditation, Breathwork, and Visualization" for some effective breathwork practices. While doing deep abdominal breathing, send breath and its healing energy up to your head when you exhale. Stay very calm, present, and mindfully focus on all the details of your sensations without a mental story about them, without resisting and fighting with what is, which makes it worse. Practice consciously embracing and even intensifying the sensations, which actually helps alleviate them. See this as an opportunity to train yourself to surrender and relax with discomfort. It is great practice for labor and life.

Please call your healthcare provider if you actually pass out, if your dizziness is severe, frequent, or not responsive to these suggestions, or if you feel like the room is spinning or moving. After other more serious conditions are ruled out, consider consulting a professional homeopath for a safe, natural remedy specific to your symptoms.

HEARTBURN AND INDIGESTION IN PREGNANCY

Heartburn and indigestion in pregnancy are caused by hormones slowing digestion and the pressure on your stomach by the growing fetus. Many pregnant mamas suffer from it. Rest assured there are plenty of holistic ways to try to prevent it and to provide relief if it occurs. Go through the list below and see what works best for you.

Strategies for Heartburn Prevention

Eat six or more small meals, rather than three large ones, each day. Eat slowly, mindfully, and chew everything well, ideally while sitting down, relaxed, and free of internal tension. Try to remain upright or walk around and be active afterwards to aid digestion.

Avoid wearing tight, constrictive clothing, bending over forward, lying flat, or going to sleep during the first two to three hours after eating a meal. Squat down instead of forward bending if you need to pick up something from the ground. Maintain a good straight posture when sitting or standing.

Sleep propped up with extra pillows to slightly elevate your upper body or sleep on your left side.

Avoid foods and other substances that trigger discomfort, such as those that are:

- Highly processed with chemicals
- Loaded with sugar and white flour

- Made with refined vegetable oils and partially hydrogenated fat
- Cow dairy
- Hot or very spicy dishes
- Coffee (even decaffeinated) and other forms of caffeine
- Alcohol
- Cigarettes
- Certain medications like aspirin and nonsteroidal anti-inflammatory drugs like ibuprofen.

Eat quality real foods that are minimally processed as given in the chapter "Nutritional Best Practices for Mom." Bland, pure and simple, minimally-processed, whole, fresh foods are usually better tolerated and much better for your health. Use only healthy fat for cooking and baking, such as organic, cold, expeller pressed extra virgin olive oil, coconut oil, or clarified butter(ghee)—goat is best.

Drink at least half of your body weight in ounces of pure water daily. This is essential, as the water raises the gastric pH, which provides relief from the pain of the stomach acid. You can add a slice of fresh fruit or mint leaves to taste.

Take a good, all-natural, whole-food-based prenatal vitamin and mineral supplements. See the chapter "Nutritional Best Practices for Mom" for my recommendations.

Before bed and periodically throughout the day, take a break to disengage your consciousness from thought and routine activity in order to center and calm yourself. Unplug from your smart phone and computer. Try simply focusing your attention on your breathing, practicing breathwork exercises, meditation, progressive muscle relaxation, yoga nidra, or gentle prenatal or restorative yoga. The chapters "Yoga During Pregnancy" and "Meditation, Breathwork, and Visualization" describe a variety of these practices that you would benefit from.

When Heartburn Occurs

If heartburn occurs, some women find relief using the "flying exercise": Sit crossed-legged or tailor style, and raise and lower your arms quickly, joining the back of your hands over your head.

Drink lots of chamomile tea and alternate with peppermint tea to see which helps more with relieving your symptoms. You can make your own chamomile or peppermint tea in a glass canning jar by steeping a tablespoon of chamomile blossoms or seven to ten whole fresh peppermint leaves in a covered cup of boiling water for 15-20 minutes. Strain and add a dash of lemon juice or honey to taste.

Try ginger tea a few times per day. You can make your own by steeping a half to one teaspoon of fresh grated ginger in a cup of boiling water for 10-15 minutes. Strain and add honey to taste.

Chew thoroughly 10-15 raw almonds and then swallow.

Drink lots of pure coconut water, which is alkaline and neutralizes acid.

Mix one to two tablespoons of raw, unpasteurized apple cider vinegar in a small glass of water, add raw honey to taste, sip throughout the day, and drink before meals.

Eat a grapefruit or drink a small glass of grapefruit juice after each meal.

Chew a healthy all-natural gum for 10 minutes after each meal.

Squeeze the juice of 1-2 lemons in a glass of water with 1-1.5 crushed fennel seeds. Add honey to taste. Boil as a tea or drink cool, a few cups per day. Bake fennel seeds and eat 1/4 of a teaspoon of them three times per day.

Try papaya enzyme chewable tablets after meals or fresh papaya fruit or juice.

You can also try slippery elm lozenges or powder, which is wonderful for relieving heartburn, as it soothes the irritated tissues of the intestinal tract. You can suck on three to four lozenges up to three times a day. It also comes in tea form, which you can drink as often as needed. To make your own tea, dissolve one teaspoon of the powdered herb into one cup of boiling water or pure almond milk. If you'd like, add a dash of honey to taste.

Take two capsules of marshmallow root up to four times per day. You can also make your own tea by dissolving one tablespoon of the powder in a cup of boiling water, then covering and steeping it for 15-20 minutes. Drink a few cups daily.

Dandelion is also a great herb for indigestion, which can be taken in doses of one dropperful of the tincture, up to four times daily or when you have heartburn. You can make your own herbal infusion-like tea. Add approximately five tablespoons of the dried root or about ten tablespoons of the fresh root to one quart of boiling water. Let it brew for three to four hours, strain into a glass canning jar, and periodically sip, totaling up to two cups per day.

Take one to two plant-based digestive enzymes after each meal.

Another helpful remedy is kudzu tea. To make, stir two teaspoons of kudzu root in 1/4 cup of cold water for a few minutes until it dissolves. Add one cup of boiling water. For a savory tea, add an all-natural bouillon cube or add kudzu to an organic miso soup broth. For a sweet tea, simply add a dash of honey.

Its considered safe to take chewable calcium carbonate known in drug stores as Tums (get their the one without chemicals or dyes), but no more than 2000 mg in 24 hours. I prefer Solgar's or other similar all natural Chewable Calcium Wafers, 500 mg. Avoid antacids with high sodium or phosphorus, such as Rolaids, Alka Seltzer, sodium bicarbonate, and those with aluminum or magnesium by themselves.

Activated charcoal can be taken in moderation for a severe case of heartburn, at least 90 minutes before meals and before taking your prenatal vitamins and supplements. You can take two tablets, and repeat only if needed and if nothing else is working. Do not worry that it discolors your tongue and makes your stool black, but stop if you feel side effects like nausea, vomiting, stomach pain, and constipation.

Take a homeopathic remedy specific for your symptoms of heartburn and indigestion. You can consult with a classical homeopath or a solid homeopathic reference book. Common remedies include Kali Mur, Nux Vomica, or Pulsatilla. Or, try Weleeda's Coleodorin, seven to ten drops, four times per day as needed, and Triplex tea. Osteopathy, chiropractic care, and acupuncture are also helpful especially for stubborn cases.

If the above remedies do not help, Mylanta, Maalox, or Riopan are okay if used only on RARE OCCASIONS and as directed. Frequent or prolonged use can cause serious electrolyte imbalances, interfere with the digestion of food and the absorption of important nutrients, such as iron, contribute to kidney stone formation, and actually cause the stomach to produce even more acid than before. Stay away from acid-blocking proton pump inhibitor medications, as they wreak havoc on your health.

If you are NOT pregnant, you can take deglycyrrhizinated licorice DGL extract (slowly chew two tablets or take half of a teaspoon of the powder in a little water before or between meals and before bedtime). Or, try Iberogast, an herbal combo with licorice, peppermint, and other herbs proven and safe to relieve heartburn and epigastric pain.

For Gas and Bloating

- Walk, move side to side while lying down, pelvic rock while in knee chest position or do a modified yoga inversion.
- Eat your foods slowly, chew thoroughly and mindfully, ideally while sitting down instead of rushing and eating on the run.
- Chew fennel seeds, drink fennel tea, or take 2-4 ml of the tincture, three times per day.

- Take a high-quality multi-species probiotic, twice daily on an empty stomach.
- Drink kefir and kombucha. Learn how to make your own.
- Take slippery elm as explained above.
- Take one to two plant-based digestive enzymes with meals.
- Limit foods that make you gassy. Common culprits are gluten-containing foods like wheat, spelt, rye, barley, and some oats, some fresh fruits and veggies, cow dairy if your are lactose intolerant, beans, carbonated liquids, and chewing gum.

You may need to experiment with cutting out a particular food, one category at a time, for a week or two, to see if your symptoms resolve. Then reintroduce the food to see if your symptoms recur. This allows you to pin down the culprit and not eliminate numerous healthy foods without definitive proof they are making you gassy.

For those with any sort of chronic heartburn or indigestion in which serious causes have been ruled out and none of the natural and allopathic remedies help, consult your healthcare provider.

LEG CRAMPS IN PREGNANCY

L eg cramps during pregnancy are quite common. They're usually felt as a sudden, painful contraction or spasm of the leg muscles, and often occur at night or early in the morning. They may also be associated with a sense of uncomfortable restlessness in your legs. Leg cramps are thought to be caused by:

- A diet too low in calcium and/or magnesium
- A diet too high in phosphorus
- Compression of nerves or impaired circulation to the area from the growing uterus
- Inadequate fluids and salt intake
- Iron deficiency
- Muscle fatigue from too much strenuous activity
- Sedentary living without adequate exercise.

Dietary Considerations for Leg Cramps During Pregnancy

Leg cramps during pregnancy are often caused by dietary factors. Make sure you are drinking plenty of pure water. My hydration recommendations are in the chapter "Nutritional Best Practices for Mom." Anemia due to lack of iron is very common in pregnancy and should perhaps be your first consideration. Please review the chapter "Anemia in Pregnancy—Prevention and Treatment" to learn more.

Calcium

Make sure your diet contains at least 1,200 mg of calcium every day. The best calcium-rich food sources include:

- Dairy products (organic, fresh, raw goat or sheep is ideal)
- Clean-water fresh fish
- Fresh dark green leafy vegetables (but not spinach)
- Ground sesame seeds (tahini)
- Blackstrap molasses
- Dried fruit (like dates, figs, raisins, and prunes)
- Nuts and pure nut butters
- Bone broth.

Certain herbs can also help as they supply a rich source of calcium and many other nutrients in a highly absorbable form. To make an infusion:

1. Combine one ounce each of nettle and red raspberry leaf in one quart of boiling water. Cover.
2. Soak them in a glass canning jar for four to eight hours, and then strain.
3. Optional: add fresh lime or lemon juice, mint leaves, or a dash of honey to taste.
4. Drink one to four cups daily.

For an additional nutritional boost, mix in one ounce of dried dandelion and half an ounce of alfalfa and/or oatstraw.

When making soup stock from bones, add two tablespoons of apple cider vinegar during the boiling process. This releases the calcium out of the bones and, thus, makes a broth rich in absorbable calcium.

Avoid alcohol, caffeine, chocolate, and an EXCESS amount of salt and protein foods that interfere with the absorption of calcium or increase the amount of calcium excreted in the urine. You need NOT LIMIT salt or protein as these are essential in pregnancy–just modify your intake if it's grossly excessive and use sea or earth salt to taste.

If you cannot consume a sufficient amount of calcium by diet alone, consider a calcium supplement like 500 mg of calcium citrate, once or twice a day with meals, to enhance absorption. The amount you need to take depends on the amount that is missing from your diet.

If you take a calcium supplement, you should also supplement with equivalent amounts of magnesium, which happens to be calming and helps with other common discomforts of pregnancy like insomnia and constipation. If you experience excessively loose bowel movements, you can cut the magnesium to half the calcium dose.

Also, reduce your phosphorus intake by reading labels and avoiding highly processed foods (like sodas, party snacks, and lunch meats) that contain phosphates.

Try eating raw foods high in vitamin E, such as cold-pressed oils, whole grains, nuts (especially almonds), and seeds (especially sunflower). You may need to supplement with up to 200 IU per day as long as you are otherwise healthy and your blood pressure is normal.

Eat foods high in vitamin C, which include raw fruits and veggies, especially green leafy vegetables, such as kale and collard greens, strawberries, citrus fruits, peppers, tomatoes, and alfalfa sprouts. Herbal sources include nettle, dandelion, rose hips, watercress, red clover, and burdock. You can supplement vitamin C with up to 1,000 mg, twice a day until 36 weeks gestation, then decrease to 500 mg per day.

Posture and Movement

Regular moderate exercise and prenatal yoga help prevent leg cramps, as well as periodic leg elevations and stretching.

Maintain a good straight posture using proper body mechanics during daily activities, such as carrying, pushing, pulling, or reaching for something. This involves engaging your abdomen (corset your ribs inward, bring your front pelvic bone toward your breast bone, your belly towards your spine), and using your leg and arm muscles instead of your back.

Refrain from prolonged sitting or standing by periodically taking a break to exercise your legs.

Avoid completely extending your foot while pointing your toe, as this can trigger a leg cramp. Make sure your foot is dorsiflexed while extended, especially during leg stretching and exercise, and make your bed loosely so your toes are not pressed down by the sheets.

Keep your legs warm with knee socks or leg warmers, especially during exercise and at night during sleep. Support stockings may help in the day.

For Immediate Relief of Leg Cramps During Pregnancy

Take a deep diaphragmatic breath by inhaling deep into your belly, expanding your ribs and chest, and really stretch the inhale to your fullest capacity. Then take a huge automatic sigh of relief on the exhale while consciously relaxing all tension. Keep up the deep breathing, and release more with each exhalation. Send breath and its healing energy to your leg cramps when you exhale. Stay very calm, present, and mindfully focus on all the details of your sensations without a mental story about them, without resisting and fighting with what is, which makes it worse. Practice consciously embracing and even intensifying the cramping, which actually helps alleviate it. See this as an opportunity to train yourself to surrender and relax with intense discomfort. It is a great skill to master for labor and life.

Also, try sitting while straightening your leg and actively flexing your toes back towards your head, using your hands or a yoga strap to help you flex your feet. This is not about bending forward and touching your head to your legs or resting it on a yoga block between them although if you already have a practice it feels nice and calming. It may help to exert steady pressure against your bed board or partner's hand, or to simply stand up with your foot flat on the floor or flexed up towards your body.

If the cramp is in your foot, roll it over a roller, baseball bat, or unbreakable bottle three inches in diameter. Some say standing on ice is effective.

Deeply massage your lower legs and feet with arnica oil, mixed with a few drops of chamomile, ginger, lemon balm, St. John's wort, and/or lavender.

Other Healing Modalities

Herbal Epsom salt foot baths—soak your lower legs in very warm water with one cup of Epsom salts, and add a few drops of wintergreen, lavender, camphor, and/or chamomile essential oils.

Heat—apply a heating pad or hot wet compress, infused with a few drops of the above mentioned essential oils, to the area of cramping.

Homeopathy—take homeopathic magnesia phosphorica alternating frequently with calcarea phosphorica several times a day until you feel relief. Consult a homeopathic reference book or a professional homeopath who can prescribe a remedy specific to your individual symptoms.

Herbs—black haw or crampbark can be taken to decrease leg cramps. Take a dropperful of either tincture as needed, up to four times daily. Herbal teas and tincture combinations that include ginger, catnip, chamomile, lemon balm, and skullcap, taken as directed on the bottle, can also help.

Acupuncture can work wonders. Consult an experienced acupuncturist.

Avoid commercial medications like muscle relaxants and quinine as they are not safe during pregnancy.

When Nothing Helps

Consult your healthcare practitioner if your leg cramps are extreme or persist in spite of following the above guidelines, if your cramps become increasingly severe or frequent, or if you notice an area of leg warmth, redness, swelling, and/or pain. Sometimes other metabolic imbalances can be the culprit, and these may need to be investigated.

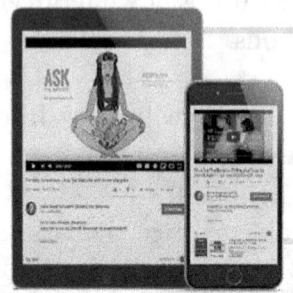

Want to learn more or have more questions?

Grab your free Book Bonuses below:
https://homesweethomebirth.com/nbsbookbonus

Pain During Pregnancy: Pelvic Area, Groin, Legs, and Back

Experiencing pain is humbling, and it can be a chance for personal growth. It can be an opportunity to practice techniques that will help with labor, birth, and life beyond. Pain provides a chance to learn patience, acceptance of normal bodily changes associated with pregnancy, and how to prioritize, delegate, let go of activities that create increased stress, and allow others to help. Pain can also be viewed as an opportunity for you to honor, listen to, and find meaning and beneficial purpose to the wise messages of your body. While I advise a variety of remedies to help you feel more comfortable, relief actually begins with relaxing into intense sensations, surrendering, being with, and befriending them.

For pregnancy-related aches and pains in the groin, back, or legs, it is recommended that you consult a reputable chiropractor or osteopath who can successfully relieve strained muscles and correct a spine or pelvis that is out of alignment. Other helpful professionals include a massage therapist (especially deep tissue, shiatsu, rolfing, and Thai) who can do wonders to release tightened, painful, or aching muscles in spasm, a homeopath who can suggest a safe, natural remedy to effectively treat your specific symptoms, or an acupuncturist skilled at directing needles on the trigger points and releasing blocked chi. Therapeutic yoga can be helpful to reduce tension and increase the strength and flexibility of the responsible muscles. Practice your mindfulness, visualization, and breathwork, and consciously send breath to areas of need.

Pain in the Groin

Sharp but short-lived pain in the groin area that can sometimes travel down into the legs is either related to the stretching of the round ligaments that hold and support your growing uterus within your abdomen, or to the pressure of the uterus or baby on local nerves. This sort of pain usually occurs while walking or moving, and can be enough to stop you in your tracks.

For relief from round ligament pain, stop to rest, bend your knees onto your abdomen while lying down, or get on your hands and knees and rock your pelvis inward and outward. Take a very warm bath with Epsom salts and a few drops of lavender or Olbas herbal combination, followed by applying Tiger Balm, then a hot or cold pack or heating pad.

To minimize strain on these ligaments:

- Take frequent breaks.
- Use full body or pregnancy pillows under your uterus and between your legs when lying down on your side.
- Roll on your side, transition through your hands and knees to use your arm, leg, and core muscles when getting up from a supine position.
- Apply gentle pressure to the area when laughing, coughing, or sneezing.
- Consider wearing a maternity support garment, like Bellefit's prenatal support wear: https://www.bellefit.com/a/12/. Use code ANNE20 to receive $20 off at checkout.
- Practice your Kegel tightening (those you use to stop the flow of urine) or even more comprehensive and effective, yoga mula bandha or root lock exercises, daily to strengthen your pelvic floor muscles that help support your uterus. Get out your yoga mat and do a modified bridge pose, supporting your sacrum on a yoga block. In this position, it is easy to practice your mula bandha by placing another yoga block between your thighs. While inhaling, tilt your pelvis up toward the direction of your face as you slowly squeeze the block and draw your entire

pelvic floor upward and inward, starting from its center. Hold it as long as is comfortable, then release and return to resting your sacrum on the block as you exhale. Let the breathing be smooth, relaxed, and deep as you do this. It takes practice, but you will get it. Start with 25 twice per day, and work up to 50 twice per day. Once you get the hang of it, you can do it in many positions, anywhere, anytime. You will also notice other benefits like easier birthing, reduced tearing, less urinary incontinence, better sex, improved exercise performance and yoga practice, and if done on a deeper level, enhanced overall wellbeing.

Sciatica Pain

Sciatica pain is caused by the pressure of the enlarging uterus or baby on nerves that pass through the lower spine into the legs. This pain can travel from the back or thigh all the way down to the feet or toes. It can be severe and associated with other strange sensations like tingling or numbness.

Back Pain

A high backache in pregnancy is related to breast enlargement and heaviness, which may produce strain in compensating back muscles, especially if your breasts are not well supported. Wear a well-fitting, comfortable, and supportive wire-free maternity bra that lifts your breasts upward and inward. Do shoulder rolls and arm exercises that tighten and release your upper back muscles, and get a regular back massage. Slouching over computers and cell phones make it worse, so minimize them and straighten your posture, as explained below. A wonderful restorative yoga heart opener that can provide relief involves lying down with a tightly-rolled yoga blanket or block lifting your thoracic spine just under your breast bone, and resting your head on another block or blanket, with your arms open like a "T" out to the sides.

Aches and pains in the lower back are related to several factors:

- Pressure on the nerves from your growing uterus or baby
- Stretching of the ligaments that connect the sides of the enlarging uterus to the lower back
- Hormonal relaxation and increased mobility of your joints, especially in the pelvis
- The shift in the center of gravity from your expanding belly, which leads your pelvis to tilt forward and your back to arch, straining the back muscles

The problem is made worse by excessive weight gain, prolonged walking or standing, frequent bending or lifting with poor posture and improper body mechanics, ill-fitting or high-heeled shoes, weak or separated abdominal muscles, or weak back muscles. Wear Bellefit's prenatal support wear or try Baby Hugger for more extensive support. They provide wonderful relief of lower abdominal pressure and an aching back from weak or stretched abdominal muscles after several pregnancies. It is also helpful for diastasis recti.

Diastasis recti can sometimes cause back pain. This is a normal physiologic separation of the rectus abdominis abdominal muscles that takes place during pregnancy for most women. More significantly, it can impact pregnancies as lax abdominal muscles do a poor job of supporting the uterus. Sometimes this causes the baby to take on a suboptimal position. The effort made to correct it postpartum is mostly cosmetic as there are rarely any major medical issues associated with mild separation, especially when the separation is less than three finger-widths. You can certainly do yoga and can learn corrective exercises to strengthen these muscles as well as bring them together. A wonderful resource for this is nurse and personal trainer Julie Tupler, of diastasisrehab.com.

General Suggestions

Watch your weight gain. Remember, under normal circumstances, you only need to gain three to six pounds during the first trimester and a half to one pound per week thereafter, for a grand total of 25-35 pounds.

You also need sufficient vitamins C, D, E, and B complex easily absorbed from a well-balanced whole-food diet, excellent hydration, as well as natural prenatal supplements to provide needed nourishment not obtained by food alone (see the chapter on nutrition for more details). If you have inflammation, especially if your pain is more chronic, you may benefit from an anti-inflammatory diet and supplements adapted for pregnancy. Load up on the tumeric in your cooking! Practice yoga postures modified for pregnancy and aimed specifically to help with the specific location of your pain. Good examples are spinal twists, hamstring stretches, and hip openers for sciatica; or down dog, forward bends, cat/cow, puppy, bridge, plank, triangle, sphinx, cobra, thread the needle, and spinal twists to stretch and strengthen your lower back.

Better Body Mechanics for Pain Reduction

Know your pregnant body's limits and pay attention to what your symptoms are telling you. Take frequent breaks or rest periods if you need to be on your feet for prolonged periods of time. Cut down on nonessential burdens in your life and be clear about your priorities. It is okay to say no or to leave the housework, piles of papers, and long to-do list for tomorrow, or better—let most of it go, and delegate it to someone else. Don't be afraid to ask family or friends to help with chores or childcare, or treat yourself to hired help and healthy take-out meals.

Avoid fatigue by making sure you are getting extra needed sleep by going to bed earlier, sleeping later, or taking naps. Rest on a firm, supportive mattress or use a bed board, and sleep with pillows positioned to straighten your back and alleviate strain or pulling. Some women find the floor or a futon helpful. Use full-body or pregnancy pillows for additional support.

Pay deliberate attention to your posture, especially when standing or walking, by lifting your abdomen up and in (bringing your pelvic bone towards your breastbone and using your muscles to corset your ribs inward), tucking your pelvis slightly up and in to minimize the arch in your lower back, and relaxing your shoulders down. Even when sitting, take care not to slump by using your abdominal muscles to lift up and keep your back straight. Sit on harder, more supportive chairs. Even better, ditch chairs and squat with your pelvis supported on a yoga block or your heels supported by a wedged yoga blanket. Use an ergonomic work station or standing desk, resting alternate feet on a foot stool while standing for extra relief on your back muscles. The foot stool will also come in handy during labor and life as a mom.

Walk barefoot while home, and wear supportive, well-fitting, comfortable flat or rocker bottom shoes when out. Save the high heels until after the baby.

Avoid heavy lifting. Spread out grocery store purchases into several bags and take more trips, carrying a lighter load instead of a heavier one all at once. Better yet, ask for help.

Watch your body mechanics by using your stronger stomach, arm, and leg muscles—not your weaker back—to lift, pull, or push something. Instead of bending at the waist or lifting abruptly, bend at the knees with a broad base and lift carefully. Instead of reaching for an object, come closer to it. Turn and twist more slowly and with caution. If a particular action feels even a bit uncomfortable, STOP!

Take extra precautions during activities requiring balance and walking on wet, icy, or slippery surfaces. Remember, your sense of balance has changed, your gait is more awkward, and you have an increased tendency to fall. Use a non-skid floor mat in the bath and shower.

If you cannot tolerate your usual exercise routine, do regular but more gentle exercise. Take a prenatal dance class, gentle yoga, or a pregnancy exercise class. A good instructor can help you maintain proper posture and teach you how to strengthen your abdominal, back, and extremity muscles. Swimming is another option, as it allows you to get great exercise without any weight on your back.

Put on a maternity support garment like Bellefit before you start each day, especially if you were out of shape before the pregnancy or have poor abdominal muscle tone after several children, if you are overweight, carrying a big baby or twins, or on your feet a lot. Many specialty stores stock lightweight maternity girdles with soft elastic fronts and an adjustable belt if you are looking for alternatives.

Stress Reduction for Pain Reduction

Emotions greatly influence nerve and muscle interaction. Try to put yourself in a more positive, joyful, and calm state by reading uplifting books, watching movies, listening to podcasts that inspire you or make you laugh, and spending time with those who bring out your finest moods.

Stress leads to increased muscle tension and pain. Although easier said than done, limit your stress and inner tension, and increase feelings of calm by following some form of the practices I suggest in the chapters on "Breathwork, Meditation, and Visualization" and "Natural Stress Alleviation in Pregnancy and Beyond." When breathing deeply and mindfully, and all is otherwise healthy and well, practice embracing, relaxing into, and even magnifying intense sensations without the mental story about them.

Can you make friends with discomfort and pain, instead of trying to escape, numb, or fight it? Is there something that they can teach you? Get curious about all of their details, including the borders or edges, and parts of you that feel good or do not have unpleasant sensations. In a meditative state, dare to visualize yourself vibrantly healthy without any pain, and really feel the emotions of relief, gratitude, freedom, and joy that would result, with the enthusiasm of a child. Yes, there are remedies to help alleviate pain. But you will be amazed at how effective these practices are and how much they will help you to better cope with childbirth, as well as with the pain that is an inevitable part of being human. It is the suffering from the pain that is optional, so you can choose not to suffer.

Home Remedies

When your back hurts, allow time to rest and get into a position that eases the pain. Some women find stretching or pelvic rocking helpful. Take slow, deep breaths in through your nose and out through your mouth, and focus on releasing your tense muscles head to toe. Most often, pain from muscle spasms heals with rest, excellent self-care, and time.

One of the most pleasant ways to relieve backache is to massage the painful area with arnica oil, mixed with a dropperful each of St. John's wort topical oil, cramp bark, and lobelia tinctures. Massage the mixture lovingly into your deep muscle, ligament, and joint aches and strains. Try any of the following and regularly use what works best for you: essential oils of ginger, juniper, cinnamon, lavender, marjoram, chamomile, lemon balm/melissa, wintergreen, spearmint, or rosemary. It can be diluted within it, alone, or in combination. You can also apply comfrey ointment, rubs of Tiger Balm, or Olbas herbal combination. Chinese herbal zheng gu shui can also help or any product that contains these soothing herbs.

After the massage, apply locally a hot or cold pack, heating pad, hot water bottle, herbal-infused hot or cold pack, or try moist heat using a hot damp towel or packs from a hydrocollator (what the professional chiropractors, massage therapists, and physical therapists use). Take a hot shower or soak in a very warm Epsom salts bath for half an hour with a few drops of any of the above essential oils or add a wonderful Swiss Olbas herbal combination.

Some find that ice packs or cool compresses help to relieve the pain, especially during the first 24 hours after an injury. For acute spasm and inflammation of your back muscles, apply an ice pack off and on for the first 12 to 24 hours. Once the pain begins to subside, apply moist heat. Complete rest in positions that feel best is essential for the first one to two days. Sometimes the only tolerable position is lying flat on your back on the floor with your buttocks up against a bed or chair and your legs raised at a right angle with your calves resting on the mattress or seat, or lying flat on your yoga mat in legs up the wall, viparita karini, position. Props like yoga blankets, bolsters, or blocks make postures more accessible, passive, comfortable, and restorative. In this case, use them to support your lower back and head, and elevate your hips. Let your legs rest straight up the wall for 10-20 minutes. It is also a great opportunity for practicing quiet meditation and focusing on slow, deep breathing and inner gazing between your eyebrows. A lavender-infused eye pillow adds to the yummy relaxation effect.

Use a TENS unit, which relieves back pain of pregnancy and can also help in labor.

Take a dropperful of cramp bark tincture every hour over four hours and then two to four times per day for no more than a one to two weeks, and one to two dropperfuls each of St. John's wort and skullcap tinctures, one to three times daily for several weeks. You can also take ginger to reduce inflammation and pain, 500-1,000 mg, once or twice per day until you feel better. Place four to five pellets of homeopathic arnica 30c under your tongue every hour while awake, every few hours the next day, then three to four times per day for a week. Discontinue topical BenGay or Tiger Balm if it lessens the effect of your homeopathic remedy.

Chamomile, lavender, or lemon balm tea are good options for relaxation and helping to soothe tension-related pain.

It is currently considered medically okay to take an occasional dose of acetaminophen (Tylenol) or an occasional ibuprofen (Advil) in the first or second trimester only. But it really is less toxic to avoid these medications altogether, which are not as benign as we have been led to believe. Do avoid other drugs before consulting with your practitioner since many have health risks and are not safe for use during pregnancy (including certain muscle relaxants, aspirin, and other non-steroidal anti-inflammatory medications). Instead, try Dr. Kelly Brogan's turmeric latte for its inflammatory benefits; curcumin (turmeric) is researched as being as effective as many common over-the-counter analgesics. Here is her recipe:

- Combine one cup of water with a half cup of organic turmeric powder in a saucepan and heat on low for about seven minutes, adding more water (up to one additional cup) if it becomes too dry.
- Remove from heat and stir in one-third cup of unrefined organic coconut oil or extra virgin olive oil, and a half to one teaspoon of black pepper.
- Store this in a glass container in the fridge.

When you are ready for a cup, do the following:

- Put one teaspoon of paste in a mug.
- Add a dash of warming spice like cinnamon, cardamom, clove (or all three!).
- Add raw honey (to taste).
- Pour about 1/3 cup of almond, coconut, or hemp milk (I love it with a Three Trees vanilla almond pistachio milk).
- Fill the rest of the mug with boiling water and stir.

Avoid hot tubs and whirlpools because getting your body to such high temperatures without allowing yourself to sweat to cool your body down may not be safe for the baby.

For SPD (Symphysis Pubis Dysfunction)

This can happen when the ligaments and joints connecting the bones of the pelvis become so lax that the pelvic bones go easily out of alignment. It can create very intense pain, especially in the pubic area, and a sense that the pelvic bones are breaking apart even though this is extremely rare and they really are not.

Typical general advice usually given to women includes avoiding activities like strenuous exercise, prolonged standing, vacuum cleaning, stretching exercises, and squatting. Women are also frequently advised to:

- Have regular chiropractic or osteopathic care
- Brace the pelvic floor muscles before performing any activity that might cause pain using your mula bandha (yoga root lock), and stabilize your pelvic bones with a support belt or belly band. You can also use a belly support garment called Baby Hugger, which uses straps and Velcro over the shoulders and under the belly to get the shoulders to assist you more in carrying the weight of the baby. This prevents the baby from resting entirely on the pelvis. I joke that the Baby Hugger is industrial-grade lingerie, especially when paired with thigh-high compression stockings, but I can attest it is helpful for SP pain.
- Rest the pelvis
- Sit down for tasks where possible
- Avoid lifting and carrying
- Avoid stepping over things
- Bend the knees and keep the legs "glued together" when turning in bed and getting in and out of bed
- Place a pillow between the legs when in bed or resting
- Avoid twisting movements of the body
- Avoid straddle movements, especially when weight-bearing
- Go belly DOWN, not UP when rolling over in bed

A sign of a true separation and not just inflammation and pain (tenderness to touch) is when walking backwards is easier than walking forwards.

If the pain is very severe, you may benefit from physical therapy. Using elbow crutches will help take the weight off the pelvis and assist with mobility. Alternatively, for more extreme cases, a wheelchair may be considered advisable.

It is usually recommended that women with SPD give birth in an upright position, with knees slightly apart, and it is often suggested that a woman tie a yoga strap to both legs to ensure that the gap never exceeds her maximum comfort zone.

Practices, such as placing the feet on the provider's hips during delivery, stirrups, and interventions such as forceps, should be avoided in the delivery room if at all possible, as they can strain ligaments further and cause long-term problems. If stirrups must be used, for example, during suturing, great care must be taken to move the legs in symmetry, maneuvering them gently into position.

It doesn't always get worse with birth, so I have learned not to be fearful about it and to use hands/knees, side-lying with knees together, or upright positions. Avoid squatting, lunging, and pushing on your back.

For those with any sort of chronic musculoskeletal pain in which serious causes have been ruled out and none of the natural or allopathic remedies help, get to the root cause and avoid getting dependent on pharmaceuticals and surgery unless absolutely necessary. Consider reading the book The Mindbody Prescription by John Sarno, MD. He is an amazing pioneering physician whose brilliant approach has helped hundreds of thousands of people heal chronic pain without drugs, physical measure, or surgery. And then consider Clarity Breathwork to release repressed painful emotions, stress, and trauma from the body stored in those areas.

Remember that not all aches and pains can be blamed on pregnancy. Consult your practitioner if:

- The above suggestions do not help.
- The pain is different than usual or is severe, persistent, or continuous.
- Pain is associated with other unusual symptoms like fever, chills, changes in bowel or bladder habits, or vaginal bleeding, leaking of water-like fluid, or anything that doesn't seem right and concerns you.
- You experience regular pelvic pressure, uterine hardening, or cramping.
- You have a local area of increased pain, swelling, and redness on your leg.
- Normal movement becomes difficult.
- You have a history of serious back problems, injury, or surgery.

Natural Remedies for Cold and Flu in Pregnancy

It's no fun getting sick, especially during pregnancy. Pregnant women are more susceptible to colds and other infections related to the effects of hormonal changes throughout the body. If you and your baby are otherwise healthy, there is no cause for alarm and you will heal with good rest, hydration, and nourishment. And there are plenty of natural remedies that will help you to feel much better and to heal sooner.

I know, mommies and midwives cannot get sick! But we do. An infection is your body's way of letting you know that your resistance is low, that you are over-stressed, rundown, and need to slow down. It's an opportunity to take a look at what in your daily life creates the conditions for illness to occur.

Do not ignore your symptoms and carry on as usual, even more so when you are pregnant. Neglected mild infections can turn into more serious and complicated ones.

Rest assured, these suggestions help whether you are pregnant or not. I am so thankful that these remedies work. I have studied them extensively and effectively used them on myself, my family, and the thousands I have guided over the many years I have been practicing as a midwife.

If You Experience Cold and Flu During Pregnancy

Allow Yourself Some Rest

Take some time off to go to bed and get plenty of rest to allow your body to heal, especially if you have been overdoing it.

Get extra sleep by going to bed early, sleeping later, and taking naps.

Reassess your lifestyle and think about ways to cut back and let go of unnecessary expenditures of energy, limit nonessential activities, and reduce unneeded stress. And please accept help from others.

Try Some Natural Remedies

Drink lots of fluids. Drink your daily dose of clean water, with additional herbal tea and broth as needed. Sip frequently. Try these recipes:

Ginger Infusion

1. Add one heaping teaspoon fresh grated ginger to one cup of boiling water.
2. Steep covered for 15-20 minutes.
3. Add manuka honey and/or fresh lemon juice to taste.
4. Drink one cup every few hours.

Ginger Plus Tea

1. Boil half a tablespoon or one inch of shredded ginger, half a tablespoon of cinnamon, and half a teaspoon of cayenne powder in two cups of water for five to six minutes.
2. Add two sautéed cloves of chopped garlic, a dash of sea salt, the juice of one lemon, and 1/4 cup of manuka honey. Steep covered 5-10 minutes. Adding one tablespoon of apple cider vinegar relieves stuffed noses.
3. Drink throughout the day.

Other powerful anti-inflammatory herbs in addition to ginger include Ceylon cinnamon and turmeric, so add plenty of them to your foods. Dr. Kelly Brogan has an excellent recipe for a turmeric latte that you can find in the previous chapter. Sweeten it with raw manuka honey and add a generous amount of Ceylon cinnamon.

Healing Broth

A fresh miso soup or bone broth with lightly cooked scallions, onions, and garlic is also very therapeutic.

1. Add five to six cloves of chopped raw garlic in one quart of boiling water, and soak covered for a half-hour.
2. Sauté a few chopped scallions, shallots, or one onion in olive oil that lightly covers the bottom of pan.
3. Dissolve one tablespoon of miso or a few organic, all-natural bouillon cubes according to package directions; then add the garlic and onions. You can also use chicken, veggie, or bone broth as a base.
4. Drink warm, up to one cup every few hours.

Kudzu Soup

Kudzu makes a wonderfully soothing and nourishing soup that lowers fever, reduces inflammation, and relieves sore throat and even stomach discomfort. When added to garlic and ginger, it can also help you heal. It is available in most health food stores.

1. Dissolve a few teaspoons of kudzu starch into 1/2 cup of cold water. Set aside.
2. Sauté two shallots or a small onion, six cloves of chopped garlic, half an inch of chopped ginger in one tablespoon of olive for a few minutes.
3. Add three cups of water and bring to a boil.
4. Cover and simmer for 20 minutes.
5. Add one tablespoon of miso paste and the kudzu mixture. Stir for 2 minutes.
6. Drink warm throughout the day.

Alternately, you can dissolve two teaspoons of kudzu in a half cup of cold water, add to two cups of boiling apple juice, then stir for a few minutes with 1/8 teaspoon of cinnamon or a cinnamon stick, and drink as often as needed.

Eat nourishing organic food. Avoid heavily processed refined flour and sugar foods, partially hydrogenated fat, refined vegetable oils, and deep-fried foods as they strain the immune system. Cow dairy and wheat products increase mucus production, so you may want to limit your intake of these foods if you are congested.

Take your daily supplements to make sure you are getting all the nourishment you need that is not supplied by diet alone. For more information on nutrition and supplements, please refer to the chapter, "Nutritional Best Practices for Mom."

Vitamin C with bioflavinoids can be taken in 500-1,000 mg doses, three to five times per day to assist your immune response. But do not take more than 2,000 mg per day in the first trimester, or 500 mg daily past the 36th week of pregnancy.

Vitamin D3 - make sure you take 1000-5000 IU daily to keep your blood levels 70 or above, which supports your general well-being and immune response.

Zinc - Take in the form of lozenges (up to 10-30 mg daily) with a meal to reduce the severity of an upper respiratory infection. Liquid drops are also fine.

Take Gaia's alcohol-free Echinacea Supreme. This is my favorite brand of echinacea, which is a remarkable and safe herb that kills all sorts of unwanted germs without disrupting the body's normal flora and strengthens the immune system's ability to fight infection. It's good to keep this herbal tincture in the house, as it works best the earlier you start to take it, just when you notice you feel like you are "coming down with something."

At the first sign of infection, take one to two dropperfuls in juice or water every few hours, and then slowly reduce the dose and frequency as you recover. Continue to take it one to two times daily for a week after your symptoms resolve. Don't worry if your tongue feels a little numb and tingly momentarily, as this is a common temporary side effect. It also comes alcohol-free, which does not make the tongue feel funny.

As a preventative tonic during the cold and flu season, after exposure to someone sick, or if you just feel rundown, take a dropperful, one to two times daily for two to three weeks of each month.

For additional protection, you can also add a dropperful of astragalus. If you cannot tolerate the liquid form, you can try capsules of supercritical or freeze-dried herbal extracts

Enjoy some garlic. As soon as you feel like you are getting sick, eat a bulb of fresh garlic daily. You can make it delicious by roasting or sautéing the whole cloves in olive oil, salt, pepper, and a dash of parsley.

If you prefer raw garlic, eat two to four cloves twice daily, crushed into your salad, or cut and swallow them as a pill. Continue until a week after symptoms have gone.

Another option is to take supercritical garlic in tablet or capsule form—a capsule several times per day.

Breathe easy. Use these suggestions to liquify thick mucus to flow more easily out of your system, keeping bacteria growth at bay and helping you breathe more comfortably.

For a cough, stuffy nose, and a hoarse, scratchy, or sore throat, use a humidifier or vaporizer in the bedroom so that you can inhale the steam. Cool mist is preferable if there are young children around to prevent burns. You can add a few drops of essential oils to the water, purchased separately or in a collection. Try a combination of two to three of the following:

- Thieves by Young Living
- Tea tree
- Peppermint
- Eucalyptus
- Sage
- Oregano
- Ginger

- Thyme
- Lavender
- Chamomile
- Rosemary.

Take advantage of inhaling steam as often as you can when not sleeping. At least several times daily, bring a pot of water to boil, then turn off the flame. Stand over it, cover your head and the pot with a towel, while breathing in through your nose slowly and deeply for relief of nasal and sinus congestion. You can breathe through your mouth with pursed lips as if sucking through a straw if your nose is too stuffed. **But be extremely careful not to burn yourself and watch that the towel is not near the hot burner!**

Alternately, you can sit in a closed bathroom with the hot, steamy shower running.

Two to three saline nose drops put into your nose will loosen thick, sticky mucus for easier removal. You can make your own by adding 1/4 teaspoon of sea salt to a quart of purified, distilled water. Tap water can also be used, but only after boiling to sterilize it.

Another method is nasal douching using a neti pot to rinse and clear the nasal passages. Tilt your head back and inhale or pour slowly the saline solution through one nostril while closing the other with your index finger, and spit the fluid out of your mouth; then repeat with the other nostril. Do each nostril several times, three to four times daily. Integrative physician Andrew Weil especially recommends this practice for sinus infections. His instructions are easy to follow:

> *"You can pour some of the salt water into your cupped hand and inhale it into one nostril at a time while closing the other nostril with an index finger. Or you can get a neti pot, a ceramic container shaped like a miniature Aladdin's lamp that allows you to pour water directly into the nose. Use enough solution to fill your nasal cavity and spill into your mouth. Spit it out and then gently blow your nose. At first, this process may seem uncomfortable and messy,*

but once you get the hang of it, you'll like what it does for your nose and sinuses."

Gargle. For a sore throat or ear congestion, gargle for a few minutes, four to five times per day, with a solution of any of the following:

- 1/2 teaspoon sea salt dissolved in one cup of very warm water
- One to two drops each of tea tree, eucalyptus, and peppermint oil in one cup very warm water
- 1/2 cup hydrogen peroxide in 1/2 cup of very warm water.

You can add a 1/2 teaspoon of goldenseal powder, or the entire contents of one capsule, to the saline solution. Remember not to swallow! Spit everything out after you gargle.

Additional Remedies for Cold and Flu During Pregnancy

Sweat for 10-20 minutes per day in a steam room or dry sauna where you will perspire freely. Intense sweating helps the body eliminate infectious toxins. Remember to drink lots of water before, during, and afterwards. Avoid immersion in hot tubs/jacuzzis in pregnancy because they make your body temperature too high for the baby and do not allow you to sweat to cool yourself and the baby down.

Manuka honey has been used for centuries to help heal infection and has been supported by research. Take one heaping teaspoon to tablespoon of UMF-rated organic raw manuka honey from New Zealand, up to four times per day. This can be added to tea or taken straight. They also come in tasty soothing lozenges.

Asian mushrooms—Host Defense makes a wonderful combination of organically-grown Asian mushrooms, used extensively in traditional Chinese and Japanese medicine for centuries to enhance immunity.

Other lozenges like slippery elm, or low dose herbal combinations, and also Ricola cough drops can also provide some relief, as do herbal throat sprays.

Other Herbs

Elderberry syrup is especially studied and is effective for the flu, but also reduces the length and severity of the common cold. It also tastes yummy! You can take two teaspoons up to four times daily.

If you are NOT pregnant, at the earliest sign of feeling sick, you can take andrographis paniculate (Ginger), easily available as the brand name Kan Jang. Take one tablet every six hours. It is reputed to be very effective at boosting immunity during the cold and flu season, and to hasten healing, as is encapsulated oil of oregano and olive leaf, Vital Nutrients' Viracon and you can take it as directed on the bottle. You can use a healing throat spray with echinacea, goldenseal, and propolis. You can take reliable pure Chinese Herbs like Traditionals' Gan Mau Ling (four every few hours) and Seven Forests Ilex 15 (six every few hours) - I am amazed how this combination works like a charm. Gradually decrease the frequency as you get better, and stop the day after you are back to yourself.

Additional well-researched, natural immune-boosting, anti-infective remedies include colloidal silver, goldenseal, cumin, rosemary, cinnamon, and elecampane to support the healing of your respiratory tract, and they kill certain common disease-causing bacteria.

Dr. Kelly Brogan in her book *Own Yourself: The Suprising Path Beyond Depression, Anxiety, and Fatigue to Reclaiming Your Authenticity, Vitality, and Freedom* also advises thymus glandular, and N-acetyl cysteine (especially to loosen mucus in a hacking productive cough) to support your immune system when sick with common infections.

Essential Oil Blends

Thieves by Young Living can be added to your tea (just a drop or two) a few times daily. You can also make it into a warm, moist compress; or dilute three to four drops of Thieves or any of the mentioned essential oils in almond oil and massage it onto your aching body, rub it onto your chest, throat, sinuses, head, or under your nose. Place it in the bath as you soak for its anti-infectious, decongestant, and immune-stimulating effects. Put three to four drops on the lightbulb near your bed and in your diffuser and humidifier.

The essential oil of tea tree may be combined with clove, cinnamon, or a few of the others mentioned, and diluted in a spray bottle of water to spray around the room to naturally disinfect and refresh the air. You can take DoTerra's On Guard essential oil pellets orally as directed. I am impressed by how effective they are!

Homeopathic Remedies

If you are within the first 24 hours of the onset of your symptoms, 30c of Belladonna or Aconite taken every few hours is usually the remedy of choice. Oscillococcinum is an excellent remedy for classic flu-like symptoms. Consult your classical homeopath or an excellent homeopathic reference book.

Cough medicines are occasionally warranted in certain situations. Hacking dry coughs that do not produce phlegm are exhausting and debilitating, especially at night if they interfere with needed sleep. Start naturally with alcohol-free tincture of mullein (one teaspoon in a little warm water every four hours). Eat fresh horseradish to help liquefy secretions.

If you absolutely need a cough suppressant medication, you can get dextromethorphan over the counter at the drug store and take 15 mg every six hours. If this does not work, ask your provider for a prescription narcotic cough medicine (Codeine or Hycodan) to use for seven to ten days. It is considered safe and well worth it for short-term use.

For productive coughs in which you are bringing up phlegm, you can use a nonprescription expectorant medication like guaifenesin immediate release tablets or in syrup form (10-20 cc every four hours). Or, extended-release Mucinex, 600-1,200 mg every 12 hours instead of a cough suppressant.

Follow These Precautions

Avoid overexposure to extremes in temperature, especially cold, to conserve your energy for healing from cold and flu during pregnancy. Allow good fresh air to circulate in the room by opening the windows occasionally. However, minimize drafts if they are causing you to feel chilled.

Be cautious about taking antibiotics, especially if you only have a viral and not a bacterial infection. Antibiotics are useless against viruses, can be quite harmful, and will only stress your system more. While in some infrequent situations, antibiotics are essential and indeed lifesaving, more often, colds, cases of flu, and other mild upper respiratory infections can safely be treated naturally without them.

Symptoms such as runny nose, sneezing, cough, and fever are your body's way of fighting the infection and ultimately lead to self-recovery. Therefore, try to avoid common over-the-counter medications that offer temporary relief by suppressing these symptoms. These drugs actually interfere with the body's remarkable capacity to heal itself, have side effects, and may be unsafe to take during pregnancy. Furthermore, they do not treat the underlying cause.

Blow your stuffed nose and cough the phlegm out of your chest regularly as needed, rather than keeping it in your system. Then wash your hands with soap and do not share your used towels.

Fever is usually beneficial as it is part of your body's first line of defense against the infection and does not need to be brought down unless:

- Your temperature is approaching 101 if you are pregnant (102 if you are otherwise healthy and are not pregnant)
- You are really uncomfortable and cannot sleep.

To Bring Down a High Fever

First, try sponge bathing in a waste-deep tub of lukewarm water. With a little cold water running, steadily to gradually lower the water temperature. You can add any of the mentioned essential oils to the water. Use a wet sponge or washcloth to bathe all exposed skin areas for 20 minutes; then allow the skin to air dry in a room free from drafts.

If you are not up to sitting in the bath, your partner, other family member, or good friend can sponge down your body with tepid water at the bedside. Expose and sponge one limb at a time until it feels cool to the touch, drying, then replacing it under the covers before going on to the next limb.

Drink plenty of fluids as needed to help cool and hydrate. Good options are:

- A cup of hot water with the juice of a squeezed lemon and a dash of manuka honey
- Peppermint or spearmint tea with manuka honey
- Coconut water
- Lots of spring or filtered water
- Pure fruit juice, fruit smoothies, and frozen fruit juice bars or popsicles
- Soup broth.

If the above measures are not successful to reduce high fever, or you are too uncomfortable to sleep, Tylenol (acetaminophen) is reportedly okay for very occasional use in pregnancy and can be taken in very limited amounts as needed and directed on the container. However, avoid aspirin, Motrin, or Advil (ibuprofen) during pregnancy, especially in the last trimester.

For Frequent or Chronic Illness

If you are susceptible to frequent or severe colds, you may want to consider having a consultation with an osteopath, acupuncturist, or homeopath.

Read *Natural Health, Natural Medicine* by Andrew Weil, MD and follow his suggestions about enhancing your immunity and limiting exposure to physical and emotional stresses that weaken your immune system and increase your risk of illness. His suggestions are well-researched, basic to holistic integrative medicine, and in sync with many similar experts in the field who have greatly influenced my practice as a professional and my own life. Prevention is key; in summary, it includes the following:

- Nourish yourself well, by eating a variety of organically-grown whole foods (lots of fresh fruits and vegetables, whole (ideally gluten-free) grains, nuts, beans, and seeds, low-contaminant fish, pastured meat, poultry, and eggs).
- Drink lots of filtered or bottled pure spring water from a reliable source.
- Avoid highly genetically modified and processed foods laden with chemicals, refined vegetable oils, cow dairy, gluten, and sugars (except raw honey and maple syrup, which are fine to use).
- Avoid personal care and cleaning products with harmful chemicals and toxins.
- Minimize milk products and foods of animal origin not naturally raised.
- Use natural plant-based cosmetics, toiletries, and cleaning products from the health food store.
- Avoid smoking, drugs, and excess alcohol.
- Avoid unnecessary use of antibiotics, non-steroidal anti-inflammatory medications, protein pump inhibitor acid-blocking drugs, and synthetic hormones and steroids unless in cases of life-threatening illness.
- Take a good multivitamin, and supplements that keep you well-nourished.
- Take natural remedies whenever safely possible, like Asian mushrooms, astragalus, echinacea, and garlic, as discussed above, to enhance your immunity.
- Unplug from the computer and smartphone as much as possible; reconnect with yourself and others in person.

- Slow down, take breaks, and limit external stressors and non-essentials on your to-do list.
- Get plenty of rest, fresh air, early morning or late afternoon sun exposure, and regular moderate exercise.
- Learn how to master your relaxation response and do things that maintain your emotional wellbeing, inner calm, and joy.
- Master your breath, and release inner stress, anger, grief, and trauma with a daily breathwork practice.
- Learn how to be your own placebo and create thoughts, feelings, and internal experiences that keep you vibrantly healthy instead of making you sick, with Dr. Joe Dispenza's books and workshops.
- Cultivate a positive mindset and do what you love as much as possible.
- Live in community.

When Your Symptoms Are Not Due to Cold or Flu

Sinus Congestion

Nasal or sinus stuffiness throughout pregnancy, without any other symptoms, is not typically due to an infection. Rather, it's related to the hormones that cause increased mucus production, blood flow, and swelling to the mucus membranes in these areas.

In this situation, simply drink eight to ten glasses per day of filtered spring, well water, or herbal tea. Drink between meals, at least 20-30 minutes before eating, or two hours after. Use plain nasal saline spray, sleep with a humidifier or vaporizer to ease breathing at night (with or without any already mentioned essential oils like eucalyptus and peppermint), and avoid over-the-counter medications such as decongestants and antihistamines.

Allergies

Seasonal or diet-related symptoms like stuffy nose, watery nasal discharge, sneezing, wheezing, coughing, skin rashes, and shortness of breath (asthma) are not due to an infectious process. Rather, they are more likely caused by allergies. Consult your healthcare provider for these symptoms and certainly before taking any medications or natural supplements in pregnancy. Alternative therapies such as mind-body work like hypnotherapy, herbs, homeopathy, breathwork, acupuncture, and osteopathic care have all been reported to be very effective in treating allergies, as well as basic lifestyle modifications. For example, a minimum 2-4 week trial of eliminating common inflammatory and allergenic foods like cow dairy and gluten products could allow you to see if your symptoms lessen or resolve; then you could introduce one gluten-type grain or dairy product at a time to see if symptoms recur (wait a few days before introducing the others, one at a time). Other possible allergenic foods to experiment eliminating and then reintroducing include soy, corn, eggs, certain nuts, and fruit.

It may also help to eat a low-protein diet, further reduce stress, avoid possible triggers, and install a HEPA home air filter. Nasal douching regularly helps with hay fever, as does the stinging nettle herb in capsules or infusion. You can make your own by steeping one large handful of dried nettle leaf in a quart of boiling water for at least four hours. Add a splash of lemon or lime juice, fresh mint, or a dash of honey to taste, and drink it throughout the day. A few weeks before your allergy season, eat foods high in quercetin like berries, citrus fruits, apples, grapes, green leafy veggies, broccoli, buckwheat, and green and black tea. If you are not pregnant, you can take quercetin in supplement form, 400-500 mg, twice a day. Or even better, take as directed, a combination formula like Natural D-Hist by Orthomolecular, which includes quercetin, bromelain, stinging nettles leaf, and N-acetyl cysteine.

Always call your healthcare provider if you have a question and certainly if these suggestions do not help and you feel worse or do not notice improvement within 48 hours of an acute infection. Use common sense. A lingering or rising fever after the first two to three days of illness, severe pain, difficulty breathing, extreme weakness, faintness, marked irritability, mental confusion, seizures, neck stiffness, prolonged vomiting or diarrhea, or any other unusual symptoms, regular uterine cramping or pelvic pressure, and/or bleeding or fluid leaking from your vagina warrants immediate consultation.

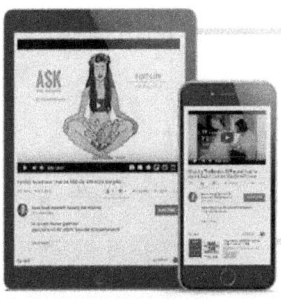

Want to learn more or have more questions?

Grab your free Book Bonuses below:
https://homesweethomebirth.com/nbsbookbonus

Stomach Bug or Food Poisoning During Pregnancy: Natural Remedies

Whether a stomach bug or temporary bout of food poisoning, having an upset stomach during pregnancy can be especially uncomfortable.

Although you may feel very sick, vomiting and diarrhea are important defense mechanisms, enabling your body to rid itself of harmful substances like toxins and germs. Therefore, it is best to allow most simple cases to run their course without suppressing your symptoms.

Make sure to get plenty of rest to enable yourself to heal.

Home Remedies for Stomach Bug and Food Poisoning

Food and Drink

The main concern with a stomach bug and food poisoning is excessive loss of body fluids resulting in serious dehydration, which in pregnancy can increase the chance of premature labor. When an acute bout of vomiting and/or diarrhea occurs, the first thing you need to do is let your irritated gastrointestinal tract heal by avoiding all food for 12-24 hours. But, try to keep hydrated by drinking frequent sips of filtered, spring, or well water, plus other clear liquids, every hour or two (1/4 cup water every 15-30 minutes is the minimum), and placing a pinch of Himalayan sea salt on your tongue to help replenish electrolytes.

After 12 hours or when your symptoms have calmed down a bit, try taking clear fluids in sips or spoonfuls as frequently as you can tolerate. The ideal is to drink your daily dose of water, and you may need more if you have been dehydrated. Avoid oily liquids and milk at this time, which irritate the intestinal tract and interfere with its healing.

In addition to filtered, spring, or well water, better choices include:

- Electrolyte-infused Smart Water
- Pure coconut water
- Diluted fruit juice
- Herbal teas with honey (like ginger, peppermint, or chamomile)
- Miso, bone, or vegetable broth
- Chicken or any other low-fat non-dairy soup stock
- Rice or barley water (drink the water used to cook barley or brown rice)
- Frozen fruit or fruit juice popsicles
- Recharge or organic Gatorade electrolyte drinks (avoid the standard chemical-laden Gatorade).

A homemade electrolyte concoction:

- Combine 1/8 to 1/4 teaspoon of Himalayan sea salt, 1/4 teaspoon of baking soda, one teaspoon of calcium/magnesium powder, one to two tablespoons of honey, one quart of spring or pure coconut water, and the juice of a fresh lemon or lime to taste.
- Drink a cup slowly, every one to two hours. Even if you vomit it up, you will still get some.

After 24 hours of only liquids and as the symptoms improve, advance to a bland diet for the next day or two in addition to frequent fluids. Good food choices include bananas, applesauce, white basmati rice, dry white toast (they have gluten-free options), white rice cakes or crackers, hot rice or buckwheat cereal cooked in water sweetened with pure maple syrup or honey, and mashed potatoes with a little salt.

Continue to avoid fats and dairy products (other than organic, live-culture yogurt), spicy or sugary food, caffeine, and alcohol. An oil that actually helps relieve diarrhea is made from flaxseed, but you may prefer to take it as directed in capsule form. For now, stay away from high-fiber foods, like most raw fruits and vegetables and whole grains. Wait 48 hours after your symptoms resolve before eating these foods and returning to your normal diet. An upset digestive tract, like any other injury, needs time to heal.

For any type of dysentery, eat unripe green bananas and basmati rice with plain organic yogurt or kefir for optimal gut health. Also eat fresh papaya with a FEW seeds, as they contain substances that kill many types of causative organisms responsible for intestinal infections. However, don't ingest more than one tablespoon of the seeds daily in pregnancy.

Herbs and Supplements

As with any infection, eat a bulb of garlic once per day. You can bake the cloves in a little olive oil, salt, and pepper, or cut them up raw and swallow a few cloves as pills, but you are more likely to tolerate taking a supercritical extract of garlic capsules. It is wonderfully effective and very mild-tasting when encapsulated in supercritical form.

You can also try Gaia's Echinacea Supreme herbal tincture, one to two dropperfuls, every few hours, daily in juice. This will help kill germs like viruses and strengthen your immune system.

Drink a strong red raspberry leaf tea, or even better, make your own infusion of red raspberry leaf by immersing one ounce of it dried in one quart boiling water, brew for a half an hour, strain it in a glass canning jar, and drink a half to one cup up to every 30 minutes to one hour, according to the severity of your diarrhea. Add fresh mint, juice of a lemon or lime, and honey to taste.

Drink kombucha, and eat lacto-fermented foods such as kimchi, as soon as you are able to tolerate vegetables. Take an excellent probiotic like Greens First, twice daily, for at least a few weeks to help resolve the diarrhea and replace healthy intestinal flora.

Slippery elm is reputed to be the best herbal remedy for soothing and healing inflammation of the bowel and/or acid reflux irritation commonly felt after vomiting. Take slippery elm capsules, three times daily, suck on slippery elm lozenges, or make your own slippery elm paste by combining the powdered form with a few spoonfuls of honey-sweetened water, applesauce, or hot cereal.

Ginger is great for relieving nausea. Try:

- Making ginger tea by boiling a tiny piece or one teaspoon of fresh grated ginger root in one cup of water for five to 15 minutes. Strain it into your glass canning jar, add honey and/or lemon to taste, and sip up to two cups throughout the day.
- Drinking all-natural ginger ale.
- Taking ginger honey tonic, one to two spoonfuls, as often as needed, plain or in tea or sparkling water.
- Sucking on ice cubes of ginger tea.
- Ingesting ginger hard candy, chewables, or candied ginger slices.
- Taking ginger root powder in capsules, 250 mg, up to four times per day (if no history of two or more miscarriages).

Dr. Andrew Weil recommends blackberry root bark as a good herbal remedy for diarrhea. Take one teaspoon of blackberry root bark tincture, every two to four hours, or make your own infusion by steeping a handful of the dried herb in one quart of boiling water for 20 minutes, straining in your glass jar, and drinking a cup every two to four hours. He also advises carob powder, which is very soothing on irritated intestines after diarrhea. Mix one tablespoon of it with applesauce and honey for taste, and eat it on an empty stomach, a half to one hour before or three hours after eating. If you have a lot of painful abdominal cramping, take an opium tincture, 10-15 drops in a small amount of water, every three to four hours, for no more than two days. But take care, as it can be quite sedating.

For diarrhea, Bentonite clay is safe for ingesting, and it has been studied to bind and rid the body of toxins and irritants, which provides effective relief of acute bouts of diarrhea. Take one to two tablespoons of it dissolved in distilled water, two to three times daily, for a few days. Another impressive complementary remedy is activated charcoal taken as directed on the bottle. It is said to be safe in pregnancy, up to 50 grams, three times daily, for no more than a week.

The essential oils of chamomile, peppermint, or geranium may be diluted and massaged into your abdomen to bring relief. Or place a few drops in your essential oil diffuser or glass spray bottle of water, and spray it near you periodically.

Dr. Aviva Romm, in *The Natural Pregnancy Book*, recommends taking two capsules of goldenseal after the first trimester, every four hours, for no more than 24 hours in cases of more severe dysentery. Stop if you feel your uterus contracting more than usual. She also writes about a wonderfully effective Japanese treatment of topical salt packs if you feel a round of vomiting approaching or if you have been vomiting frequently. To prepare it:

1. Heat a half cup of sea salt in a pan for three minutes.
2. Put the salt in a pillowcase or cloth bag.
3. Fold it into a rectangular pad or small square, and wrap it in a towel if too hot.
4. Apply directly to your stomach (not belly).

Always remember to wash your hands with soap after going to the bathroom, and use separate towels.

Consult with a classical homeopath, or refer to an excellent homeopathic reference book for a remedy most specific to your symptoms. The remedy that works best for me is arsenicum. Others report much success with Weleeda's homeopathic combination Nausin (seven to ten drops four times per day), especially for nausea.

Do not take any medications (even over-the-counter ones) without consulting with your practitioner, as many are not safe to use in pregnancy, slow your body's attempt to heal, or mask important symptoms and give a false sense of reassurance.

Contact your practitioner if these suggestions do not help and there is NO IMPROVEMENT in 24-36 hours, especially if:

- Diarrhea and/or vomiting is incessant and you cannot keep anything down.
- You have severe abdominal pain.
- Your temperature is over 101.
- The vomiting material or stools is unusual (bloody, black tarry, grey, white, or resembling coffee grounds).
- There is yellowing of your skin or eyes.
- You experience dark-colored urine.
- You have unusual fatigue for more than a few days, and your discomfort is in the right side of your abdomen.
- There is evidence of dehydration: your mouth is without saliva and your eyes are without tears, your eyes appear sunken and your normal skin texture is lost (if you pinch up some skin and it does not immediately snap back into place), and/or urination has reduced or stopped.
- Your symptoms occurred after an injury or ingestion of a drug or poison.
- Other family members or close contacts have been diagnosed with hepatitis.
- You suspect a bacterial or parasitic infection (like Shigella, for example).
- You experience regular uterine cramping or hardening, a new pattern of lower abdominal or back ache or pressure, or vaginal bleeding or leaking of amniotic fluid.
- Your baby is not moving as much as usual.
- You are worried that something isn't right.

BLADDER INFECTION DURING PREGNANCY AND BEYOND: NATURAL REMEDIES

Bladder infection is one of the most common ailments in women. Also known as cystitis, lower urinary tract infection, or UTI, it can occur more frequently from bodily changes during pregnancy. Prevention and prompt treatment of early symptoms are the safest courses, as the untreated infection can spread to the kidneys and then the bloodstream, and cause serious illness as well as preterm labor. Simple bladder infections can be treated successfully with natural remedies, and, thereby, you avoid the overuse of antibiotics and the cycle of multiple antibiotics.

Early warning signs of a UTI include feeling an urgent and frequent need to urinate but only a little comes out; burning during and after urination; cloudy, odorous, or blood-tinged urine; pelvic pressure and aching or cramping in the lower abdomen. Some women feel exhausted and unwell while others do not notice many symptoms at all.

Frequent trips to the bathroom (especially at night) are common in the first and third trimesters of pregnancy from the pressure of the growing uterus and baby on the bladder, so that isn't necessarily due to infection.

Other predisposing factors in bladder infection besides pregnancy include:

- Sexual and hygienic practices that bring bacteria from the bowel towards the urethra
- Frequent or traumatic sexual intercourse

- Use of public whirlpool baths or hot tubs
- Bubble baths
- Perfumed soaps
- Use of the contraceptive diaphragm in some susceptible women
- Coffee and other caffeinated drinks
- Dehydration
- Cigarette and alcohol addiction
- Diabetes
- Menopause
- Urinary catheterization
- Kidney diseases and other illnesses.

To Prevent and Treat Bladder Infections

Hydration

Drink your daily dose of water to dilute the urine and increase the force of flow. Filtered tap, well or spring water is preferable to hydrate, but adding herbal tea, soup broth, some citrus drinks, and unsweetened cranberry juice are fine. The last two help acidify the urine, discouraging bacterial growth.

You can limit the intake of fluids and natural diuretics, like juicy fruits and vegetables, during the evening to minimize waking in the middle of the night to urinate.

In the third trimester, recline on your side for a bit before going to bed. This relieves the pressure of your uterus on the major vessels and thus allows the increased fluid that has been trapped in your lower body during the day to return to the heart and kidneys, allowing you to urinate this additional amount out before sleep.

Urinate as soon as you feel the urge, or at least every two to three hours while awake, as bacteria grow more easily in concentrated urine held back.

Diet

Eat a well-balanced whole, real food diet. Please see the chapter "Nutritional Best Practices for Mom" for my diet and supplement recommendations. Do avoid bladder irritants such as alcohol, caffeinated drinks, spicy foods, red and black pepper, food colorings, cigarettes, and alcohol.

Also be sure to read the chapters "Natural Stress Alleviation in Pregnancy and Beyond" and "Natural Remedies for Cold and Flu in Pregnancy" to learn how to reduce stress and strengthen your immunity.

Hygiene

Always wipe from the front (vagina) towards the back (rectum), ideally using plain, unscented toilet paper. Wash the rectal area with water and soap or hypoallergenic wipes after a bowel movement until clean.

Wear all-cotton underwear or no underwear, and avoid tight, synthetic clothing, as bacteria thrive in the moist heat created by this. If you need to wear pantyhose stockings, use those with a 100% cotton crotch. Likewise, change into dry clothing after swimming and sweat-inducing exercise.

Change sanitary pads and tampons frequently, at least every time you go to the bathroom. Use the organic brands of tampons and/or pads, or use a menstrual cup instead.

Avoid bubble baths, perfumed soaps, and bath oils, as they can change the delicate acid-base balance and cause inflammation of the urethra. Even colored toilet paper and certain laundry detergents have been known to aggravate UTIs in sensitive individuals.

Women who get frequent bladder infections and use the diaphragm may need to be fitted for a smaller size or one with a less rigid rim, or switch to a different contraceptive. Some women react to the spermicide used with the diaphragm, as well as with sponges, condoms, and foam, and may need to consider alternative methods.

Avoid traumatic sexual or anal intercourse and repeated episodes of sex in a short time. Have a tall glass of water before intercourse to dilute and flush out possible bacteria. Urinate and wash with cool water afterwards, as sex may transfer bacteria from the bowel forward towards the urethra (the tube where the urine comes out).

Drink a strong nettle leaf infusion every day to strengthen the kidneys if you are prone to UTIs. To prepare your own herbal infusion of nettles:

1. Steep a handful of the dried herb in a quart of boiling water for at least four hours.
2. Strain to a glass canning jar.
3. Add a splash of lemon or lime juice, fresh mint leaf, or a dash of honey to taste (optional).
4. Drink one to three cups daily.

At the First Suspicion of a UTI

In addition to upping your hydration, drink eight fluid ounces of UNSWEETENED cranberry juice every two hours, which has been studied to prevent bacteria from adhering to the bladder wall by acidifying urine and making it hostile to the causative bacteria, thus effectively treating bladder infections. You can make your own by using cranberry juice concentrate diluted in water or other juices to reduce the sour taste, or by adding powdered cranberry, as directed, to your smoothie, applesauce, yogurt, or oatmeal. You can also take an encapsulated powdered cranberry, 800-900 mg, or the studied brand Cranactin, one to two capsules, every three to four hours with plenty of water until symptoms resolve. Dr. Aviva Romm reports the most success with a cranberry d-Mannose supplement, two capsules twice per day. If you are prone to frequent UTIs or are going on a honeymoon get-away weekend with your partner, you can take a half of a dose of any of the cranberry supplements daily and drink extra water for prevention.

Take 500-1,000 mg of vitamin C with bioflavonoids, every four to six hours, for three to five days or until a few days after you are better, but limit the dose to 500 mg daily once you are past 36 weeks of pregnancy.

Eat a bulb of fresh garlic cloves daily. You can make it delicious by sautéing them in olive oil, salt, pepper, and a dash of parsley. If you prefer raw garlic, eat several cloves twice a day. You can crush it into your salad or cut it and swallow it as a pill. Eating it with parsley reduces the odor. Another wonderful option is to take a capsule of mild-tasting, supercritical garlic, one to two capsules daily, as directed, with eight ounces of water per capsule until the UTI resolves. Garlic is a powerful natural antibiotic that safely kills unwanted germs while preserving the healthy flora that normally reside in the body.

To boost your immunity, fight infection, and reduce inflammation, take Gaia's Echinacea Supreme, one to two dropperfuls in juice or water, every few hours and then three times daily for a week after your symptoms resolve.

Take marshmallow root as directed if you need to soothe the pain of inflammation in your urinary tract.

Drink even more fluids (up to 14 glasses a day, or a glass of water every half to one hour) to further dilute the bacteria and flush them out. Try drinking two tablespoons of apple cider vinegar with juice, three times daily, to acidify urine and kill the infectious bacteria.

Drink a cup every half hour of barley water with lemon juice. To make this concoction, simmer a handful of whole barley and cut pieces of a lemon in plenty of water for 40 minutes, strain off, and drink daily.

Drink kombucha and eat more lacto-fermented probiotic foods. Take a high-colony-count mega-probiotic like Green's First Women's Probiotic that survives obstacles like stomach acid (two to four capsules, twice daily, until symptoms resolve; then continue with one to two capsules per day) to increase the amount of normal bacterial flora to offset the imbalance that created the infection. This is especially important if your gut microbiome has been disrupted from antibiotics, other medications, and chronic inflammation from stress, food culprits, and toxic exposures.

Try homeopathic remedies. Start with a common effective remedy like Cantharis 30c; take three to five pellets under your tongue every few hours for the first day, but if you get no relief, you may need a different remedy. Consult an excellent homeopathic reference or a professional classical homeopath if you need more personalized support. You can also drink Weleda's sarsaparilla tea, at least twice per day.

Take a daily bath or use a sitz bath to direct the healing where it is most needed, and add to the warm water a few drops of essential oils of bergamot, lavender, and/or sandalwood. Use the mixture in your peri-bottle to wash yourself after urination, squirting your genitals towards the back while on the toilet. Both the sitz bath and peri-bottle will come in handy postpartum as well.

Get extra rest and keep warm with additional clothing or blankets as needed to avoid feeling chilled.

If You Are Passed the First Trimester or Are NOT Pregnant

Take a short course of an encapsulated extract of uva-ursi while temporarily stopping the cranberry, which blocks its effect. Dosage recommendations are one to two capsules, 400-800mg tablets, or one dropperful of the liquid tincture, three to four times per day, up to three to five days. You can also make your own herbal infusion by adding a handful of the leaves of uva-ursi to a glass canning jar filled with water, brew it for a few hours, and strain and drink it. Dr. Aviva Romm advises drinking it hot or cold, 1/4 to one cup, every four hours, increasing the dose depending on the severity of your symptoms. For bladder pain, spasm, and cramping, she recommends one to two dropperfuls each of cramp bark and wild yam tincture, every 2-4 hours for the first 24 hours, then every 4-6 hours for the next 24 hours. You can also take oil of oregano, one capsule, three times daily to treat the infection.

When to Call

Consult your practitioner if you do not notice any improvement by 24 hours and full resolution of symptoms within three to five days after following the above suggestions or if you start to feel ill and develop such symptoms as:

- High fever
- Shaking chills
- Sweats
- Muscle aches
- Marked weakness and exhaustion
- Low back or flank pain
- Severe abdominal pain
- Headaches
- Nausea and vomiting
- Increased burning pain or persistent blood in the urine.

Under these circumstances, you may need antibiotics for a more serious infection. Always contact your practitioner if you feel consistent cramping, contractions, or hardening of the uterus (over four per hour), lower back ache or pelvic pressure, or bleeding or fluid leaking from the vagina, as these may be signs of labor.

Healthy nonpregnant women may wait 48 hours of trying the natural remedies before reaching out to a professional if the burning pain is slight, the frequent urination is mild, and there are no other symptoms.

Ideally, get a urine culture before medical treatment to not only confirm or rule out a urinary tract infection, but also to determine what organism is responsible and what antibiotic it is sensitive to. If you must take antibiotics, take the full course even after you feel better. Eliminate sugar intake and eat, drink, and take probiotics that contain Saccharomyces boulardii, two capsules, twice daily, for six to eight weeks after you finish the antibiotics to restore the balance of healthy bacteria in your body, prevent a vaginal yeast infection, and minimize stomach upset. And continue to follow the above suggestions. Drink kombucha, eat lacto-fermented natural probiotic foods and the prebiotics that they feed on (like simple vegetable starches such as white rice and potatoes, and beans). You may need to eliminate inflammatory foods like gluten, sugar, cow dairy, and those that are genetically modified. Others require additional dietary changes and supplements like aloe, beta-glucan, curcumin, licorice in the form of DGL and L-glutamine. Avoid exposure to certain medications that can disrupt the gut and its balance of flora such as non-steroidal anti-inflammatories (like ibuprofen), hormonal contraceptives, stomach acid-blocking drugs (like Prilosec) and additional antibiotics, unless in cases of life-threatening infections.

Do another follow-up urine culture after you complete the natural treatment or prescription medication and every trimester if you are pregnant or have a history of recurrent UTIs to make sure the infection has been successfully eradicated and does not recur (which can happen, even though you do not feel symptoms).

VAGINITIS: NATURAL PREVENTION AND TREATMENT

Just about every woman is susceptible to vaginitis, or vaginal infection, at some point in her life. But not every vaginal symptom is related to an infection. Sometimes it is simply a sign of normal changes in a woman's cycle or pregnancy. Other times it is related to temporary inflammation, local irritation, allergy to latex condoms, or another cause. There is much to learn about your vagina and how to keep it healthy and feeling well.

Discharge changes in response to the changing hormonal environment throughout the menstrual cycle. For example, women notice an increased amount of clear to cloudy, odorless, slimy, egg-white discharge around the time of ovulation to help the sperm reach and fertilize the egg. The hormones of pregnancy also cause an increase in normal vaginal discharge, as well as an alteration in the acid/base balance of the vagina. This can lead to an imbalance of normally occurring microorganisms and, thus, an increase in susceptibility to vaginal infections (especially yeast).

The normal reduction of hormones during breastfeeding, and more dramatically after menopause, cause the vaginal walls to become thinner and dryer. This makes the area more prone to becoming sore (especially during sexual intercourse), irritated, and prone to yeast infections. Allow time for the normal increase in vaginal secretions during sexual arousal before penetration, and use all-natural, water-soluble lubricants or Astro-glide. Menopausal women may want to consider the option of bioidentical all-natural hormonal vaginal cream.

Possible Culprits for Vaginitis

The vaginal area is sensitive and can easily become irritated (look red, burn, and/or itch) for a variety of reasons. Most commonly, this is from substances within a new product that you or your sexual partner is using, such as:

- Detergent, fabric softener, or bleach
- Chemically scented body soap or bath oil, powder, or lotion
- Douches, deodorant, vaginal sprays, and perfumes
- Tight clothing
- Synthetic underwear or pantyhose
- Colored or perfumed toilet paper
- Conventional pads and tampons
- Vigorous and frequent sexual intercourse (more than three times in 24 hours)
- Foreign objects in the vagina, such as contraceptive devices, spermicidal cream, foam, jelly, medication applied locally, dildos, and vibrators
- Bubble baths, hot tubs, and prolonged or frequent immersion in a swimming pool
- Hanging out in a wet bathing suit
- Horseback riding or cycling.

Eliminate these irritants one by one to see if your symptoms improve. Buy a mild natural detergent without bleach (such as those made for infant clothes), or use an extra rinse in your laundry cycle. Use cornstarch rather than talc-based powder to keep dry. Buy white, unscented toilet paper, and avoid perfumed toiletries and feminine hygiene products. Try using a menstrual cup or go organic and green with your pads and tampons.

Imbalance of normal bacteria another common cause of vaginal infections that is often associated with frequent sexual intercourse and other factors that upset the normal balance of the vaginal flora (such as routine douching and medications like antibiotics, steroids, and synthetic hormones) and results in an overgrowth of organisms like

Gardnerella (bacterial vaginosis). It occurs in all women, even those in a mutually monogamous relationship, as it is not believed to be sexually transmitted. It is often associated with sex, and a gut lining disruption and healthy gut flora imbalance (from inflammatory foods, toxic exposures, chronic stress, and medications such as those above, plus non-steroidal anti-inflammatory drugs, and protein pump inhibitors that block stomach acid)

Conventional medicine recommends bacterial vaginosis should be treated with prescription medication in pregnancy as it has been implicated in the premature rupture of membranes, preterm labor, and uterine infection postpartum. It carries risks for all women, namely increased susceptibility to other more serious sexually transmitted and genital tract infections, as well as reproductive disorders from ectopic pregnancy and fertility issues, to pelvic inflammatory disease. Men generally do not have symptoms, same-sex partners can absolutely have symptoms, but all partners should be treated simultaneously, so they do not reinfect their spouse. A vaginal antibiotic is preferable to an oral antibiotic to minimize aggravating gut dysbiosis, but both are short-term Band-Aids that may or may not work, and recurrence is common, so it is important to address root causes and follow the prevention and natural treatment suggestions of lifestyle medicine below for a more effective long-term solution.

A vaginal infection caused by the trichomonas protozoa is most often sexually transmitted when there is more than one sexual partner. However, less commonly it can be caused by anal-vaginal contact, sitting on a dirty, wet toilet seat, being splashed with dirty toilet water, using communal baths or hot tubs, and sharing moist, contaminated clothing, washcloths, or towels.

This type of infection also needs treatment in pregnancy as it has been associated with complications similar to bacterial vaginitis. Your sexual partner should be treated simultaneously to avoid recurrences in you, even though they may be without symptoms. If you have a trichomonas infection, you should be screened for other more serious sexually transmitted infections and protect yourself by having a mutually monogamous sexual relationship, abstinence from intercourse if you or your partner are not monogamous, or at least by using latex or effective latex--free condoms (with spermicide containing nonoxynol-9 if you want to prevent pregnancy as well).

Vaginitis Prevention

Unless you have an actual vaginal infection or are prone to one, you should avoid routine douching (especially in pregnancy), as it washes out the natural secretions and organisms that normally reside in the vagina. Further, it alters the delicate acid-base balance there that actually protects you from infection. The only exception is if you are **NOT pregnant** and **treating an actual confirmed infection,** or are **prone to recurrent vaginal infections and nothing else is working.**

If you are pregnant, you can certainly acidify your system by drinking unsweetened cranberry juice diluted in other fruit juices to reduce the sour taste or add a scoop of cranberry juice powder to your smoothies, oatmeal, or yogurt. You can also take powdered cranberry juice concentrate in capsule form, like Cranactin (one capsule, twice daily). Combine one tablespoon of apple cider vinegar, the juice of half a fresh lemon, and honey to taste in a cup of hot water, and drink several cups daily.

Calendula cream or diluted tincture, or aloe vera gel applied morning and night helps strengthen vaginal tissues, heal minor abrasions, relieve pain, and discourage infection. You can spread some of the gel onto a menstrual pad and wear it throughout the day.

Change tampons and pads at each bathroom visit, and do not wear one for more than eight hours at a time. Avoid tampons during scant menstrual flow and a vaginal infection. Or switch to menstrual cups.

Wear cotton crotch stockings, loose clothing, and organic cotton underwear changed daily. Even better, skip the underwear altogether and go panty-free, especially during sleep, to allow for air circulation and to keep the area dry and hostile to infectious organisms. As soon as practical, change out of wet bathing suits and sweaty clothing.

You and your partner each need to wash the genital area daily with a mild soap, rinse, and dry well. Always wipe yourself from the front (vagina) towards the back (anus) to avoid contamination from the bowel. Avoid painful or abrasive sex and sexual practices that involve the anal/rectal area.

Don't share unwashed bathtubs, towels, washcloths, contraceptives, or douching equipment. Avoid reinfection by not reusing washcloths, towels, and underwear that have not been laundered. And don't sit on public toilets, either squat or put paper on the seat before sitting.

Maintain health and general resistance to infection by staying well-hydrated and eating a nourishing and wholesome diet as discussed in the chapter on nutrition. If you are prone to recurrent vaginal infections, you may find the best results by completely avoiding cane sugar, fruit juices, dairy, gluten, and alcohol, in additional to other gut-disrupting inflammatory foods.

Eat more fresh garlic (a few cloves daily sautéed, baked, crushed into salads, or added to cooked vegetables) and Asian mushrooms (like shiitake, reishi, and maitake) to boost your immune system. Take a good all-natural, food-based multivitamin, mineral, and probiotic supplement to ensure you are getting full nourishment beyond what is supplied by diet alone. Limit exposure to harmful chemicals and toxins (this also includes those found in drugs, cigarettes, food, water, cosmetics, toiletries, and household products). Please refer to the chapter "Nutritional Best Practices for Mom" for specific diet and supplement recommendations.

Be sure to get enough sleep, and exercise for 30 minutes, 5 days per week.

The mind, body, and heart are intricately connected and when out of balance, dis-ease can result: physical or emotional. Make a conscious effort to improve your emotional state and reaction to stress by mastering your ability to keep internal calm no matter what the circumstances (especially when there is no imminent danger). Surround yourself as much as possible with people, things, sounds, and places that inspire, relax, and restore you and limit your exposure to things and people that agitate your mind and create negativity.

Natural Treatment for Vaginitis

If you develop an unusual change in the amount, color, consistency, or odor in your vaginal discharge with itching, burning, and/or soreness, you may have a vaginal infection. The following natural remedies are quite effective against vaginal infections and are often safer than prescriptions (especially in pregnancy). They can certainly be used in the early stages of your symptoms without having to know the responsible organism. Many of the treatments mentioned below can be adapted to your sexual partner.

It is best to avoid intercourse and oral sex until the vaginal infection has cleared up, as the area is uncomfortable, irritated, and needs time to heal. And it is possible to pass the infection to your partner unless you are using condoms.

Wash the genitals after urinating and after sex as the associated fluids can aggravate the situation (squirt yourself from front to back with a peri-bottle filled with warm water and any of the herbs or herbal combinations mentioned below). Wash undergarments in hot water, disinfect tubs, and soak your diaphragm, douche equipment, and sex toys in vinegar.

If you are not pregnant, while reclining in the empty bathtub, use a vinegar douche once daily until the symptoms improve, for seven to ten days. You can make your own by mixing 1/4 part apple cider vinegar with 3/4 part warm water in a reusable douche bag. A douche of cranberry juice concentrate (one tablespoon to one quart of water) is also very effective to acidify the vaginal environment and discourage the growth of infectious organisms, as is a solution of pure, all-natural grapefruit seed extract used as directed. If the acidic applications are too irritating, try douching with two tablespoons of baking soda to one cup of water instead. A douche of 1.5 tablespoons of tea tree oil to one cup of warm water, two to three times per day is a very effective anti-fungal, as are tea tree oil vaginal suppositories.

If you are prone to recurrent yeast infections, especially after sex, antibiotics, or a known trigger, you can use a lower dose vinegar douche once to ensure the vagina is mildly acidic and hostile to unwanted bacteria. To make the douche, combine two tablespoons of apple cider vinegar, white vinegar, or pure lemon juice with a pint of warm water. Again, routine douching for general hygiene is not recommended, as it is actually harmful and increases the risk of genital tract infection.

If you are pregnant or simply prefer not to douche, you can acidify the vagina with a vaginally inserted ActiGel, Vitanica vaginal suppository, or you can put a few cups of pure apple cider vinegar in your bath water or a 1/2 cup of vinegar in a warm sitz bath. Either way, soak for 15-20 minutes several times a day. Another effective option is to apply 600 mg of encapsulated pharmacy-grade boric acid suppositories inserted high in the vagina for one to two weeks (although ideally not during pregnancy).

Add Aveeno powder (oatmeal) or a few drops of the essential oils of calendula, chamomile, or lavender to the bathwater and sitz bath to help soothe symptoms of itching and irritation, and to the peri-bottle of water for use after the bathroom. You can also add tea tree, sandalwood, and/or thyme oil to help fight the infection.

One of my integrative OB/GYN role models, Dr. Christiane Northrup, in addition to many other holistic functional medicine practitioners, advises increasing certain fermented foods rich in healthy bacteria for both bacterial vaginosis and yeast vaginitis, to restore your gut and vaginal flora. Drink kombucha and eat lactose-fermented foods like kimchi, sauerkraut, and pickles with simple prebiotic starches like white rice, potatoes, and beans. Take a multi-organism, high-colony-count probiotic for women orally as directed that includes the strains Lactobacillus reuteri and Lactobacillus rhamnosus. A reputable brand is, Greens First Female Women's Health Probiotic. You can also place one to two capsules high in the vagina in the morning and before going to sleep for two weeks. If you are not pregnant, a few live culture tablets can be dissolved in one quart of water to be used as a douche once daily for a week, then every other day for a week, then twice weekly for a few more weeks (you can alternate this with your vinegar douche).

Apply plain live-culture yogurt to the affected areas and vagina as needed to help relieve itching, inflammation, and restore the normal bacterial environment in the vagina. Put a few tablespoons of yogurt on your finger and smear it inside the walls of your vagina and around your cervix, or use a vaginal applicator to insert the yogurt. Repeat twice daily during an infection and a few times weekly if you are prone to recurrences. You can also dilute 16 ounces of yogurt in the water for a sitz bath (Yuck! But it works!).

Garlic suppositories are also effective. To use, insert a peeled, un-nicked clove lubricated with olive oil high up into your vagina for a few weeks before bed and in the morning. You can wrap it in a thin layer of gauze with a tail for retrieval, but it is not necessary as it will eventually come out itself in your discharge. Don't worry—it can't get lost or travel further up past your vagina, which is a dead end.

Wet compresses of burrows solution can be soothing to irritated skin— apply externally only. Comfrey root powder, slippery elm powder, and marshmallow root powder will also soothe dry, itchy vaginal tissue, relieve irritated and inflamed tissue, and promote healthy skin growth. Goldenseal root powder is effective for treating the actual infection and enhancing your immune response. You can apply each powder or an equal part mixture directly to the vulva and vagina daily for one to two weeks. You can make your own healing compress by mixing one tablespoon of any of the herbal powders with one cup of warm water. Dip gauze pads in to make the compresses and apply. You can also soak a menstrual pad and wear it throughout the day.

Apply healing and soothing salves that contain chickweed, calendula, and/or plantain to relieve itching, reduce inflammation, and discourage infection. Also, use topical vitamin E oil to decrease itching and help heal sore inflamed skin.

Some find it helpful to apply fresh raw honey for its anti-fungal properties and to moisturize and heal tender tissue (Sticky!).

You can drink burdock root, chickweed, and dandelion root teas, but an herbal combination infusion or tincture is more effective to reduce inflammation and infection. You can make your own by steeping a handful of each dandelion root, chickweed, and burdock root into a quart of boiling water, brew covered for a few hours, strain in a glass jar, and drink one to two cups daily. You can add fresh lemon or lime juice, mint leaves, or a dash of honey to taste. If you prefer the tincture, take one to two dropperfuls each of burdock root, chickweed, and dandelion root tinctures, one to three times per day.

For any infection, you can always use Gaia's Echinacea Supreme tincture (one to two dropperfuls every few hours), Host Defense's combination of Asian mushrooms (one to two capsules each daily), and garlic to kill unwanted germs as well as stimulate your own immune system. Take them at the earliest sign of infection. Make sure your diet and multivitamin are sufficient in vitamins C, E, D, B complex, and A with mixed carotenoids, selenium, and omega-threes.

If you are not pregnant, you can take additional immune-boosting supplements:

- Vitamin C—1,000 mg, three to four times per day
- Zinc—25-50 mg, every day
- Vitamin E—400-800 IU, each day
- Vitamin B complex—50 mg, three times daily until the infection has cleared
- If you are prone to frequent infection, you may want to consider daily supplements in addition to a multivitamin to enhance immunity. Good options are encapsulated oil of oregano, olive leaf, goldenseal, as well as oral, all-natural grapefruit seed extract, as directed. If you are pregnant, the remedies and doses in the cold and flu chapter are a safer option to combat infection and boost immunity.

For those who have recurrent vaginal infections not helped by these suggestions, at the first onset of symptoms and around the time you usually get the symptoms (for example, after sex, antibiotics, your period, swimming, certain stresses), apply vaginally as directed RePhresh vaginal gel (up to every three days) or a vaginal Prebiotic.

Natural Treatment Specific for Yeast and Bacterial Vaginosis Infection

Yeast and bacterial vaginosis infections both occur more frequently under the following circumstances:

- During pregnancy
- After menopause
- With increased stress
- Use of certain medications that disrupt gut lining and the healthy balance of flora (such as antibiotics, steroids, hormones, and even acid-blocking and non-steroidal anti-inflammatory drugs)
- A diet high in simple sugar, refined carbohydrates, alcohol, and inflammatory foods
- Frequent or regular douching
- Wearing synthetic, tight underwear, thongs, pantyhose, and using conventional menstrual products laden with toxic chemicals and synthetic fragrances
- Toxic exposures to chemicals in our food, water, body and cleaning products, anemia, obesity, diabetes, and other medical conditions that increase blood sugar and/or alter the normal environment in the gut and vagina, cause chronic inflammation, or suppress the immune system.

As mentioned, avoid cane sugar, dairy, gluten, and synthetic yeast, and limit fruit juice and jam until the problem has cleared up. Eat more fresh vegetables (especially the dark green ones, raw garlic and onion, turnips, and cabbage), quality protein, and complex carbohydrates (like brown rice, quinoa, kasha, and millet). Some report success by following the yeast-free or anti-candida diet, which is very strict and unclear that it makes a difference or worth the trouble. And do a healthy full-body detox, like with Bentonite clay. See a naturopath or holistic nutritionist for additional guidance.

For vaginal candida, you can take homeopathic Yeast Guard internally, insert homeopathic vaginal suppositories or Yeast Arrest by Vitanica vaginally as directed and apply it externally as well, all safe in pregnancy.

Consult a classical homeopath who can prescribe a homeopathic oral remedy specific to your individual symptoms if you are without relief or you get recurrent infections.

Drink pau d'arco tea (three cups per day), use the superfood powder in cooking, and/or insert tampons soaked in the extract vaginally and change every 12 hours. It has antifungal and antibacterial properties. If you are not pregnant, take pau d'arco capsules, 500mg, two to four, once or twice daily. You can also use it in your douche (one part strong tea to three parts warm water) or douche with a half teaspoon of goldenseal powder to one cup warm water, one to two times per day.

Dr. Aviva Romm and many integrative practitioners recommend supplements to support your adrenals and stress response, especially if you are getting recurrent infections related to increased stress and overwork so common in modern times.

If all else fails, for yeast, you can use diluted gentian violet painted locally for more stubborn cases (yes, it temporarily stains everything bluish purple), or contact your provider for prescriptive medications (ideally after the first trimester of pregnancy). Frequent use of antifungal creams such as Monistat and Gyne-Lotrimin sold over the counter in grocery or drugstores is discouraged, for they are not strong enough and can promote the growth of less common yeast strains, leading to recurrent or persistent infections. Your sexual partner will need treatment only if symptomatic or if you are otherwise healthy but suffer from chronic or repeated episodes.

Please consult your practitioner if the above-mentioned suggestions do not help or if your symptoms become worse, do not clear up after one to two weeks, or recur frequently. And certainly if you develop:

- Lower abdominal pain
- Fever
- Vaginal bleeding or spotting
- Heavier or more painful periods
- Unusual lumps or sores

- Sexual contact with someone suspected of having syphilis, gonorrhea, chlamydia, herpes, warts or HPV, or HIV infection
- Bleeding, regular contractions or cramping, low pelvic or back pressure, or leaking fluid with pregnancy.

Aside from being uncomfortable, untreated yeast infection is not dangerous, but if it occurs close to delivery, it can increase the chance of newborn thrush and subsequent yeast infection of the breastfeeding nipples.

CONSTIPATION DURING PREGNANCY: RELIEF MEASURES AND NATURAL REMEDIES

Constipation during pregnancy is caused mainly by:

- Hormones slowing down digestion
- The growing uterus pressing on the intestines
- Dehydration
- Certain medications
- Some iron supplements such as ferrous sulfate
- Lack of exercise
- Internal tension
- Lax abdominal muscle tone
- A diet made up of mostly refined, highly processed carbohydrates (white flours and sugars), refined or partially hydrogenated vegetable oils, and not enough natural fiber.

Establishing regular bathroom habits and responding to the urge to have a bowel movement, instead of ignoring or delaying, will help train your body for proper elimination. Set aside uninterrupted and unrushed bathroom time. Elimination normally follows the morning meal by half an hour. Plan accordingly so you do not have to rush. Ensure an ample supply of reading material by the toilet to enhance relaxation.

Support your feet on a low stool while sitting on the toilet and avoid straining, which can lead to hemorrhoids. Squat with your feet on the toilet seat or a squatting stool.

Get regular exercise for at least 30 minutes, 5 days per week. Try to do specific exercises to tone your abdominal muscles a few times each week. Good options are prenatal yoga, Pilates, Julie Tupler's Maternal Fitness Program, and gym equipment modified for pregnancy.

A Significant Factor in Constipation: Your Diet

Consider making some dietary adjustments to ease your constipation. Try to eliminate from your diet refined grain products made with white wheat, spelt, or rye flour (like white bread, noodles, cookies, cakes, pretzels, and cold cereal), white rice, and canned or overcooked fruits and vegetables without edible skins. Eat more fiber-rich foods such as organic, sprouted whole-multi-grain bread, cereal, and pasta, and fresh, raw, lightly steamed, or sautéed vegetables, fresh or dried fruits (with edible skins when possible), nuts, seeds, and beans.

People who shift to mostly whole-plant foods are often amazed by the great improvement in their bowel habits.

During an episode of constipation, mix two tablespoons of 100% unprocessed ground flaxseed and two to three tablespoons of wheat or oat bran into hot cereal, applesauce, or yogurt. Daily snack on prunes, raisins, and figs, and add a large portion of fresh leafy greens to your lunch and dinner. Enjoy your greens lightly steamed, sautéed, or raw in a tossed salad.

Drink plenty of pure water each day.

Juice fresh vegetables, including a variety of leafy greens, especially spinach.

A natural laxative home remedy can be made by soaking or stewing four to six dried pitted prunes in one cup of boiling apple or pear juice. Add one tablespoon of ground flaxseed or gluten-free oat bran, and let sit for 15 minutes. Ingest the mixed combination one to two times per day, when you get up in the morning and early evening.

Hot tea or other warmed liquids on an empty stomach or between meals does wonders. Try:

- Warmed prune juice
- A half to a whole lemon squeezed in water sweetened with a dash of honey or a tablespoon of blackstrap molasses
- Hot soup broth
- One cup of green or black tea
- One cup of caffeinated coffee (only occasionally)
- One cup of Smooth Move tea if you are not pregnant. It's delicious and very effective.

Breathwork for Constipation During Pregnancy

Try taking brief breaks at least three times per day to practice relaxation techniques, such as meditation, breathwork, visualization, and yoga nidra/progressive muscle relaxation. Make it a regular part of your daily routine to practice them, even just for 15-20 minutes. This will help disengage your consciousness from thought, increase inner calm, and lessen inner tension. See the chapters on breathwork and stress reduction for more details.

Support Digestion with Herbs and Supplements

Natural supplements that have harmless laxative effects include vitamin C with bioflavonoids, 1,000 mg (safe in this amount until 36 weeks of pregnancy, then reduce to 500 mg per day) and magnesium glycinate or citrate, 400-600 mg. Floradix makes a tasty liquid magnesium, one capful, one to two times per day as needed. Peter Gilham's powdered Natural Calm is another tasty form of magnesium that you add to hot water. The benefit of the liquid or powder is that you can adjust the dose a little lower if your stools are too loose and frequent, or higher if you do not feel the laxative effect.

If you are anemic and an iron supplementation is needed, use herbal sources, such as red raspberry and nettle infusions, Floradix iron, or yellow dock root. Avoid ferrous sulfate found in most pharmacies, as not only is it not well-absorbed or tolerated, it is very constipating. Refer to the chapter on anemia for more details.

Here's a recipe for an effective herbal remedy for anemia and constipation:

1. Add a generous pinch each of dandelion and yellow dock root to a quart of boiling water.
2. Soak for at least four hours.
3. Strain in a glass jar.
4. Add one to two tablespoons of blackstrap molasses.
5. Add the juice of lemon or lime, fresh mint leaves, cinnamon, or honey to taste.
6. Drink several times throughout the day, or boil it down to make more of a syrup, chill in fridge, and take one to two spoonfuls daily as needed.

If you are not pregnant, try an Indian herbal capsule of three fruits called Triphala.

If necessary, try over-the-counter bulk laxatives, such as Citrucel, Metamucil, or powdered psyllium seed husks. If your bowel movements are very hard, painful and straining, causing hemorrhoids or making them worse, try a stool softener like docusate sodium (Colace), 100mg, one to three times per day. This is only a temporary fix without addressing the root causes, as the solution will come by the lifestyle and diet changes recommended here, when you are otherwise healthy.

Avoid reliance on enemas, laxatives, and colonics, as they can lead to dependency, vitamin deficiencies, and abdominal cramping among other problems, and may stimulate labor prematurely. If you are desperate and not pregnant, you can try a natural laxative like rhubarb root commonly found in the health food store.

Avoid smoking and other stimulant drugs, as well as addictive regular caffeinated coffee drinking.

Take a homeopathic remedy specific for your symptoms of constipation. Consult with a classical homeopath, or refer to an excellent homeopathy reference book.

Other alternatives that are especially helpful if none of the above suggestions work include biofeedback and acupuncture.

If none of the above remedies prove to be helpful, if you have not had a bowel movement in over four days, you have severe or unusual pain, your constipation is alternating with diarrhea, you have rectal bleeding, or your stools are the color of old blood, call your provider.

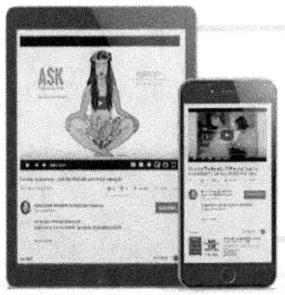

Want to learn more or have more questions?

Grab your free Book Bonuses below:
https://homesweethomebirth.com/nbsbookbonus

Varicose Veins and Hemorrhoids in Pregnancy: Natural Remedies and Relief

Varicose veins are enlarged and often prominent, bluish, and bulging vessels that have been stretched and weakened, such that blood accumulates in them rather than flowing back to the heart. They can often result in dull aching cramps and a sensation of heaviness in the legs.

Varicose Veins in Pregnancy

In pregnancy, varicose veins are caused by a combination of:

- Hormones that relax the vessel walls and increase blood volume
- The pressure of the growing uterus, impairing the return of venous blood to the heart from the lower body
- An inherited tendency or history of weakness of veins and their valves in previous pregnancies
- Inactivity and poor leg muscle tone
- Prolonged periods of sitting or standing
- Excess weight gain and obesity.

Simple Tricks and Tips

Avoid strong spices, such as cayenne, mustard, black pepper, hot sauces and curries, coffee (even decaffeinated), alcohol, smoking, and sweet clover tea, as they can aggravate the problem.

While sitting or lying in a comfortable, quiet place, take some slow, deep abdominal breaths until your mind is quiet. Then visualize your blood flowing easily through your veins in your legs, back up to your heart, without any resistance. Imagine your varicose veins getting smaller and smaller, then eventually resolving. See yourself as healthy and strong. This can be easily added to your regular meditation practice.

A daily five-minute leg massage, working hard, deep, and up with the flow of the veins does wonders for prevention. But NEVER massage the leg if you have significant varicosities, or you notice an area of hardness, heat, redness, or swelling.

Body Positioning

Avoid prolonged periods of standing still or sitting, especially with your legs crossed. If you need to be sitting for a long time, take frequent breaks every hour to get up and walk around, squat, rotate your feet, and point and flex your toes.

If you need to be sitting or on your feet for a while, periodically rest with your legs elevated above the level of your chest while keeping your back straight. Or lie down on your side at least for 30 minutes, twice a day.

Don't sit on chairs that press into the backs of your thighs. Make sure your feet can be flat on the floor, a stool, or a book, with your thighs completely free while sitting.

Raise the end of your bed six to eight inches with bricks or a block of wood to create a slight elevation and help drain your lower body of excess blood volume when you sleep. Or you can simply put a few firm pillows under your feet.

Exercise regularly for 30 minutes, 5 days per week to develop healthy muscle tone in your legs and keep the blood circulating, in addition to helping you maintain a normal weight. Inverted yoga postures, such as bridge, legs up the wall, headstand, and shoulder stand, modified for pregnancy, are also helpful in relieving pressure on the lower veins. You can use the wall for support. Props like yoga blankets, bolsters, or blocks can be used to make the postures more accessible, passive, comfortable, and restorative.

Clothing Considerations

Wear loose clothing, and avoid restrictive pants and knee highs that go partway up the leg and constrict the flow of blood back to the upper body. Wear low-heeled or flat, comfortable shoes.

Each day, apply maternity supportive compression leggings or stockings before getting out of bed in the morning and after elevating your legs a bit. Women with significant varicosities need to wear open-toed porous stockings that supply at least 30 mmHg and up to 50 mmHg of graduated pressure. Start using them early in pregnancy before the problem worsens and continue through six weeks postpartum. Some stockings come with gloves to help put them on. If not, a little cornstarch on the legs and dishwashing gloves may help slide them on.

Diet

Every day eat a variety of foods that nourish the blood vessels such as:

- Dark leafy greens
- Kelp
- Beets
- Okra
- Citrus fruits
- Strawberries and blackberries
- Apricots
- Black currants
- Plums and prunes
- Grapes
- Cherries
- Cantaloupe
- Broccoli
- Asparagus
- Avocado
- Alfalfa sprouts
- Tomatoes
- Green peppers

- Carrots
- Squash
- Sweet potatoes
- Fresh parsley
- Buckwheat
- Oats, wheat germ, quinoa, and other whole grains
- Nuts
- Brewers or nutritional yeast
- Eggs
- Fish
- Organ meats.

Use lots of fresh garlic, onions, ginger, and turmeric in your cooking.

Avoid excessive weight gain and constipation, as this will aggravate varicosities.

Eat clean, whole, organic foods and avoid the toxic, highly processed products as discussed in the chapter on nutrition.

Limit excess sodium by simply salting to taste and avoiding processed foods that are high in sodium additives.

Eat a bulb of fresh garlic daily. You can make it delicious by roasting or sautéing the whole cloves in olive oil, salt, pepper, and a dash of parsley. If you prefer raw garlic, eat two cloves twice daily, crushed into your salad or cut and swallow as a pill and continue until a week after you are all better.

A great way to incorporate olive oil and raw garlic into your daily foods is to peel and soak a crushed bulb in one cup of cold expeller-pressed extra virgin olive oil, and let sit for a couple of days. The final product can be used on salads, veggies, beans, sprouted whole-grain breads and pastas. Another option is to take a capsule of supercritical fresh, organic garlic, one to two capsules daily as directed with eight ounces of water per capsule.

Herbs and Supplements

If you are interested in herbs, take a standardized extract of horse chestnut, or in higher doses for more severe cases, like Venistat, use as directed on the bottle. If you are not pregnant and otherwise healthy, take butcher's broom as directed on the bottle.

Nettle and oatstraw are herbs known to strengthen the vascular system, lessen varicosities, and prevent them from feeling uncomfortable and swollen. Drink one to four cups daily of the organic combination in an infusion, according to how severe and extensive your varicosities are. To make your own infusion:

1. Soak a generous handful of dried nettle leaf and a large pinch of oatstraw in one quart boiling water for two hours.
2. Strain to a canning jar.
3. Add a dash of honey, lemon or lime juice, or fresh mint leaves to taste.
4. Drink hot or cold.

Alternate the following herbal external applications, two to three times daily. Some find cold or frozen compresses more helpful than warm or room temperature as it causes constriction of the blood vessels. Drench a washcloth or towel in witch hazel and wrap the affected areas for 20 minutes and alternate with a cloth or towel soaked in raw apple cider vinegar. If you prefer the frozen option, you can make several in advance and store them in the freezer.

You can add to your compresses comfrey, yarrow, oak bark, calendula, don quai, bayberry bark, and/or mullein to help relieve aching and swelling, and tighten the distended veins. There are wonderful herbal combination salves for varicose veins and hemorrhoids in many health food stores and holistic apothecaries like mine. Experiment with one at a time or in combination, and use what works best for you. Take the homeopathic remedy hamamelis 30 c, three times per day.

Make sure you are taking your daily supplements including whole-food prenatal multivitamins, minerals, and essential fatty acids to ensure that you are getting all the nourishment you need that cannot be derived by a healthy diet alone, covered more extensively in the chapter on "Nutritional Best Practices for Mom." In addition, each day take:

- 1,000-1,500 mg of vitamin C with bioflavonoids until 36 weeks pregnant, then reduce to 500 mg
- 500 mg of rutin, one to two times per day
- Whole-food B-complex or 50 mg of vitamin B6, one to two times per day
- 500 mg of evening primrose, borage, black current, or flaxseed oil after the first trimester
- Kelp powder or capsules as directed on the container if you do not have hyperthyroidism or a sensitivity to iodine
- 200-600 IU of vitamin E until the seventh month if you are otherwise healthy, then taper to 400 IU
- 400 mg of magnesium.

For Varicose Veins in the Vulva (Genital Area)

Wear cool packs in your underwear as tolerated.

Support the area with a specialized supportive garment such as the belly band for vulvar varicosities. For added relief, place two frozen sanitary pads saturated with witch hazel held in place with the support band. You can add any of the above-mentioned herbs to your compress. Make up a bunch and store them in the freezer.

At work, take frequent rest periods to sit with your buttocks on a pillow and your hips elevated, or lie on your back against the wall and use the wall to elevate your legs and lower back as you walk your legs up it.

When home, get out your yoga mat. Using props to elevate your hips while in bridge or legs up the wall is especially helpful for vulvar varicosities. Legs up the wall or viparita karini is done lying down flat on your back with your buttocks all the way to the wall, or elevated on a folded yoga blanket, bolster, or block. Let your legs rest straight up the wall for 10-20 minutes. It is also a great opportunity for practicing quiet meditation, focusing on slow, deep breathing, and inner gazing between your eyebrows. A lavender-infused eye pillow adds to the yummy relaxation effect.

Do modified bridge alternating with legs up the wall, supporting your sacrum on a yoga block, for 10 minutes, twice a day. While doing bridge, practice strengthening your pelvic floor muscles using your mula bandha, or root lock, which is similar to kegel exercises but much more comprehensive and effective. As discussed previously, place another yoga block between your thighs. While inhaling, tilt your pelvis up toward your face as you slowly squeeze the block and draw your entire pelvic floor upward and inward, starting from its center. Hold as long as is comfortable, then release and return to resting your sacrum on the block as you exhale. Let the breathing be smooth, relaxed, and deep as you do this. It takes practice, but you will get it. Start with 25, twice per day, and work up to 50, twice per day.

Do lively and energetic pelvic tilts for 5 minutes, once or twice a day. Get on your yoga mat, and in the middle, lay a folded yoga blanket for extra knee padding. Tilt your pelvis up and down or forward and backward like when you do yoga cat and cow movements. But, focus more on the pelvis. It is very helpful to coordinate the movements with your breathing, such as inhaling when you do cow, exhaling when you do cat, or vice versa. Gradually make the movements stronger and faster, using your core by drawing your belly inward, corseting your ribs, and isometrically pulling your front pelvic bone towards your breastbone to protect your back. You can also circle your hips in both directions and do figure eights. You can do them lying on a rug or while standing by tilting your pelvis back and forth in the same way. Include some belly dancing-like figure-eight movements of your pelvis and have fun with it. Some good dance music can help you get into the rhythm!

When pushing during childbirth, make sure to be on your hands and knees, kneeling, or side-lying. Avoid squatting to lessen pressure on your veins.

For all types of varicose veins, consider consulting a professional homeopath or acupuncturist skilled in traditional Chinese medicine, osteopathic, or chiropractic care, especially if none of the above suggestions help and your problem is chronic.

Contact your provider if nothing seems to work or your leg has an area of hardness, heat, pain, redness, and/or swelling, as this could indicate inflammation or a clot formation.

Hemorrhoids in Pregnancy

Hemorrhoids during pregnancy are so common as to be considered normal, unless they cause symptoms that bother you (such as itching, pain, and bleeding). Here are some tips and tricks for preventing and reducing those irritating symptoms, and you can also refer to the above general suggestions and remedies for varicosities.

That is because hemorrhoids are varicose veins (enlarged blood vessels) that develop inside or just outside the anal area. They are caused by a combination of factors:

- Increased pressure on veins in the pelvic area from the growing uterus
- The hormones of pregnancy, which increase blood volume and relax the vessel walls, allowing them to distend and become congested
- An inherited tendency
- The pressure of gravity from being overweight or excessive weight gain in pregnancy
- Constipation and straining to push out a bowel movement

Hemorrhoids During Pregnancy—The Dos

ONE: Do eat the foods listed already in this chapter because they nourish the circulatory system. Follow the guidelines about eating lots of garlic and staying well hydrated.

TWO: Do keep moving. Exercise regularly for at least 30 minutes, five times per week.

For relieving pressure on the lower veins, do one of the inverted yoga postures and exercises explained above for 10-20 minutes, twice per day (come on, they're fun and a time for you to relax!).

THREE: Do take supplements. Please refer to the supplement recommendations already given in this chapter.

FOUR: Do try and relax and use the power of visualization.

While sitting or lying in a comfortable, quiet place, take some slow, deep abdominal breaths until your mind is quiet. Then visualize your blood flowing easily through your veins in your anal area, back up to your heart, without any resistance. Imagine your varicose veins or hemorrhoids getting smaller and smaller, then eventually resolving. See yourself as healthy and strong. This can be easily added to your regular meditation practice.

FIVE: Do try some home remedies.

When experiencing a hemorrhoid flare-up, there are a number of natural home remedies available to ease your discomfort.

Wear a small soft icepack held in place close to the affected area by a belly band for vulvar varicosities.

Applying local herb-infused compresses to the area can be very soothing and healing. You can make your own by soaking a small cloth or round pad to make a compress with the essential oils of lavender or frankincense. Make a bunch in advance and freeze them In a storage container. Also, try applying these and do regularly what feels best for you:

- Wet or dry baking soda to relieve itching
- Lemon juice or raw apple cider vinegar to reduce swelling or bleeding

- Raw potato to ease swelling and pain
- Garlic oil or a peeled clove of garlic inserted into the rectum overnight to reduce swelling
- A regular black tea bag, steeped in a little water for a few minutes, then squeezed to remove the water; apply it several times daily as a poultice to your hemorrhoids
- Pure aloe vera gel to reduce bleeding
- Herbal ointments containing comfrey to help reduce swelling, bleeding, and pain
- An herbal combination of plantain and yarrow ointment or salve to relieve pain and shrink hemorrhoids quickly
- Horse chestnut can be purchased in liquid form and made into a compress, especially in combination with plantain, witch hazel, and even pilewort and yellow dock root, which can be applied locally as often as needed. You can also add to your compresses yarrow, oak bark, calendula, don quai, bayberry bark, and/or mullein to help relieve aching and swelling, and tighten the distended veins. Any combination of these herbs can be used topically as a gel, salve, cream, or ointment
- Herbal combination creams like Dr. Cole's Hemorrhoid Treatment ointment that contain some of the above-mentioned herbs soothe and relieve hemorrhoids
- Already-made witch hazel compresses (known as Tucks in the pharmacy or Hamamelis as a homeopathic remedy in the health food section) to reduce inflammation and swelling
- Homeopathic or herbal hemorrhoidal ointment or cream throughout the day and before bowel movements to ease their passage

You can also wipe yourself with these compresses after a bowel movement instead of toilet paper, or moisten the toilet paper with liquid witch hazel. Smear the hemorrhoids with cream or soapy water and try to gently push them back inside. Then tighten your perineal muscles, your mula bandha, and practice kegel or pelvic floor exercises to help them stay in.

Try a soothing warm sitz bath for 15-20 minutes, followed by 1 minute of a cool sitz bath, four to six times per day. A sitz bath is a special shallow container designed to sit in that fits on most toilets and directs the water and healing herbs to the perineal and anal area.

You can add the above mentioned essential oils, herbs, or Epsom salts to the water. Most hemorrhoids will shrink after a few days of frequent herbal sitz baths. This herbal sitz bath will come in handy postpartum as well, to cleanse, soothe, and hasten healing.

Shine a red heat lamp to the affected area.

Use a pillow or cushion when you need to sit.

Sleep on your side.

Make sure when pushing during birth, to be on your hands and knees, kneeling, standing leaning forward, or side-lying, which lessens pressure on your hemorrhoids.

Hemorrhoids During Pregnancy—The Don'ts

When dealing with hemorrhoids, there are some foods and activities to avoid. For example, avoid the following:

- Excessive weight gain and constipation, as they will aggravate and contribute to rectal and anal varicosities
- Straining on the toilet or sitting in the squatting position for prolonged periods, as it increases pressure in the area and encourages hemorrhoids
- Highly processed and refined white flour products, foods that are high in sugar, refined vegetable oils, or partially hydrogenated fat and chemicals.
- Long periods of sitting or standing (try to rest on your side with your hips and legs elevated three times daily)
- Sitting on hard surfaces (instead, use an inflatable seat or cushion)
- Squatting or lithotomy position while pushing in labor.

Consuming the following can aggravate hemorrhoids:

- Cayenne
- Mustard
- Black pepper
- Hot sauces and curries
- Coffee (even decaffeinated)
- Alcohol
- Cigarette smoke.

Consult a professional homeopath or acupuncturist skilled in traditional Chinese medicine, osteopath, or chiropractor, especially if none of the above suggestions help and your problem is chronic.

Contact your provider if nothing seems to work or if you have severe pain, persistent bleeding, or firm lumps. Also, check with your provider before using any over-the-counter medication, as most drugs relieve symptoms without healing the problem and contain toxins like mercury or other substances that are not safe during pregnancy.

Natural Measures for Headache Treatment and Prevention

Nearly everyone gets a headache at one time or another. In fact, headaches account for more doctor's visits than any other health condition. The tension headache is the most common variety, which usually begins in the early afternoon or evening, and feels like a steady tight band around your head. The pain can sometimes radiate up your neck and the back of your head.

Headaches are common in pregnancy, as well as before your period, related to the effects of the changing hormones within your body. However, many women claim that pre-existing headaches like migraines often improve when they are pregnant.

On rare occasions, a headache can be caused by a serious health problem, especially when persistent, severe, or following an injury. If you are pregnant and developing high blood pressure, a headache could be a sign of a potentially dangerous condition known as preeclampsia, which must be prevented, ideally, and addressed promptly by your provider. However, in the majority of cases, a headache signals your body's reaction to a variety of stresses, such as:

- Overwork
- Emotional upset or worry
- Muscle tension
- Too much time on the computer or smart phone
- Not enough sleep
- Too much sleep
- Eye strain

- Improper posture
- Teeth grinding
- Strong sun or bright light
- Irritating stimulation like too much noise or a strong, unpleasant smell
- Feeling too hot or too cold
- Stuffy rooms
- Fluorescent lighting
- Motion sickness
- Nasal or sinus congestion
- Infection
- Low blood sugar
- Poor diet or overeating
- Dehydration
- Sensitivities to certain foods
- Exposure to toxic substances like tobacco, alcohol, caffeine, certain drugs and medications, chemicals, food preservatives, gases, fumes, pesticides, and even household cleaning and body products.

Headache Prevention

Minimize time online, especially time spent with addictive, stressful apps, social media, and computer games. Avoid things (like certain agitating movies, blasting hard rock, heavy metal or angry rap music, and the news) and people (like those who are angry, stressed out, negative, down, fearful, critical, or demanding) that agitate your mind and raise your internal tension. Surround yourself, as much as possible, with calm, centered people, things, sounds, and places that inspire you, relax you, allow you to feel at ease, and restore you to inner peace and serenity. For some, this means being around nature, beautiful art, soothing music, or close family and friends.

Learn how to recognize early sensations of emotional and muscular tension so that you can:

- Get out of the stressful situation for a few minutes until you are feeling calmer, and activate your relaxation response.
- Do some stretching and exercise activity like dancing to release the built-up tension and move emotional energy through the body.
- Practice slow, deep breathing or any of the breathwork exercises in the chapter on breathwork, as well as meditation, Qi Gong, Tai Chi, yoga (especially yin, prenatal, gentle, and restorative), progressive muscle relaxation techniques (yoga nidra), or prayer.
- Take a walk outside.
- Use natural light as much as possible, or lamps, and dimmer lighting when indoors.
- Take a relaxing bath with a few drops of lavender oil.
- Watch a funny movie or video.
- Read the chapter "Natural Stress Alleviation in Pregnancy and Beyond."

Conscious Relaxation

Notice habits of increased muscle tension, especially around your upper back, shoulders, neck, forehead, and jaw, and make an effort to release these tightened muscles while doing slow, deep abdominal breathing. Ask someone to massage these areas or treat yourself to regular massage therapy.

Get in the habit of taking a "healing interval" to do meditative breathwork for a few minutes several times each day using any of the techniques in the related chapter. It would be very beneficial to you if you could learn how to relax the muscles that are tensing up on your own. It is an essential skill for labor and can be used in any stressful situation. Set aside a 10-15-minute time slot, like during one or two of your "healing intervals," to focus on releasing all of your muscles.

Awareness and Care

Keep a written record of your headaches to increase your own awareness of situations in your life that precede your headaches, and make needed changes if possible. Sometimes it's as simple as:

- Taking a daily nap or just lying down for a few minutes with your eyes closed in a quiet room
- Getting a mother's helper for the afternoon or morning rush
- Making sure you don't forget to eat breakfast or lunch
- Deleting foods with monosodium glutamate and other chemical additives
- Getting some fresh air or moving away from cigarette smoke
- Saying "No," or "I'm sorry, but I can't help you this time," when you are overworked
- Having your eyes checked and getting new glasses.

Notice your posture when standing as well as when sitting. Make sure your back is straight and lifted, using your stomach muscles, your pelvis is tilted forward, and your shoulders are relaxed and down. Avoid high heels.

If your headaches are related to awkward posture and chronic muscle straining, you may benefit from osteopathy, acupuncture, and/or the Alexander or Rolfing deep massage technique, in addition to regular yoga practice.

Pay attention to your diet and don't skip meals, especially if you are pregnant. Drink plenty of clean water daily. Eat enough of a variety of healthy, ideally organic whole foods. Make sure you are eating at least 80 grams of protein daily. Avoid foods with lots of chemical additives, unhealthy fats, cane sugar, coffee, even decaffeinated, and all other products with caffeine, like soda, chocolate, and certain over-the-counter medications. Salt your food to taste with quality mineral-dense sea salt.

Small, frequent meals that include quality fat and protein and fresh whole foods are preferable to fewer large binges, to keep your blood sugar stable. If you are eating a carbohydrate like a fruit, starchy vegetable, like squash or sweet potatoes, or a grain, eat it with a protein or fat, like nuts, nut butter, meat, or dairy, to prevent the rapid rise, then drop in blood sugar that can cause headaches from eating high sugar and white flour foods. Take your prenatal supplements—including fish oil—to ensure you are getting the additional nourishment you need beyond what a healthy diet can provide. See the chapter on nutrition for more details. Make sure to take iron if you are anemic and prevent constipation as advised in these respective chapters so that you are having daily bowel movements to release, rather than reabsorb, toxic waste that can cause headaches and trigger migraines.

Get at least 30 minutes of moderate exercise, 5 times per week

Ensure you are getting 7-8 hours of sleep if not pregnant. If you are pregnant, aim for more sleep by going to bed earlier and/or waking later, as well as taking a short daily power nap. Even if you cannot sleep, lying down in *savasana* (yoga's corpse pose), focusing on your breath and gazing internally between your eyebrows for 20 minutes, will do the trick. Decrease length of naps if that's the culprit.

Natural Treatment for Headaches

Sinus Headaches

If your headache is related to a mild, infectious illness or the flu, refer to the chapter "Natural Remedies for Cold and Flu in Pregnancy." This includes a sinus infection, which is indicated by:

- A steady pain in your forehead
- Pain around your eyes and nose
- Postnasal drip
- Cough with thick sometimes yellow or green nasal congestion.

In this case, pay particular attention to increasing your fluid intake and liquefying your secretions with a humidifier or vaporizer during sleep, steam inhalation with essential oils, and nasal douching with a neti pot. Use plain nasal saline spray. Strengthen your immune system with lifestyle modification, herbs, supplements, and homeopathy. At the start of sinus trouble, put hot wet towels over your upper face for 15 minutes, three to four times per day, eliminate milk and all other dairy products, and avoid smoking. If your sinus headache is triggered by allergies, take stinging nettle herb in capsules or via infusion. You can make your own by steeping one large handful of dried nettle leaf in a quart of boiling water for at least four hours.

If the natural remedies do not help and your symptoms worsen or do not improve, please contact your practitioner. If your sinus headaches are chronic, they may be due to allergies, which are not covered in this chapter. However, osteopathy, acupuncture, homeopathy, and mind-body work can be very helpful, as well as working with an integrative or holistic physician.

Migraine Headache

If you get migraine headaches, which are usually felt as one-sided, severe, throbbing pain, often preceded by an "aura"-like visual disturbance and associated with nausea and vomiting, as well as intolerance to light, noise, and motion (and many other variant symptoms), there are things you can do to prevent them:

- Eliminate all coffee and caffeinated products during headache-free intervals.
- Note what else triggers your headaches and avoid them. Common triggers include:
    - Chocolate
    - Red and white wine
    - Strong-flavored aged cheese
    - Processed meats with nitrites
    - Fermented foods like soy sauce and miso, especially with monosodium glutamate

- Sardines, anchovies, and pickled herring
- Artificial sweeteners like aspartame
- Strong synthetic fragrances in perfumes, body care products, and incense
- Certain medications.

Keep a headache journal to help become more aware of what triggers your migraines, what makes them worse, and what makes them better, so you can be more aware and empowered to prevent them or treat them most effectively. You may benefit from doing an elimination diet for three weeks to see what common foods might be responsible.

At the first sign of a migraine, drink one to two cups of strong coffee, and drink a turmeric latte (recipe is the chapter about pain in pregnancy) and fresh ginger tea (recipe is in the chapter on nausea). Take 250 mg of ginger capsules up to four times daily. You can take 300-600 mg of curcumin if you are not pregnant, up to three times a day. Lie down in a dark room focusing on slow, deep breathing. For maintenance, Dr. Andrew Weil recommends taking the following daily for 1.5-2 months to notice your response:

- Magnesium—500 mg, one to two times per day
- Calcium—500 mg, one to two times per day
- Vitamin B2—400 mg daily
- Coenzyme Q10—100-150 mg, one to two times per day.

Get biofeedback training to master your autonomic nervous system and increase the temperature of your hands (a wonderful technique you can use to abort an attack). Do hypnotherapy with a trained professional to go beyond what is conscious and experience effective healing.

If you are NOT pregnant, take Petadolex's supercritical freeze-dried extract of butterbur, 50-100 mg, one to two times per day, that is free of toxic PAs, and feverfew, at least 100-150 mg, with at least 0.2% parthinolides, or a combination formula of these herbs. Dr. Aviva Romm additionally advises trying either melatonin, 3 mg or hydroxytryptophan, 200 mg every day, ideally taken before bed. It may take several weeks to months to notice the full benefit.

Dr. Andrew Weil suggests changing the way you think about your migraines: "View them as electrical storms in the head, violent and disruptive, but leading to a calm, clear state in the end. Let yourself have a headache once in a while. Be with your headache, as it's a good excuse to drop your usual routine and go inward, letting accumulated stress dissipate. As you come to accept them in this way and see them as serving a purpose in your life, you may not have them as often."

The Occasional Headache

To remedy the occasional headache...

- Eat a nutritious, wholesome snack with complex carbohydrates, protein, and a healthy fat.
- Drink 1-2 cups of pure water
- Get off the computer or smart phone and get some sun and fresh air.
- Lie down in a quiet place with your eyes closed, and take a nap if possible.
- Apply an iced or warm pack or a cool or warm dampened washcloth to the area that hurts.
- Rotate your head slowly and evenly around in each direction, lift your shoulders high and then lower them.
- Massage your aching muscles.
- Drink a relaxing herbal tea with lemon or lime juice, mint, or a dash of honey to taste. Repeat as needed throughout the day. Good choices include chamomile,lavender, lemonbalm, motherwort, hops, skullcap, catnip, and passionflower.

Massage your jaw, neck, shoulders, and temples with Tiger Balm alone, or almond oil blended with a few drops of each or any combination of your favorite essential oils of chamomile, vanilla, melissa, lavender, rose, geranium, frankincense, jasmine, marjoram, basil, citrus, sandalwood, rosemary, eucalyptus, peppermint, and/or neroli. You can also add them to your diffuser, into your relaxing, very warm Epsom salt bath by candlelight, in a spray bottle to sprinkle in your space, and onto your pillow if needed.

Try this healing visualization:

1. Choose a comfortable spot to sit or lie down for at least 15-20 minutes.
2. Close your eyes and focus internally between your eyebrows. Block out light with a soothing weighted lavender eye pillow, and mute sound with a noise-reducing earmuff headset.
3. Breathe in slowly from your abdomen, expanding your ribs and lungs up to your collarbone to a count of three or four.
4. Pause, then exhale to a count of three or four, and release all the tension in your body.
5. Repeat this cycle a few times, each time releasing more with each exhale.
6. Then, with each inhale and exhale, mentally direct your breath to your head, consciously healing your headache.
7. Imagine the pain and tension melting away down into the ground, or imagine a spiritual light shining on your head, filling you with light and releasing all the tension and head discomfort out into the surroundings.
8. Then imagine yourself sitting, reclining, walking, or floating on a cloud blissfully in your favorite place, where you feel the most joyful and relaxed, without any headache. Really visualize what it is like to be there and feel such relief, using all your senses.
9. When you feel calm and more comfortable, hang out there as long as you want.
10. When ready to return, transition slowly back to a peaceful, alert state of being.

Helpful herbs include the following. Try one at a time as indicated and see what works best for you. Tinctures are taken best in a small amount of water or followed by juice:

- Passionflower—you can take capsules with at least 0.8% flavonoids, as directed on bottle, two to three times per day as needed, or one to two dropperfuls of tincture, one to two times daily (after the first trimester)

- Ginger—especially effective at the earliest sign of a migraine or daily as prevention. Take one 250 mg capsule up to four times daily, or one to two dropperfuls of the tincture, once or twice per day.
- Skullcap tincture—one to two dropperfuls, capsules as directed, especially if your headache is keeping you from sleep.
- Chamomile tincture—one to two dropperfuls.
- Lavender oil—can be taken in capsule form or one to two dropperfuls of the tincture, if not pregnant.
- Lemon balm—in one higher dose for sleep, as directed on the bottle, or in lower doses of 200-300mg early evening and before bed. This can be quite sedating, so take precautions.
- Motherwort—a half to one dropperful of the tincture, no more than every two hours, or up to three times per day for tension headaches, after the first trimester.
- You can take the CBD from hemp oil, as it is gently calming and can relieve headaches without the potential risks of the THC component of cannabis on the developing fetus. Make sure it is absolutely pure and from a reputable source who can recommend proper dosing or from pharmacies licensed to dispense it. It is usually taken as several drops under the tongue.
- Renowned herbalist, midwife, and physician Aviva Romm recommends Jamaican dogwood tincture, 15 to 20 drops, every four hours, up to four times for the occasional severe headache.
- In her book *The Natural Pregnancy Book*, for more severe tension headaches, Dr. Romm suggests St. John's wort (a half to one teaspoon), black cohosh (1/4 teaspoon every four hours), and cramp bark (a half teaspoon every four hours) alone or in combination. She also advises another herbal medley in adjunct to support liver and digestive functions for more mild but recurrent headaches: dandelion root and leaves, yellow dock root, blue vervain (after the first trimester), and burdock root. Take any of these tinctures, up to a half teaspoon alone or in combination, three to four times per day.

Definitely get osteopath or chiropractor treatment to gently restore anything out of alignment.

If you are pregnant and nothing else helps, you can take an occasional Tylenol (acetaminophen), 500 mg tablets, every four hours until you feel better. But consult your practitioner before taking any other medication since many products sold over the counter contain substances that are not safe to take during pregnancy (like aspirin or ergot), and regular use can actually worsen your headaches.

If you are NOT pregnant, you can very occasionally use over-the-counter medications containing ibuprofen, aspirin, or acetaminophen as directed if the more natural measures are not effective and you do not have any other health problems that would contraindicate their use. But before reaching for these medications, try 1-2 grams of curcumin (turmeric), a natural herb studied to be as effective for pain relief as most of these over-the-counter synthetic analgesics without their associated potential risk of toxicity.

Contact your practitioner if your headache is not relieved by these suggestions and:

- It persists beyond 24 hours.
- It occurs frequently.
- Is getting worse.
- It is unusual for you or severe.
- It occurred after suffering head trauma or taking prescribed medication (like birth control pills).
- It is accompanied by other unusual symptoms such as a stiff neck or high fever, unexplained vomiting, weakness of part of your body, difficulty speaking, lack of coordination, visual disturbances, dizziness, increased swelling around your face, hands, or legs, pain in the middle of your chest/upper abdomen, or sudden weight gain (especially if you are pregnant and/or have high blood pressure).
- It is chronic and painful, and none of the remedies help.

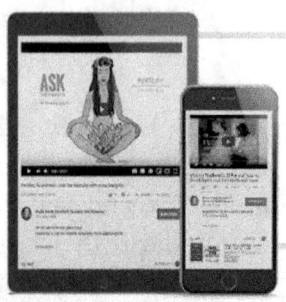

**Want to learn more or
have more questions?**

Grab your free Book Bonuses below:
https://homesweethomebirth.com/nbsbookbonus

Swelling in Pregnancy

S welling during pregnancy can be alarming and uncomfortable. But it's also totally normal and a healthy sign, especially when mild to moderate, and changes based on your activity.

The fluid retention and increased amount of body fluids in the tissue space outside the blood vessels reflect the normal hormonal changes of a healthy pregnancy. Many women notice a slight puffiness or swelling in their fingers, hands, and face. However, the additional fluid typically congregates in the lower part of the body, namely the feet, ankles, and genital area. This is related to the pull of gravity and the pressure of the enlarging uterus on vessels that bring blood back to the heart. It's called "dependent edema" and usually temporarily decreases after rest and elevation or a night's sleep on your side.

Swelling during pregnancy is made worse by:

- Prolonged periods of sitting or standing
- Carrying a large fetus or twins
- Being overweight
- Hot weather
- Increased perspiration leading to loss of salt
- Inadequate intake of fluids, protein, or salt
- Anemia.

How to Decrease Swelling During Pregnancy

While swelling during pregnancy is common, many women find it uncomfortable and unsightly (not to mention it can make it hard to get your shoes on!). However, there are a number of ways to reduce the amount of swelling.

Diet

Avoid salt excess, but don't restrict your intake either. Salt your food to taste, as you need a minimum of two to three grams of sodium daily. Sea salt is high in minerals and is preferable to table salt that has chemical additives.

Make sure your diet includes 60-90 grams of protein every day. You can boost it with an organic pastured gelatin in a protein-powdered drink.

Avoid curbing your fluid intake, as this will actually aggravate the problem. Drink your daily dose of pure water.

Remedies

Check if you are anemic. If so, increase your intake of iron with food and/or an herbal supplement like Floradix Iron and Herbs or yellow dock, and follow the recommendations given in the chapter "Anemia in Pregnancy: Prevention and Treatment".

Drink one to two cups of a nettle and dandelion herbal infusion each day. To prepare it:

1. Soak one ounce of each herb in one quart of boiling water for three to four hours.
2. Strain in a glass canning jar.
3. Add a dash of honey, fresh lemon or lime juice, or mint leaves to taste.

Alternately, take a dropperful of each herb in tincture, twice daily, or the dried encapsulated form, one to two caps, two to four times per day.

Avoid diuretic medications. Safe and gentle herbal diuretics include:

- Hawthorne berries—try the encapsulated, freeze-dried extract, 500 mg per day or one to two caps, two to four times per day
- Cornsilk tea—one cup, two to four times per day
- Black tea—(if you are not a regular drinker of caffeine).

Consult a professional homeopath to suggest a remedy specific for your symptoms or refer to a homeopathic reference book.

Movement

Avoid prolonged periods of sitting or standing, and lying on your back during the third trimester.

Flex or bend your feet back towards your body several times at frequent intervals if you have to sit or stand for a long time.

Do regular exercise for at least half an hour, five days per week.

Inversions are wonderful yoga postures to reduce swelling and are especially helpful and calming at the end of the day when swelling is usually at its worst. A great one that is easy to do is viparita karini, otherwise known as "legs up the wall." Lie down on your back, with your buttocks all the way to the wall, flat on the floor, or elevated on a folded yoga blanket, bolster or block. Let your legs rest straight up the wall for 10-20 minutes. It is also a great opportunity for quiet meditation, focusing on slow, deep breathing and inner gazing between your eyebrows.

A lavender-infused eye pillow adds to the delicious relaxation effect. Use the props to help you feel more comfortable and modify the postures to suit your needs. They are a great asset for your yoga practice and will help in labor as well.

An alternative is to lie flat with your head and shoulders supported on folded blankets, and elevate your legs on one, or even better two, yoga bolsters.

Rest and Comfort

Don't stand if you can sit. Even better is to squat, and don't cross your legs while sitting.

Take frequent breaks to lie down on your side, or sit with your back straight and your legs elevated above the level of your torso (ideally for half an hour, four times daily, depending on how much swelling you have).

Avoid tight, restrictive clothing from the waist down, especially socks, knee highs, tight pants, and girdles.

Wear comfortable, flat shoes instead of high-heeled or ill-fitting ones.

Put on elastic maternity support stockings before you get out of bed in the morning, but raise your legs first to empty them as much as possible of excess blood.

Get a regular foot and leg massage with arnica oil while you lie on your left side. Your partner can do this each night!

Soak your legs in a warm bath using one cup of Epsom salts, and add a few drops of wintergreen and lavender essential oils.

When It Might Be More Serious

Call your midwife or doctor if these suggestions do not help or if the swelling:

- Becomes severe, excessive, or generalized throughout your body.
- Becomes pitting, in which pressing the puffy area leaves a temporary indentation mark.

- Increases, especially in your hands and face.
- Is only affecting one arm or leg, not both.
- Is as bad in the morning as it is at the end of the day and does not lessen with rest and elevation.

Seek help if you experience sudden weight gain (five pounds or more in less than one week) not related to diet changes or reduced activity, and if your swelling is associated with headaches, dizziness, lightheadedness, you see spots before your eyes or experience blurry vision, changes in mental status, chest or abdominal pain, shortness of breath, or other unusual symptoms.

Keep in mind that, for most people, swelling in pregnancy is just a common side effect that will quickly be relieved with the birth of your beautiful baby.

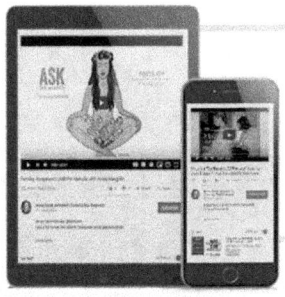

Want to learn more or have more questions?

Grab your free Book Bonuses below:
https://homesweethomebirth.com/nbsbookbonus

HIGH BLOOD PRESSURE IN PREGNANCY: PREVENTION AND NATURAL TREATMENT

About 6-10% of pregnant women develop consistently high blood pressure while pregnant. Typically, if mild, by itself it's usually harmless. But, if not monitored or controlled, it can be dangerous, and it may lead to a more serious condition known as preeclampsia, which poses a threat to the health of you and your baby.

Always remember that blood pressure varies widely in healthy individuals and is normally sensitive to moment-to-moment changes in activity, posture, nutritional status, and emotional factors. It can even be a response to a fear of being checked, of having high blood pressure or being diagnosed with a complication! It is the steady and consistent increase that is concerning.

To Prevent High Blood Pressure in Pregnancy

Regular aerobic exercise involving moderate exertion throughout pregnancy is one of the best ways to maintain health and prevent high blood pressure. Some good options are brisk walking, dancing, and swimming. If you are a beginner, build up gradually to the ideal goal of at least 30 minutes, five times per week. Gentle forms of meditative movement like Tai Chi, Qi Gong, and yoga (especially yin, gentle, prenatal, and restorative) also help maintain normal blood pressure. Below are more tips for preventing high blood pressure during pregnancy.

Consider Your Diet

Avoid stimulants, such as spicy or peppery foods, caffeinated products, nicotine products, cocaine, diet pills, and other stimulant herbs and medications.

Eat a highly nutritious, whole-food, organic diet, high in fiber and quality protein to prevent hypertensive disease and to avoid excess weight gain. And avoid foods that are highly processed, laden with sugars, white flour, and unhealthy refined vegetable oils. Eat lots of fresh organic fruits and vegetables, and at least 80 grams of protein, which you can boost with protein powders or organic pastured powdered gelatin.

Take your prenatal supplements, so you get the nourishment you need for your pregnancy that is not supplied by diet alone. Refer to the chapter on nutrition for more details on healthy eating and supplements. Especially important are an excellent whole-food prenatal vitamin and omega-three essential fatty acids. Be sure to include foods high in calcium, like raw or cooked greens (except spinach), sesame seeds/tahini, salmon, sardines, and dairy. You may need additional calcium to get 1,200-1,500 mg of it daily.

Substitute refined vegetable oils with healthy fats like organic, cold expeller-pressed extra virgin olive, clarified pastured butter (ghee), or coconut oil in your cooking. You can salt your food according to taste with Himalayian sea salt, but avoid excess and processed foods high in sodium.

Drink lots of pure water each day, so you are well hydrated.

Drink more whole juiced veggies. Add one to two tablespoons of powdered spirulina to your daily smoothie or take as directed in capsule form.

Drink strong nettle, red raspberry, and dandelion teas regularly, as well as decaffeinated green tea. When feeling stressed, drink some strong calming chamomile, lemon balm, lavender, passionflower, or skullcap tea. Add honey, fresh mint, or the juice of a fresh lemon or lime to taste.

Reduce Stress

Cut down on the stress in your life. This is easier said than done, but this is an important time to be clear about your priorities. If you feel very stressed and pressured and your blood pressure is on the rise, your body is sending you early-warning signals to rearrange your schedule and increase your rest periods in order to protect your health and that of your growing baby. Don't be afraid to ask family and friends to help with chores or child care. Even better, treat yourself to hired help. And be sure to rest on your side three times a day for 30-60 minutes. Especially learn to master your reaction to outside stress and relax yourself from the inside, which relaxes your blood vessels and lowers blood pressure.

For my complete recommendations on reducing stress, consult the chapter "Natural Stress Alleviation in Pregnancy and Beyond".

Natural Remedies for High Blood Pressure in Pregnancy

Once you have been diagnosed as having pregnancy-induced hypertension (PIH), you will get lots of extra attention in the interest of monitoring how mild or serious your condition is and to protect your health and that of your baby. You will be asked to go to your provider's office more frequently to check your blood pressure and the baby's heartbeat, as well as to check for excess swelling, protein in the urine, and labs that signal developing complications like preeclampsia.

Periodically take your blood pressure in your own home when you feel relaxed and secure. You can buy an easy-to-use digital blood pressure monitor. Sometimes there is an artificial elevation in blood pressure in the office due to anxiety about being examined and having your blood pressure reading be too high.

Continue to use the preventative suggestions, but increase the amount of time you are resting on your side as much as possible. Depending on your individual situation, you may need to maintain a stricter rest on your side most of the day–this means no housework or errands–but often this is not necessary.

Increase the frequency and duration of your breathing and relaxation exercises. Visualize your blood vessels dilating for five minutes, several times daily, while thinking and feeling that your blood pressure is now normal.

Watch comedy. Laughter is extremely healing, reducing internal stress that is reflected in lower blood pressure.

Be in tune with your baby's movements. Make sure you count at least ten moves in one hour during the times your baby is most active, which is usually after you eat and when resting.

Take biofeedback training to lower your blood pressure.

Take several warm baths daily with Epsom salts and a few sprinkled drops of the essential oil of lavender.

Time to Consider Supplementation

Again, if you aren't already taking a natural prenatal vitamin and mineral supplement, now is the time to start. Also consider additional calcium and magnesium. Take 500 mg of each in the morning, afternoon, and at bedtime. If you experience loose stools, you can experiment with skipping the magnesium dose in the morning.

Eat more potassium-rich foods, which includes most fresh fruits and vegetables, for example, starchy roots, potatoes, dark leafy greens, bananas, oranges, and cream of tartar. Renowned herbalist Susaun Weed advises drinking a mixture of the juice of half of a lemon or lime with two teaspoons of cream of tartar and a half cup of water once daily for three days. Take 1,000-2,000 mg of vitamin C daily up until 36 weeks gestation, then reduce to 500 mg. Also take 400 IU of vitamin E and 2-3 mg of methyl folate to boost your antioxidants.

Make sure to take at least 300-400 mg of DHA/EPA omega-three essential fatty acids found in contaminant- free fish oil, twice daily. You can take a vegetarian source, but they aren't as ideal. However, some benefit can be derived from eating two tablespoons of ground flaxseed every day. You can add it to your cereal, salad, baked goods, or yogurt. Alternatives are 1,000 mg of flaxseed oil taken in capsule form or using one tablespoon of uncooked flax oil in your salad or other cold foods, twice daily; or taking 500 mg of black currant or evening primrose oil each day.

Eat a bulb of fresh garlic daily. You can make it delicious by roasting or sautéing the whole cloves in olive oil, salt, pepper, and a dash of parsley. If you prefer raw garlic, eat two to four cloves, twice daily, crushed into your salad or cut and swallowed as a pill with a spoon of honey and a glass of water or citrus juice, which minimizes garlic breath and stomach upset. Another option is to take encapsulated garlic several times daily. Infuse your olive oil with garlic by soaking all the cloves from a bulb in one cup of olive oil for a few days. Use this garlic-infused olive oil for delicious and health-enhancing meals and on salads, veggies, beans, and sprouted whole-grain breads and pastas. Eat more onions, parsley, fresh beet juice, cucumber and its juice, watermelon, and turmeric.

Prepare your own herbal infusion:

- Steep up to one large handful of dried nettle leaf and/or red raspberry leaf and dandelion root in a quart of boiling water for at least four hours.
- Strain in a glass jar, and drink several times throughout the day.
- You can add a splash of lemon or lime juice, fresh mint, or a dash of honey to taste.
- Drink two cups daily.

Take one to two dropperfuls of tinctures of passionflower, skullcap, and lavender, one to three times per day, especially if your increased blood pressure is due to stress and anxiety. Alternately, passionflower capsules can be taken as directed, twice daily.

Drink hops tea before bed during the last few months of pregnancy.

If you are interested in more healing herbs specific to your situation, you can take dandelion (a natural diuretic) and hawthorn berry (a natural vasodilator). The herbs should ideally be supercritical or encapsulated freeze-dried extracts. Take one to two capsules of each, two to four times per day or one dropperful of each liquid tincture of dandelion and hawthorn berry, two to three times per day.

Dr. Aviva Romm, in The Natural Pregnancy Book, recommends adding equal parts cramp bark, black cohosh, and motherwort after the first trimester, as they relax the nerves and muscles, and dilate the peripheral blood vessels, thereby reducing high blood pressure. Take a dropperful of each tincture up to a few times daily as needed, depending on your blood pressure. But stop if you feel a pattern of preterm contractions (four per hour or every 10 minutes before 37 weeks). She also advises mixing together the following herbal tonic tinctures to support the liver and kidneys, especially to prevent worsening preeclampsia, and taking one teaspoon of the mixture, one to two times daily:

- 3 teaspoons each of nettle leaf, schisandra, American ginseng, dandelion root, and burdock root
- 1.5 teaspoons each of passionflower and linden.

Call your provider immediately if you have any of the following symptoms: sudden severe swelling of your feet, legs, hands, or face; a severe headache; pain in your upper abdomen or uterus; spots in front of your eyes; blurry vision, dizziness, or light-headedness; vaginal bleeding; a sense that your baby is moving less than usual; regular contractions; or your water breaks.

Skin Changes in Pregnancy

Skin changes in pregnancy can be a nuisance, but there are a number of home remedies available to alleviate discomfort and improve appearance. However, it begins with embracing all the normal changes as beautiful marks of blessing, wisdom, and transformation, to not only appreciate but also to celebrate.

The hormones in pregnancy cause a variety of skin changes, such as:

- Darkening of your nipples and areola
- Darkening of existing moles, freckles, and birthmarks
- The development of dark patches on the face
- A dark line in the center of the abdomen, from your pubic area upward
- Stretch marks
- Red palms
- Spider veins
- Dryness
- Sweating
- Itching
- Increased sensitivity to irritants.

Skin Discoloration

To minimize skin discoloration, avoid tanning salons and excessive sun exposure, especially between 10 am and 2 pm. During these peak hours, apply low-dose natural sunscreen containing an SPF of 15 to 30. Protect yourself with a big-brimmed hat and light clothing as needed.

Make sure you eat foods high in folates, such as whole grains, fresh fruits, vegetables, and liver. Alternately, you can take a prenatal herbal supplement that provides 1 mg of methylated folic acid, which has other benefits as well, like prevention of fetal neural tube defects. It also comes in chewable form.

Avoid hydrocortisone cream and coal tar preparations.

Red palms may be caused by a deficiency in vitamin B6, which is unlikely if your diet is healthy and well-balanced, as B6 is found in fresh fruits and vegetables, whole grains, and protein-rich foods, as well as in prenatal vitamins.

Consult your dermatologist if a mole develops and changes other than simply darkening, such as becoming larger, irregular, discolored, or irritated.

Stretch Marks

Stretch marks are made worse by increased weight gain and skin stretching, like with large babies or twins. If you have a tendency to develop stretch marks, you can help to prevent or minimize them with a regular massage to the vulnerable areas with equal amounts of the essential oils of argan, bitter almond, gotu kola, pomegranate, lavender, bitter orange, rosehip, vitamin E, and dragon's blood extract diluted in a container of almond, coconut, and/or wheat germ oils.

Try experimenting with creams said to help, such as Earth Mama Organics Belly Butter, or those containing cocoa butter or shea butter, elastin, vitamin E, and any of the above essential oils. Massage them slowly into your body with love and honor for your goddess self, looking for and admiring the beauty inside and out. Take time to breathe in a sense of deep gratitude for the blessings in your life, including the ability to bring a new baby into your family.

Wear a supportive bra and a good maternity girdle, and watch your weight. Remember, you only need to gain 3-6 pounds during the first trimester and 1/2 to 1 pound per week for the remainder of your pregnancy, for a grand total of 25-35 pounds.

Thirty minutes a day, five days per week, engage in moderate exercise as well as muscle toning through floor work exercises, light weights, Pilates, and/or prenatal yoga.

Drink eight to ten glasses of water daily. And eat lots of fresh vegetables, fruits, whole grains, beans, nuts, seeds, and quality protein. Avoid highly processed products laden with chemicals, white flours, sugars, and unhealthy refined vegetable fats.

Be sure to supplement your diet with prenatal vitamins, minerals, essential fatty acids, and other nutrients needed to sustain a healthy pregnancy. See the chapter on nutrition for a more in-depth discussion of a healthy diet and advised supplements.

You can also try homeopathic remedies called calcarea fluorica, graphites, and/or silicea to prevent stretch marks. It is usually given in low doses, several pellets of the remedy most specific to your symptoms, a few times daily. If without relief, consult a classical homeopath, or refer to a solid homeopathy reference book.

Most skin changes resolve during the early postpartum months, but stretch marks are often referred to as a mark of motherhood, as they never completely disappear. Try to think of them as reminders of the gifts that have been bestowed upon you, to be thankful and appreciative of your ability to bear children. Try to see the beauty in a pregnant belly. As one wise African midwife once remarked at a midwifery conference, there are many infertile women who would do anything just to have those stretch marks.

Dr. Aviva Romm in "The Natural Pregnancy Book" views stretch marks as "silvery jewelry on the belly of a woman adorning her and reflecting her ability to grow and change." She further states that contrary to the values of American society, we need to "take pride in our individual form, shape, and markings ... to love ourselves with awe and admiration at the amazing accommodation your body is giving to your growing baby." I couldn't agree more!

Rashes and Itching

If you develop a local itchy rash, it may be the result of a mild allergy to something that never bothered you before. You need to experiment by paying attention to everything that comes in contact with the affected area of your skin. Eliminate possible culprits one at a time. Common causes include:

- Bath soap
- Laundry detergent
- Synthetic cosmetics and body products
- Chemically laden household and workplace cleaning products
- Environmental toxins
- Synthetic clothing
- Metal on watches and jewelry
- Poison ivy or poison oak
- Certain foods (like cow dairy, gluten, soy, certain fruits, nuts, or chemical additives).

Keep cool with loose, comfortable all-cotton clothing.

Watch for improvement after switching to all-natural hypoallergenic products available at most health food stores, wearing only cotton close to your skin, putting the laundry through an extra rinse, taking off your metal, gardening with gloves and protective clothing and avoiding certain plants altogether, or cutting out a specific food item for a few days. Given the common reactions to these foods, allow a month for going completely dairy-, soy-, and gluten-free, and marvel at the results.

Try to avoid scratching as this makes the rash worse. If your skin is irritated, take a hot or cool water bath as often as you need and add a packet or a half cup of Aveeno colloidal oatmeal or cornstarch to the water. Once your skin is completely dry, apply aloe vera gel, a few drops of lavender oil or calendula salve, or a herbal combination lotion or cream to the affected areas. Ointments or creams containing Tigar Balm,

Ben Gay, or vitamins A, E, and C may also help, as well as a homeopathic remedy specific to your symptoms (but do not use at same time as products with strong odor like Ben Gay and Tiger Balm, which can interfere with its effectiveness). If you touch poison ivy or oak plant, you have 20-30 minutes to wash the oil off with soap and water, or up to 24 hours to wash it off with Tecnu lotion or Zanfel, which is more effective.

For itchy skin **without** a rash, make sure your diet is high in organic, whole foods, with plenty of fresh fruits and veggies, nuts, seeds, and beans. Avoid processed, refined, chemical-laden, and deep-fried foods. Also try a month off gluten, soy, and dairy. Drink at least a half-gallon of water daily. Follow the recommendations in the chapter on nutrition.

Apply calendula oil or rub cocoa butter on the itchy part of your body. Prevent skin dryness with almond or coconut oil. You can add to the oil a few drops each of the essential oils of lavender, rosehip, bitter orange, and pomegranate.

Try aqueous cream with aloe vera and/or collagen, and consult your homeopath for a remedy that most closely matches your symptoms. Supplement with 1,000-1,500 mg of evening primrose oil and 400-600 mg of DHA/EPA essential fatty acids commonly found in fish oil tested free of common pollutants.

A wonderfully effective herb that helps with generalized itching and is one of the finest nourishing tonics in pregnancy is stinging nettles. You can make your own tea by adding a handful of the dried herb to one quart of boiling water. Steep, covered in a glass canning jar for four to eight hours, and drink several times daily. Or, you can take one to two of Gaia's capsules of freeze-dried nettle extract every two to four hours as needed.

Another effective remedy recommended by Dr. Aviva Romm in "The Natural Pregnancy Book" is made by combing 1/4- to 1/2-ounce each of bulk echinacea root, burdock root, licorice root (only if blood pressure is normal and not high), and dandelion root. Steep in one quart of boiling water for four hours, strain, and drink a half-cup, twice daily until your condition improves. You can try adding lemon or lime juice, fresh mint, or honey to taste. Women who suffer from chronic allergic skin complaints often find that they clear up in pregnancy, but occasionally they do get worse.

If you have eczema that is not improving, try eliminating all cow's milk and gluten products from your diet for two to four weeks to see if that helps. If you see improvement, resume dairy or one grain at a time for a few days and note if the symptoms recur. If so, you will need to avoid that food completely. But, if they do not recur, then you can safely eat that particular food item. Other common allergen triggers to experiment with eliminating and resuming one at a time include soy, corn, eggs, and yeast.

Increase your intake of other foods high in calcium (like dark green leafy vegetables, sesame seeds or tahini, and wild, clean-water salmon and sardines) or take supplemental 500 mg of calcium citrate with magnesium, two to three times per day. Cook with fresh turmeric and ginger. Dr. Andrew Weil recommends taking 500 mg of evening primrose or black currant oil to get a fatty acid hard to obtain through diet called GLA (gamma-linolenic acid), twice daily, and applying chaparral salve or aloe vera gel to the affected areas when the skin is still moist after bathing.

Reduce inner stress and increase inner calm with a regular practice of yoga, meditation, and breathwork, and do what you can to reduce stressors in your life. This includes unplugging from your smartphone and computer as much as possible to connect more with life, yourself, and others, and doing what you really love. Doing this is probably the most important remedy, as the mind and body are exquisitely connected, and inside stress is a major cause of health problems, especially chronic allergic skin issues.

If you have psoriasis that is not improving, increase sunlight exposure to the affected areas. Weather permitting, spend at least 20 minutes in the early morning or late afternoon sun. Take two tablespoons of ground flaxseed daily. You can add it to hot or cold cereals, baked goods, smoothies, or yogurt.

Take a good prenatal multivitamin and mineral supplement with omega-threes and GLA, says Dr. Weil. In his book *Natural Health, Natural Medicine* he also advises applying topical applications of aloe vera or chaparral lotions or salves and taking additional antioxidants that include:

- 10,000-20,000 IU of mixed carotenoids (a safe source of vitamin A)
- 400-800 IU of vitamin E
- 200 mg of vitamin C
- 100-200 mcg of selenium
- 60 mg of coenzyme Q10 softgel capsules.

And you can try two capsules of milk thistle, twice per day if needed. Allow at least three months for optimal effects.

For both psoriasis and eczema, explore wonderfully effective alternative modalities such as hypnotherapy, visualization, breathwork, guided imagery therapy, and traditional Chinese medicine and acupuncture. Read Dr. Andrew Weil's Natural Health, Natural Medicine, which provides information on improving nutritional habits and practical ways in which you can reduce inflammation, as well as internal tension, and enhance your own health and wellbeing safely and naturally.

Increased Sweating

If you perspire a lot, make sure you replace fluids by drinking extra water. Bathe or shower, one to two times daily as needed. Wear all-natural roll-on deodorant from the health food store, or melt and combine equal parts each of shea butter and coconut oil, add baking soda, scented as you wish with a few drops of your favorite essential oil. Allow it to cool in a glass or stainless steel container. Avoid antiperspirants, as you do not want to interfere with the sweating your body needs to do. You can simply apply arrowroot or corn starch to keep you feeling more dry, or add equal parts of one of them to your homemade concoction.

Sweating is made worse by being overweight, as well as over-dressing and wearing clothing made from synthetic material like nylon and polyester instead of cotton. Dress in layers of loose cotton clothing, and eliminate coffee and other sources of caffeine from your diet.

Slippery elm bark powder or marshmallow root powder can be applied to your skin creases to reduce chafing or to rashes from heat or increased sweating.

Consult your provider if your skin changes become severe or associated with other unusual symptoms not related to pregnancy. For instance:

- Your rash looks like a bull's eye, is tender, swollen and/or exuding pus
- Your rash is spreading all over your body.
- You experience general itching without a rash, especially on your palms and soles.
- You have a sudden appearance of hives and your throat feels constricted.
- You develop a fever, chills, and/or muscle aches.
- The above-mentioned suggestions do not help, and your symptoms persist or worsen.

Shortness of Breath in Pregnancy

Pregnant women often have a heightened awareness of their breathing, have mild breathlessness, or feel a slight shortness of breath. This is related to normal conditions of pregnancy such as:

- Hormonal changes
- Added demands on the heart
- Increased oxygen needs
- Pressure of the growing uterus on the diaphragm breathing muscle

Shortness of breath after exertion is worse in women who smoke or are not physically fit due to a lack of exercise or a sedentary lifestyle.

To keep or get in shape and build your stamina, do an aerobic form of exercise for at least 30 minutes, 5 times per week. If you're not accustomed to exercise, start lightly and build up slowly. But, listen to your body, modify as needed, and avoid overexertion. And, of course, quit smoking right away.

Feeling stressed, which is so common in the modern world, contributes to shallow breathing and worsens the feeling of being winded and tense. Conscious breathwork is literally key to your salvation. It will transform your life and can certainly make a huge difference in labor too!

If You Experience Shortness of Breath in Pregnancy

There are a number of methods shown to reduce shortness of breath in pregnancy. Try some of the ideas below and find what feels right to you.

Focused Breathing

Periodically check in on your breathing. If you're breathing fast, slow it down. If it's shallow (just from the chest or not a full abdominal breath), try to take deeper, fuller breaths down into your belly. Regularly make yourself yawn several times.

Practice breathing exercises for 10-20 minutes a few times daily. Ideal moments are before going to bed at night, before rising in the morning, and throughout the day. Draw on these techniques whenever you experience:

- Stress or internal tension
- Anger or feeling triggered
- Depression or sadness
- A break in activity (for example traveling, bathing, or waiting in line—let these be opportunities to practice and perfect your skills).

Take frequent short breaks throughout the day to reduce inner tension and increase feelings of centeredness and tranquility. Spend time outside in nature as much as you can. Practice meditation, mindfulness, and progressive muscle relaxation, releasing all the muscles in your body from head to toe. This is especially helpful if you are nervous about your breathing. For more details, refer to the chapter on meditation, breathwork, and visualization.

For acute attacks, pause to rest, breathe slowly and deeply, exhaling through pursed lips, and try standing with your hands stretched up towards the ceiling.

Posture

The way you hold your body can make a significant difference in your ability to take a full breath. Yoga and dance help with this tremendously. Periodically check your posture, especially during the second half of pregnancy. Make sure you are standing or sitting straight using your abdominal muscles and that your shoulders are down, but not slumped forward.

Sleep with some extra pillows to keep your head or shoulders elevated, or lie down on your side. Wear loose, comfortable clothing so you aren't restricting your movement or your body's ability to expand with each inhale.

Self-Care

Be sure to take good care of yourself in general. Eat a diet that is healthy and well-balanced, including a variety of whole foods and choose organic whenever possible.

Drink lots of water daily to stay well hydrated. Add berries, a few squeezes and slices of lemon, lime, orange, grapefruit, or fresh mint leaves to taste.

Other Tips

Make sure you are getting enough sleep and rest periods for the added demands of pregnancy. Go to bed earlier, sleep later, and/or take daily naps.

Cut back on unnecessary demands if you feel you are doing more than your body can handle.

Avoid self-medicating with alcohol, drugs, or tobacco.

Consult an acupuncturist with expertise in shiatsu treatment.

Contact your physician or midwife if your breathlessness:

- Becomes severe.
- Occurs especially during rest.
- Interferes with your ability to carry out routine household chores.
- Is associated with other unusual symptoms like chest pain or palpitations, severe fatigue or weakness, fainting, or blood-tinged sputum.
- Occurs with signs of an infection such as fever, coughing, or congestion.
- Is in addition to history of asthma or other respiratory problems, heart disease, or smoking.

Numbness and Tingling (Paresthesia) During Pregnancy

Numbness, tingling, pain, and other unusual sensations in the fingers and toes during pregnancy are quite common. Termed "paresthesias," these sensations are related to the pressure on local nerves from the growing uterus, fluid retention, and/or your altered posture.

To Reduce the Frequency of Paresthesias in Pregnancy

Periodically check the way you are sitting and standing, making sure that you are erect and using your abdominal muscles instead of your back muscles. Keep your pelvis tilted forward so that your back is straight, not arched, and your shoulders relaxed down but not slumped.

Pay scrupulous attention to good body mechanics, meaning that you should use your arms, legs, and abdominal muscles to do your work, never your back. Get close to an object to move it rather than pull or pick it up towards you.

Exercise regularly, at least 5 times per week for 30 minutes.

Try a prenatal class yoga class to help you to work on correct posturing, flexibility, and the building of muscle strength. Exercise, stretch, elevate, and massage the affected extremity as often as you can.

Avoid movements that are jerky or painful, and make sure you are also getting regular daily rest periods off your feet. Sometimes lying down, pelvic tilts on your hands and knees, or assuming a prenatal, yin, gentle, or restorative yoga posture may help.

Drink lots of clean, live water daily. This is especially important if your hands and feet are a bit swollen with fluid.

Make sure your diet is healthy and nourishing. Use plenty of fresh ginger and turmeric in your cooking. Avoid highly processed, white flours, sugary foods, and unhealthy refined vegetable oils.

If the sensations are mainly in your hands, this is often termed "carpal tunnel syndrome." Periodically elevate your arms, flex and extend your fingers, and roll your shoulders to see if this brings relief. Try hanging your arms out of bed at night. Avoid or modify repetitive activities like typing. Try wearing a special wrist brace. Take 100-200 mg a day of vitamin B6.

Practice authentic yoga regularly to ensure proper body alignment and full use of your lung capacity. Poor posture and shallow breathing have a ripple effect and negatively impact your health, even carpal tunnel syndrome.

Do the following wrist exercises several times per day. When home, get out your yoga mat and support your body with props like blankets, bolsters, or blocks as needed.

Wrist Flexes

Sit or stand straight and hold your arms out in front of you with palms facing down. Flex one wrist so that your fingers point towards the floor, and use the other hand to increase the stretch. Hold for 20-30 seconds, then repeat on the other side. You can also hold your hands in a namaste or prayer position; in this position, move each hand forward and backward using the other hand for resistance. Then press the palms and fingers firmly together in front of your chest and hold for a few minutes. Finally, reverse your hands so that the back of your hands are pressing together, fingers pointing down. Hold as is comfortable.

Hand Circles

Circle your fisted hands in each full circular direction; then shake them out for 15-30 seconds.

Wrist Stretch

Place a folded yoga blanket in the middle of your mat for extra knee padding. Get on your hands and knees, with your feet flexed, and your fingers facing backwards towards your knees. Press down evenly on your hands as you move your hips back enough to feel the wrists stretch. Stretch for as long as is comfortable.

Then switch it up so the backs of your hands are on the floor, palms facing upward, with your fingers now facing forward. Lift up as you evenly press the backs of your hands into the floor, and move your body to feel the stretch in your wrists. Again, hold for as long as comfortable. You can also do this with your fingers pointing inwards, and again with your fingers pointing outwards, palms up, and palms down.

Seek out a classical homeopath to find a remedy specific to your symptoms. A chiropractor, osteopath, acupuncturist, massage or physical therapist may also be helpful.

If none of these suggestions work for you or your paresthesias becomes severe, persistent, or worrisome, or it is associated with other unusual symptoms, consult a specialist in orthopedics or neurology.

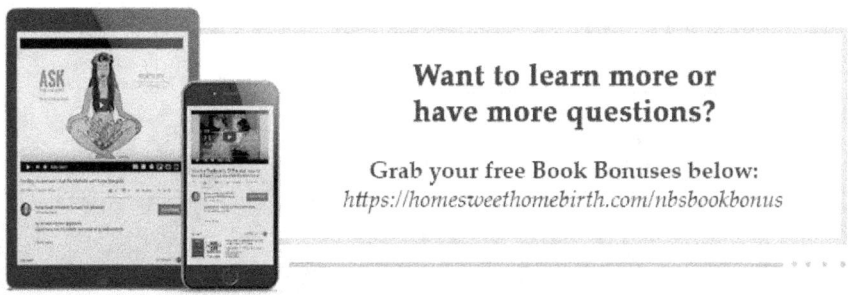

Want to learn more or have more questions?

Grab your free Book Bonuses below:
https://homesweethomebirth.com/nbsbookbonus

POSTERIOR POSITION: PRACTICAL STEPS FOR PREVENTION AND REMEDIES

A baby in a posterior position is facing your abdomen, and the baby's back is towards your back. Some babies are born easily in the posterior position with the baby facing mama's face "sunny side up." This is especially if mama:

- Has given birth before.
- Is carrying a baby of average or smaller size.
- Has an adequate-sized pelvis.
- Is committed, relaxed, and prepared.
- Is able to be upright, move, and change positions at will.
- Has the ability to eat and drink freely.
- Is supported by providers who are patient, calm, and trained to help the baby turn.

Other babies in a posterior position can be more challenging, creating problems like not going into labor, water breaking prematurely before labor starts, slower, more difficult labor progress, exhaustion, and labor felt mostly as back pain that can be harder to cope with. All of these factors increase the risk of complications, interventions, and cesarean if the baby cannot be safely born vaginally.

Epidurals increase the incidence of posterior babies, as well. But sometimes in prolonged labor, when mama is exhausted and can no longer cope, the compassionate use of an epidural can help her give birth vaginally.

The modern sedentary lifestyle of slouching in chairs over smart phones and computers, sitting back in sofas and car seats with associated poor posture, stress, and tension in our bodies contributes to the rise in babies presenting in the posterior position. Many of us in the west are no longer as active as our ancestors and as indigenous cultures around the globe. We are not often leaning forward doing manual work, which helps a baby's heavier back come forward into the anterior position, unless we are doing activities like gardening.

Ideally and actually most often, the baby will be in an anterior position, facing your spine at term, or they might turn anterior during labor for childbirth. It is important to know when your baby moves into the optimal anterior position, so you can encourage the baby to stay there, which usually means an easier and shorter labor.

You can learn on your own what position your baby is in with belly mapping. A wonderful resource for that is spinningbabies.com. But if you are unsure, ask your practitioner for help figuring it out. Then try to pay attention to your baby's position, without getting needlessly obsessed about it. This is easier to do when your baby moves or when momentarily you are lying on your back. It may take a lot of concentration to understand what is what at first, but soon you will get the hang of it.

When your baby is posterior, your tummy may look flatter and feel more squashy, and you may feel arms and legs and kicks all over the front towards the middle of your tummy. The area around your belly button may dip to a concave, saucer-like shape, and you may also experience long and painful practice contractions with a more severe lower backache as your baby tries to turn around to the anterior position to engage down into the pelvis.

When your baby is anterior, the back feels hard and smooth and rounded on one side of your tummy, and you will usually feel kicks on the other side under your ribs.. Your belly button will normally poke out and feel firm.

Pay attention to your posture and positioning at the time when your baby may be starting to descend into your pelvis, which is during the last six weeks of your first pregnancy, and the last two to three weeks of your subsequent pregnancies. The goal is to make room for your baby to assume the optimal position for birthing.

The baby's back is the heaviest side of its body and will, thus, gravitate towards the lowest side of your abdomen. So, if your tummy is lower than your back (such as sitting on a chair leaning forward), the baby's back will tend to swing anterior towards your tummy.

If your back is lower than your tummy (such as reclining back in an armchair with your feet up), then the baby's back may swing towards your back into a posterior position. With this in mind, when you are 34 weeks onward, avoid any position where you are spending time leaning backwards with your knees higher than your pelvis.

Ideally, ditch the chairs. If you do need to sit on one, make sure your knees are lower than your pelvis and your trunk is tilted slightly forward. If you need to work at a desk, consider a standing one at least some of the time, resting an alternating foot on a step stool.

Watch TV, read, and lounge while kneeling on the floor, over a beanbag, birth ball, cushions, an ergonomic chair, or sitting backwards on a straight-backed dining room or kitchen chair, facing and leaning on its back.

Practice yoga to be in shape for the lunges and varied positions used to help your baby come down and out. Use yoga positions like bound angle (badha konasana), which entails sitting with your back upright and with the soles of your feet together, or on your hands and knees while curving your back up like a cat, followed by dropping your spine down in an arch and/or wiggling your hips from side to side. Get out your yoga mat and support your body with props like blankets, bolsters, or blocks as needed.

Avoid crossing your legs, as it reduces the space in front of your pelvis and opens up the back. Sit on a wedge cushion in the car, so your pelvis is tilted forward, and keep the seatback upright.

Avoid deep squatting until your baby is anterior and well down in your pelvis or when needed in labor. Deep squatting opens up your pelvis and encourages the baby to move down, so refrain from it until your baby is in the anterior position. You can squat on a low stool or yoga blocks instead, keeping your spine upright or leaning forward.

Rest and sleep on your side, with two pillows under your bent right knee, which should be jackknifed up towards your chest, and keep your left leg straight out.

Swim with your belly downwards, doing the front crawl and breaststroke. The leg movements with the breaststroke, in particular, are great for opening your pelvis and encouraging your baby into an optimal anterior position.

If Your Baby Is Posterior

Continue the above-mentioned positions, and add the following exercises for 20-30 minutes each, three times daily while watching something inspirational, romantic, or funny or while listening to music:

- Maintain a knee-chest position, with your buttocks sticking up in the air to tip the baby back out of the pelvis, so there is more room to turn around to the anterior position.
- Sway your hips back and forth, and do the pelvic rock up and down while in knee-chest or on your hands and knees.
- Crawl around the floor on your hands and knees, or hands and feet like an elephant.
- Scrub your floors or do some gardening.
- Swim belly down, kicking with straight legs only. Avoid frog-leg movements.
- Lie on a slant board (using an ironing board or see-saw), with your head down and your legs up, or lie with your pelvis and legs on the top stair landing or sofa and rest on your hands or

forearms on a lower stair so you are at a similar incline. Jiggle your pelvis as you do this.

- Try resting and sleeping on your tummy using lots of pillows and cushions for support.
- Sit on a kneeler-rocker, which is a kneeling stool that sits you in an upright position with your knees lower than your chest and has a rocker underneath for movement that encourages your baby to rotate. There are several types. See what is best for you.

When your baby turns to the anterior position, you can encourage descent further into your pelvis by walking around upright, gently massaging the baby's buttocks downward, deep squatting, and swimming, this time using lots of breaststroke frog-leg kicking.

If you have lax abdominal muscles from several babies or don't do toning exercises, use a supportive maternity binder to keep baby in place.

If Going Into Labor with a Posterior Baby

Starting in early labor, try the following movements involving altering the level of your hips, which help wiggle the baby down through your pelvis:

- Walk up and downstairs, sideways if you need to.
- Rock and dance from side to side.
- March or tread in place.
- Step on and off a step stool.
- Climb in and out of the birth pool.
- Lie on your side, so the part of your belly where your baby's back is can lean forward almost over the sofa or bed, with your upper knee resting on a lower chair.
- Consider having your midwife help to rotate the baby using a variety of external techniques, or if needed, by manually lifting your baby out of your pelvis during a contraction.

During the pushing stage of labor:

- Kneel on all fours, with the other leg up in a lunge. Switch legs periodically. You can do this standing, alternating one leg up on a chair, and moving towards and away from it.
- Maintain a supported high squat in a birthing stool or hanging from a dangling squatting rope or your partner, with your bottom at least 18 inches off the floor.
- You can rest on your side with one leg straight out and the other leg bent up towards your chest, supported with pillows.
- Avoid lying back, semi-reclining, sitting, or semi-sitting.

For more information online, visit Spinning Babies, Association of Radical Midwives, or the Gentle Birth archives for Suboptimal Fetal Positions.

When Your Baby Is Breech or Transverse

I f you've been told that your baby is breech, don't freak out. There are many ways to gently and lovingly ease your baby into vertex.

Towards the end of pregnancy, the baby settles into their favorite position. Ideally, this position will be vertex, meaning that their head is down towards your pelvis and their bottom is high up in your abdomen.

Less commonly, the baby is breech (with its head up and its bottom down towards your pelvis). Even more rarely, the baby sits in a transverse position (with its head and bottom on either side of your abdomen).

It's not always known why a baby is breech or transverse. Sometimes it has to do with:

- The relationship between the shape of the baby and the shape of mom's uterus or pelvic bones
- The location of the placenta
- Issues with the umbilical cord
- Excessive amniotic fluid
- Lax abdominal or uterine muscle tone

Labor and delivery carry more risk of complications when the baby's head is not down towards the pelvis, even though breech is a variation of normal. So, when a baby is breech or transverse by the 32nd week of pregnancy, they should be encouraged to convert to the ideal vertex position. That said, the majority do turn by themselves at the beginning of the ninth month.

What to Do When Baby Is Breech or Transverse

If your baby is breech or transverse at 32 weeks, consider doing a couple of the following exercises for 10-15 minutes, two to three times each day until your baby turns.

1. **Belly massage.** Massage your abdomen GENTLY in the natural direction the baby will turn. But stop if you meet any resistance, and never attempt to forcefully turn the baby yourself.
2. **Visualization.** Close your eyes and imagine your baby with their head moving down in your pelvis and staying there.
3. **Coaxing.** Play classical or relaxing instrumental music by your pelvis, so that the baby will turn towards the soothing sound. Or shine a flashlight by your pelvis, so that the baby may move towards the light.
4. **Go for a swim.** Swim laps and do some handstands in the pool.
5. **Pelvic rocking.** Shift your pelvis up and down and side to side while on your hands and knees.
6. **Act like an elephant.** Walk around the house on your hands and feet.
7. **Bridges and inversions.** If you have an established yoga practice, go upside down with any of the inversions, using props, including the wall, for supportive modifications. Headstands and downward-facing dogs work wonders.

Beginners should start with bridges. To do this, simply lie on your back with your feet flat on the floor, approximately 1.5 to two feet apart, and your knees bent. Elevate your hips 9-12 inches higher than your shoulders. You can support yourself in bridge with a yoga block under your sacrum.

Alternatively, lie on your front in the same "upside down" position, keeping your weight on your forearms and knees wide, with your bottom in the air. Lying on three pillows or a beanbag chair can help further elevate your hips.

Alternatively, lie bent over the edge of a sofa or top of a staircase with your legs on the floor and your body lying down the sofa or stairs. Support your body with your hands or forearms so that your torso is inclined upside down.

Gently roll your hips side to side while in any of these positions.

Taking homeopathic Pulsatilla 30C will help the above exercises be more successful. Allow four to five pellets to dissolve under your tongue, three times daily for three to five days. As with any homeopathic remedy, avoid eating or drinking for 15-20 minutes before and after.

Natural Medicine for Breech and Transverse Babies

In addition to exercises that help your baby move into the best birth position, there are a few techniques that can be administered by care providers. If you've tried the above suggestions without success, look for a practitioner that practices one of the following.

Moxibustion

Find an acupuncturist or doctor of traditional Chinese medicine who has had success turning breech babies to vertex with moxibustion. The technique involves burning a certain herb called moxa close to the skin at specific acupuncture points.

Webster Technique

A chiropractor trained in the Webster Technique can use this sacral adjustment to help facilitate the pelvic alignment needed for your baby to get into birth position.

Manual Turning

If all else fails, you can opt for having your baby turned manually if the right conditions are met (such as no lower segment uterine fibroids, no cord around the baby's neck or short cord, adequate amniotic fluid, and a healthy baby as detected on ultrasound with a normal fetal heartbeat). Sometimes, this can be easily done in your birth practitioner's office at 36-38 weeks, especially for a woman who has delivered vaginally before, while carefully assessing the baby's heartbeat.

Experienced midwives can turn breech and transverse babies. Most obstetricians prefer to do it in the hospital, often with medication to relax your uterus, ultrasound guidance, continuous fetal heart rate monitoring, and access to life saving interventions if needed.

Ask for a wedge pillow to support you in a tilted pelvic lift position or a bed that can be placed at an angle, with your legs higher than your head to help the baby out of the pelvis.

Once the baby is turned to the head-down position, stop inverting yourself and wear an abdominal binder at all times to prevent the baby from turning back to breech. Bellefit makes a fine one.

If your baby insists on being breech as you approach your due date, discuss your options with your provider. If they are not supportive of your choices for a vaginal breech birth, find a different practitioner, optimally one who has the essential skills and philosophy of birthing breech babies vaginally when appropriate and safe to do so.

A baby lying in the persistent transverse position, however, can only be delivered safely by cesarean section.

Braxton Hicks and "False" Labor

There is no such thing as "false" labor. The uterus contracts sporadically throughout the entire pregnancy as the uterine muscle cells stretch and prepare for the "real" labor contractions that will open and thin your cervix and push your baby out during childbirth. A better term for these sensations would be "warm-up" labor.

These sporadic contractions or tightening sensations are referred to as Braxton Hicks contractions. They are experienced as occasional lower abdominal, menstrual-like cramping in early pregnancy. But, as your pregnancy progresses, you can actually feel your uterus ball up and harden, often from the top downward before it softens again.

While not painful, Braxton Hicks can feel like uncomfortable sensations in your abdomen and groin area. They are usually brief and irregular, occurring without any rhythm or pattern. However, they do happen with increasing frequency, length, and intensity as your pregnancy advances - especially more frequent with each subsequent baby. This can sometimes make it hard to distinguish them from actual early labor.

To Relieve Discomfort from Braxton Hicks Contractions

Make sure to keep well-hydrated with pure water. Dehydration can cause the uterus to become irritable and tighten more often.

Frequent Braxton Hicks contractions may also be your body's message that you are doing too much and need to slow down, so take heed. Braxton Hicks contractions usually subside when you stop what you are doing and change your position, get up and walk around, or sit or lie down.

During a contraction, stay mindful and fully aware of whatever is happening in the present moment. Get curious about and lean into your internal sensations without the story. Practice slow, deep breathing while consciously relaxing any tense muscles. Breathe into the most intense sensations you are feeling. This enables you to hone coping techniques for labor and for life's challenges! When you shift your mindset in relation to discomfort and pain, especially when everything is normal (but also when it's not), miraculous transformation occurs. Start by welcoming it all, and look for the deeper message in your symptoms. Your body is brilliantly wise and has reasons for its behavior. This not only helps lead to relief, but also minimizes suffering, as well as pointing you in the direction of root causes that you need to address.

Master your breath and concentration by doing your breathing exercises on a regular daily basis (see the chapter "Breathwork, Meditation, and Visualization" for more details).

While breathing into your belly and baby, visualize what the tightening sensations are doing to "ripen" your cervix as they help it to soften, come forward, shorten, become thinner, and possibly dilate or open a little in preparation for labor at term. Be reassured that a ripe cervix often responds more readily to actual labor contractions, meaning a shorter and, thus, easier time getting to the point when you can push your baby out.

If you are bothered by these contractions and nothing seems to help, consider homeopathy specific to your individual symptoms. I have had great success with cimicifuga or caulophyllum 30c, particular to each person's unique presentation. You can consult with a classical homeopath or refer to an excellent reference book.

Herbs can also help you relax, sleep, lessen the pain, and either discourage your contractions or encourage them if you are term. If you are interested in herbs, there are several options to try alone or in combination.

For persistent irregular uterine cramping that is not associated with labor, make sure you are getting plenty of calcium and magnesium in your diet. Start by eating lots of green leafy and seaweed veggies, ground sesame seeds (tahini), wild-caught fish from non-polluted waters like wild Alaskan salmon, almonds, whole grains, and organic yogurt and cheese (ideally from goat or sheep). Avoid excessive cow dairy intake, coffee, soda, and even spinach, which decreases calcium absorption. You may need additional supplementation. Take at least 400 mg of magnesium and 1,200 mg of calcium daily in two to three divided doses, or make your own infusion of nettles and red raspberry leaf tea.

Also, helpful herbs to reduce cramping are cramp bark, black haw, and wild yam. You can experiment with one of them at a time, or use them all together in combination. Take 1-5 ml of each tincture every 30 minutes to few hours, depending on how often and intense the cramping is (particularly if it is interfering with your sleep each night in the last several weeks of pregnancy).

Prior to 37 weeks, you need to drink two large glasses of water, lie down, and contact your midwife or doctor immediately if you experience any of these potential warning signs of premature labor:

- A feeling of your uterus tightening or cramping in a pattern of every 15 minutes
- Cramping becomes closer, longer, and stronger
- Dull lower backache that feels different than usual (not related to position or strain)
- Pressure or fullness in your pelvic area like something is going to fall out
- An increased amount of discharge, fluid, or bleeding from your vagina
- Persistent diarrhea or intestinal cramping
- A sense that something isn't right.

As Things Progress

Toward the last several days to weeks of pregnancy, Braxton Hicks contractions can be frequent enough to feel like early labor and can, thus, lead to frustration and exhaustion, especially if they are keeping you from sleeping.

In this case, it is important that you encourage them to go away at night, so you can sleep well. Unplug from the computer or smartphone after dark, dim the lights, and go to bed early. For more support winding down, take a warm bath with your favorite essential oils, ask your partner to give you a soothing massage with a few drops of lavender in almond oil, read a calming book or watch a light drama or a comedy, and drink a glass of warm milk. But if you need something stronger and do not have a history of alcohol addiction, drink a glass of wine or beer, or take two shots of whiskey in juice before going to bed. Or try alcohol-free hops. Sufficient rest is essential to give you the needed strength for the hard work of labor to come.

Common herbs taken alone or in combination to ease discomfort once you are in early labor are:

- Motherwort tincture—1/4 to 1/2 of a dropperful up to every few hours
- Skullcap tincture—1/4 to 1/2 of a dropperful up to every hour
- St. John's wort tincture—a dropperful up to every hour

For sleep, you can try a great mineral combination of magnesium and calcium in approximately equal amounts like 400 mg each, or doubling the magnesium dose. Magnesium is also available in tasty powder form like Natural Calm to make a warm drink.

If you are interested in herbs, take two capsules of herbal valerian standardized extract (400-900 mg) or hops (300-600 mg). Using these herbs together in a lower dose combination can be more effective.

Also, try pure, reliably sourced CBD oil, several drops under the tongue, and repeat every few hours as needed.

During the day, you have the choice of carrying on as usual and letting nature take its course, or encouraging the contractions to develop into a progressive early labor pattern by:

- Taking a long brisk walk alternating with climbing stairs
- Engaging in another sort of upright but gentle exercise activity like dancing—do both slow, sensual dancing with or without your partner, and more upbeat, funky, hip hop, belly, or African styles. Turn on the music that speaks to you, get lost in it, and move like no one is watching
- Getting romantic and sensual, and having sexual intercourse
- Rolling and pulling on your nipples as a baby would do during breastfeeding
- Using a breast pump

Continue these activities until you get regular contractions every 5 minutes lasting at least 45-60 seconds, but there is no need to end the walking, dancing, and being sensual and romantic - you can do that throughout your labor and birth when all is well. In any case, make sure to drink lots of fluids and eat small, frequent meals of nourishing food (especially whole grains, nuts, seeds, beans, fresh fruit and vegetables, and healthy protein) as an athlete does who is running a marathon. Do something that you enjoy and/or organize a pleasant change of scenery, express your fears and emotions with your partner, a close friend, or family member, and try to surrender to the process. Remember your body knows what its doing, we just need to get out of its way.

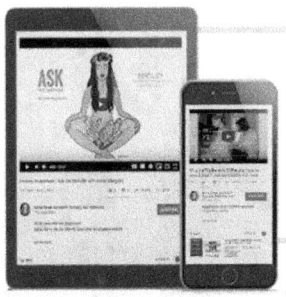

Want to learn more or have more questions?

Grab your free Book Bonuses below:
https://homesweethomebirth.com/nbsbookbonus

"Overdue" Baby: What to Do If Past Your Due Date

Although it's totally normal to have an "overdue" baby, it can be very frustrating. The ideal is to prevent it early on by knowing when you conceived and getting accurate pregnancy dates. There is a five-week timeframe around the estimated due date, when babies are considered term, in which it is normal and most common for moms to go into labor. In a well-nourished, healthy woman whose pregnancy has been accurately dated, the actual time of delivery often extends 1-2 weeks past the estimated 40-week due date. This is especially true with first-time moms. Only a small percentage of women give birth on their due date, and most babies are, indeed, born at the perfect time for them.

A pregnancy is actually "postdates" when it exceeds the 42nd week of gestation. In this case, it is usually best to wait for labor to occur naturally, assuming:

- Your baby is still as active as usual.
- The amount of amniotic fluid is adequate.
- Your baby has a normal heart rate, with reassuring postdates testing.
- The size of your baby is estimated to be compatible with the characteristics of your pelvis.
- You are healthy, and there are no other pregnancy complications.

Monitoring a Postdate Baby

There is an increased risk of complications associated with postdate pregnancies, mostly related to an aging placenta that ceases to function as well as it did earlier or to a baby that continues to grow to an exceptionally large size. Therefore, there will be a need to monitor you and your baby more closely after 41 weeks. Rest assured, though, that the majority of postdate babies do just fine.

Fetal Movement Counts

Fetal movement demonstrates adequate nourishment and oxygen from a healthy placenta. A baby will significantly decrease its movement as the condition of the placenta deteriorates. With that in mind, a wonderful way you can monitor the continued wellbeing of your baby throughout the third trimester is to do daily fetal movement counts.

Pick a time when your baby is usually most active; often this is after meals, when resting, or at night when you are lying in bed. Make sure you count at least ten distinct moves in an hour. If you notice less, the baby may be sleeping. Try again a little later after drinking two large glasses of fruit juice, a cup of coffee, and eating a complex carbohydrate and natural sugar meal, such as a peanut butter and jelly sandwich on sprouted whole-grain bread. Lie down after 30-40 minutes, and count the number of moves. If the baby is not moving after this, or you still feel that the baby is moving less than usual in a 12-hour period, contact your practitioner right away. The baby needs to be evaluated, and if in trouble, will need to be delivered as soon as possible.

In-Office Testing

Two tests commonly done in the office to monitor the condition of the placenta and a baby's wellbeing are the twice-weekly NST (non-stress test) and the weekly BPP (biophysical profile sonogram).

The NST uses an external electronic fetal monitor to note the character of the baby's heart rate and its response to fetal movement. The desired response is a fetal heart rate that varies from beat to beat within the normal range and increases at least twice when the baby moves, 15 beats per minute for at least 15 seconds within 20 minutes. Out-of-hospital midwives are asked and can use a fetoscope or doppler to check fetal heart rate and record accelerations manually, but it is less accurate, without a recorded tracing, not the standard of care, nor evidence-based; it is also not supported by modern medicine or by most of the collaborative obstetricians whom midwives work with.

The BPP uses ultrasound to examine the fetus and its environment in utero by assessing a variety of parameters including the baby's movements, muscle tone, the placenta, and the amount of amniotic fluid. The ultrasound can also provide estimates on the baby's growth and weight, but they are only estimates and not always accurate at this late stage of pregnancy. Try to schedule this test during a time the baby is usually active and moving the most. On the day of the test, make sure you are drinking your usual daily eight to ten glasses of water, so the baby has plenty of amniotic fluid. 30-40 minutes before the test, make sure to have two large glasses of fruit juice and a natural sugar/carbohydrate meal or other foods that usually wake the baby up and cause lots of movement. You can even have a cup of coffee or tea just in case the baby is still sleeping after the meal. The test is somewhat dependent on the baby moving, and we would not want a false report of no fetal movement indicative of fetal stress when the baby was just sleeping healthfully.

Natural Measures to Help Prevent Problems Related to Postdates

These recommendations are especially helpful if you had complications from postdates in prior pregnancies, you are attempting a vaginal birth after a previous cesarean, or you have other complications, such as diabetes or high blood pressure, and it is not advisable to let the pregnancy extend past term. Research on natural induction methods is sparse, but growing. Sometimes, one remedy or a combination of them does the trick, and all is well. Sometimes, no matter what we do, we cannot get labor started. Nothing works consistently, including the medications used in hospitals. Unless there is a scheduled cesarean birth, when a baby comes into the world is ultimately not in our human control. Meanwhile, try to keep yourself occupied by doing things you enjoy, continuing to exercise as tolerated, and planning some daily pleasurable activities to keep your morale upbeat and positive.

Know Your Status

If you are planning a pregnancy, keep an accurate record of your cycle and know the first day of your last menstrual period. Or better yet, the day of conception around the time of ovulation. If there is a question about your dates (if you are breastfeeding, recently miscarried, went off the birth control pill, or have long or irregular cycles), an early first trimester ultrasound can accurately date your pregnancy. This will prevent a lot of aggravation later on, like unnecessary testing, pressure to deliver, and induction based on miscalculated dates. Refer to the chapter "Fertility Awareness and Pregnancy Dating" for more details.

Eat Right for Your Baby

Drink lots of pure water and maintain a healthy, well-balanced diet as described in the chapter "Nutritional Best Practices for Mom." Limit your intake of fruit juice, and avoid refined white flour and sugary products. Aside from being unhealthy and fattening, they grow big babies that are harder to push out.

Make sure to eat plenty of dates and pineapples—some swear by them to encourage labor. I am not convinced, but there is no harm in trying.

Prepare Your Mind

Prepare for a deeply positive childbirth experience. It is very important to enter labor and birth with positive feelings, trusting your body and the whole birth process.

It is helpful to write a positive birth vision, what you wish your labor and birth to be like from start to finish, and include the role and involvement of all persons who will be there. This is something you and your partner can think about and write together. You may write as little or as much as you like, but enjoy thinking about this special time in your life.

There are a number of methods to help you get ready for the amazing experience to come:

- Childbirth classes. See the chapter, "Childbirth Classes—What's the Scoop?"
- Hypnosis for birth in adjunct
- Gentle, prenatal, and restorative Yoga. Refer to the chapter, "Yoga During Pregnancy and Labor."
- Breathwork, meditation, and progressive muscle relaxation techniques (yoga nidra). Read the chapter, "Meditation, Breathwork, and Visualization."
- Watching positive birth movies
- Listening to inspiring podcasts and birth summits
- Reading books. My online course has a comprehensive list of all my favorites, but some top picks are:
    - *Mindful Birthing* by Nancy Bardacke
    - *Orgasmic Birth* by Elizabeth Davis and Debbie Pascale Bonaro
    - *Ina May's Guide to Childbirth* by Ina May Gaskin
    - *Baby Catcher* by Peggy Vincent
    - *Bountiful, Beautiful, Blissful: Experience the Natural Power of Pregnancy and Birth with Kundalini Yoga and Meditation* by Gurmukh Karma Kalsa.

Accept and express feelings that might be holding you back, such as anxiety or fear about childbirth or becoming a mother, uncertainty about your changing role as a person or relationship with loved ones, and hesitation about giving up the special attention you've enjoyed while being pregnant. Do not hesitate to talk with a close friend, family member, childbirth educator, therapist, or transformational life coach, as labor and birth are heavily influenced by your emotions. Often, simply sharing and releasing ambivalent or troubling feelings does wonders to help you open up, let go, and give birth. When that does not help, try releasing it from your body with breathwork.

Practice the following thoughts daily while doing slow, deep breathing in a quiet meditative space:

Spend some time saying goodbye to your pregnancy and inviting your baby to come out. Tell yourself that you and your baby are ready for labor and birth to occur. Imagine your uterus contracting. Visualize your cervix softening and opening, and picture your baby descending through the birth canal, so you can cradle your beautiful newborn child in your arms. Affirm that you will surrender, let yourself be relaxed and open so that your body will do what it was perfectly designed to do— give birth to a new human being.

Herbal Support

Drink fresh infused red raspberry leaf tea regularly. Among its many benefits, it encourages more effective uterine activity and, thus, an easier birth. It is optimal to make your own by adding a generous handful of the dried herb to one quart of water. Let it soak in a glass canning jar for approximately one hour, then strain. You can add honey, fresh mint leaves, and/or lemon juice to taste. Drink it several times per day.

Dr. Christopher's Birth Prep herbal formulation is designed to cause an increase in toning contractions in late pregnancy and prepare your body for labor and birth. It can be taken during the last six weeks of pregnancy under supervision by your provider. The recommended cycle is one capsule per day at week 34-36; two capsules per day at week 37; and two capsules, twice per day at week 38 onward, until you have your baby.

Make your own wonderful late-pregnancy herbal tonic to be used 37 weeks onward. Combine one dropperful each of red raspberry leaf, partridge berry, blue vervain, and cramp bark with 1/4 of a dropperful each of wild yam and motherwort in a separate tincture bottle, and shake to mix well. Take a half of a dropperful of the mixture a few times daily. You can double the dose in the last week before your due date.

You can take evening primrose oil capsules, 500 mg daily, as early as 36 weeks to help ripen the cervix.

At 38 weeks gestation, start inserting six to eight capsules of evening primrose oil deep inside your vagina behind the cervix, every 8-12 hours if:

- This is your first baby OR
- You have a history of post-dates babies (babies that were diagnosed at birth as being post mature, especially associated with complications).

At 41 weeks gestation, start inserting evening primrose at the dose above if:

- Your cervix is still not ready for labor as measured by internal exam AND
- Your bag of waters is intact.

You should have a ripe cervix within a few days. At 41 weeks, you can also increase the oral 500 mg dose to three times daily.

Get in the Mood

As long as your bag of waters is still intact and you do not have a history of premature labor, engage in frequent sexual intercourse, especially after 36 weeks. Semen contains prostaglandins which can help ripen the cervix for labor, and reaching climax can bring on uterine contractions that may stimulate labor if the cervix is ripe and the baby is ready. The same energy that gets the baby in, gets the baby out, so turn up the sensual and make lots of love.

Get Moving

Likewise, if you do not have a history of preterm labor, engage in regular moderate exercise for at least 30 minutes, 5 days per week. As you get closer to term, moving around while upright uses gravity to help get the baby in an optimal position for birth, as well as pressing on the cervix and causing it to ripen and stimulate contractions.

As women get closer to the term, it is common to feel an increased frequency, length, and intensity of Braxton Hicks contractions so the uterine muscle can warm up for labor. These contractions are felt as occasional lower abdominal, menstrual-like cramping in early pregnancy. But, as you get closer to term, you can actually feel your uterus ball up and harden, often from the top downward before it softens again. They are usually brief, painless, and irregular without a pattern, and they increase with activity and resolve with rest.

If you do not feel such uterine activity beginning at 39 weeks, you can do nipple stimulation every ten minutes for an hour, three times per day, to stimulate contractions. To do this, roll the end of your nipple between your fingers and compress and pull slightly as a suckling baby would do. Alternately, you can use a breast pump, which will come in handy postpartum.

Natural Ways to Bring on Labor

Do get regular chiropractic care or special physical therapy, and acupuncture with an experienced provider who has high success rates. This often works like a charm.

Only use the below methodologies if you have reached or passed your due date and you have discussed options with your practitioner.

Increase nipple stimulation to every five minutes for two hours, four to five times per day. It may take several hours, but with a little persistence, this can get labor going. Nipple stimulation causes a release of your body's own oxytocin, the hormone that ripens the cervix and stimulates uterine contractions. Don't stop until labor is progressing on its own.

Take homeopathic cimicifuga 30c, four to five pellets, alternating with caulophyllum 30c, four to five pellets, every hour for 12 hours. Repeat for two days. This gently stimulates your cervix to ripen and labor contractions to begin.

Massage your uterus with castor oil until you get a contraction, and then repeat every five minutes until a labor pattern is established on its own.

If all else fails and your cervix is ripe, you can try drinking castor oil. This induces labor by stimulating your bowels, so be prepared for the possibility of diarrhea. Take two ounces of Castor oil in orange juice every hour for a total of three times. Two ounces of vodka, brandy, or bourbon can be added to this mixture to loosen you up psychologically if needed. After each drink, go for a walk around your house (staying close to a bathroom!) and then take a hot shower, letting the water flow onto your nipples and persistently massage your belly with some of the castor oil.

If still no labor, there are other thing that you can do like an enema, asking your midwife to gently stretch and strip your your membranes (separating the membranes from their attachment to the lower uterine wall), or as a last resort, breaking your water if baby's head is low enough and/or medication if your baby needs to be born without delay.

Labor and Birth

Choosing Your Birth Setting

Homebirths: In the Home or the Hospital

Homes and hospitals–they might not seem to have a whole lot in common, except for the fact that they both begin with the letter H. But homebirth and hospital birth can and do co-exist though that is sometimes hard to reconcile. We are so accustomed to categorization in our society–something has to be either/or, this or that. And oftentimes those two choices are seemingly opposing ones. Why? Must there be conflict and judgment at every turn, especially when we are talking about tiny, precious babies and their awesome parents-to-be?

Personally, I don't think so. I believe we should be framing birth in the context of generational wisdom, evidence-based practices, and ultimately, the sacredness of little ones coming into the world. All of these things can and should be applied to every kind of delivery setting, whether it's a home, birth center, or hospital.

Some women who would like to have a homebirth don't have legal access to care in their states. Some need to deliver in a hospital for medical reasons. Some choose to deliver in a hospital but desire–to the best of their abilities–a homebirth-like experience.

Women interpret that phrase in different ways. For some, a homebirth-like experience means being surrounded by treasured items that remind them of the comforts of home. For others, it means being cared for by midwives and having a beautiful and respectful natural birth. For one client of mine, whom I'll call Jackie (not her real name), it meant birthing without unnecessary medical intervention.

Jackie and her husband both came from long lines of doctors who felt very strongly that a woman should have her baby in a hospital with an OB/GYN. Although she wanted to give birth at home, Jackie decided it wasn't worth the familial turmoil and chose a doctor for a hospital birth. But she didn't take these tasks lightly. She selected a care provider whom she felt would really honor her preferences and who would chart them so that they were on record. She took a comprehensive childbirth education course, which taught her to be prepared and open-minded, and made it abundantly clear to the nurses upon admission that, though she was aware pain medication was available, she did NOT want it to be offered. Lastly, Jackie had faith in herself and in the birth process.

Of course, labor is completely unpredictable, and women who are very firm about their birth visions have the right to change their minds at any given time. In addition, many hospitals are, in fact, set up to intervene, because they are based on a model that considers labor and birth for even low-risk mothers a medical condition, not a physiological process. Of course, these potential challenges had crossed Jackie's mind. But she was determined.

As Jackie's midwife consultant, I certainly had faith in her. And I knew her husband was going to be a terrific and loving support partner. But I was silently concerned about those who would be attending her during labor. Would Jackie's nurses respect her preferences? Would another care provider in the practice (in case the doctor she really liked wasn't on call at the time) do the same?

Fortunately, Jackie's nurse was fabulous and agreed to her requests. Every once in a while, she would come in and marvel at how Jackie listened to her body and just allowed labor to happen. When Jackie went into transition, this nurse came in, gently approached her, and whispered, "You are doing such a fabulous job! But I have to chart that I offered you pain meds, even just once." Jackie nodded, confirming that she heard the nurse and said, "No thanks." Then the nurse gave me the thumbs up and quietly left us.

Shortly thereafter, Jackie's beautiful baby came into the world without any medical management in the most highly interventive hospital in the county. Jackie was over the moon at the sight of her gorgeous baby boy and proud that she had done it her way. In no small part, she was able to accomplish this because she found people to care for her who really listened and supported her choices.

In the end, it's not that any one comfort technique, any one protocol, or any one approach is right or wrong. What counts is a truly healthy baby and mom, whose preferences and needs are recognized throughout pregnancy, labor, and birth.

There are lots of things you can do to maximize your odds for having the kind of birth you envision. You can start by building your support team with people who believe in you. An aligned mom-provider philosophy is a great place to start. You may ultimately have to make some compromises, but the value of a mutually respectful relationship can be immeasurable.

Watch my video about how to have a homebirth-like experience in the hospital: https://homesweethomebirth.com/nbsbookbonus

Can *All* Women Have a Homebirth? Do You Encourage All Women to Do So?

First and foremost, I believe in a woman's right to be empowered, informed, and supported in however she chooses to birth. I promote a homebirth model of care in all settings. This means that I support physiologic birth without disturbance when all is well; I do things as naturally and holistically as possible, without intervention unless medically necessary. The care is sensitive, kind, personalized, family-centered, and evidence-based. The setting is as close to home as a woman desires, and most importantly, one in which a woman feels supported, heard, and her choices respected.

A woman brings her sensuality, ways of coping, and spiritual practices to her birth. She is free to eat, drink, vocalize, and move in a way that helps her labor and feels good to her, and she is being treated with compassion and care. A physiological birth is advantageous to a woman and her baby, so I promote a birth and healthcare provider who encourages this.

Not all women are candidates for a home or freestanding birth center birth. Some women may have a health condition like high blood pressure, seizures or insulin-dependent diabetes, have preterm labor that cannot be stopped, or the baby is found to have a heart defect that makes birthing out of hospital inappropriate or unsafe, as it would pose a risk to the mom or the baby during or immediately after childbirth. In these cases, I suggest they give birth under the guidance of a healthcare professional in a hospital setting, which is well- equipped to handle the situation and potential risks involved. But these mamas and babies will still benefit from the homebirth model of care in the hospital, a model of care I am passionate about for all settings.

Some women don't feel comfortable birthing at home or even in a freestanding birth center. When I meet a woman for the first time, I never try to convince her to have a homebirth or where to birth. I ask that she convinces me, because a woman needs to feel safe and committed to this experience in a way that will best serve her as she labors and brings her baby into the world.

If a well woman is experiencing a healthy pregnancy, like most women, she is a candidate for a homebirth or freestanding birthing center. She will most likely do well birthing out of hospital if she is well-prepared and takes responsibility for her health, feels comfortable with her midwife and support system–a doula, other close family members and/or friends of her choosing to mother her–and a general conviction about wanting to have her baby at home or a birth center.

Regardless of the birth setting, I am passionate about restoring humanity to the childbearing experience and to maternity and newborn care. I am devoted to promoting homebirth-like care at home, birth centers, hospitals, and the offices and clinics where mamas go for their prenatal and postpartum visits. Any woman, no matter where she births, can take the philosophies and practices of a homebirth, create a birth plan she feels empowered by, and have a homebirth-like experience in the hospital. I help mamas locally and around the world make this happen.

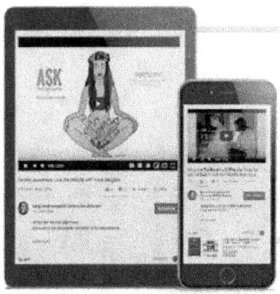

Want to learn more or have more questions?

Grab your free Book Bonuses below:
https://homesweethomebirth.com/nbsbookbonus

Understanding Epidurals and the Benefits of a Natural Birth

Though modern medicine today encourages epidurals, this doesn't make epidurals inherently bad. They are simply being misused and overused. It is time we tell the truth about epidurals. Epidurals can be literally life-saving in a dire situation when a cesarean birth or medical induction of labor is needed, and there are times when they are indeed warranted, but there are serious concerns about their use in a childbirth process that is proceeding normally and healthfully, when their risks outweigh their benefits. I aim to give you an enlightening look at the different sides of epidurals, including the situations when they are very necessary, so you can make an informed decision for yourself.

How Do Epidurals Work?

An epidural is an injection of a large needle in the lower back that pierces the covering of the spinal cord. Medications are injected through a tiny catheter threaded through the needle into the space surrounding the spinal cord where they then infuse the nerves nearby. These medications usually consist of a regional anesthetic and an opiate.

The anesthetic drugs temporarily block the sensory nerves, which usually create the numbing that, in turn, inevitably blocks the motor nerves with some degree of temporary paralysis. The opiates are included because they increase the effectiveness of the anesthetic, allowing for a smaller required dose, while working to decrease the blockage of motor nerves at the same time.

The Cons

The true downturns of using an epidural occur in a birth that is perfectly healthy and normal are many, according to the research. Using an epidural is found to lead to a cascade of other risky and potentially dangerous interventions, just by taking a drug in which there is no need for in the first place. As pointed out by physician, neonatologist, and researcher Michael Klein in his three-part Science and Sensibility blog analysis of the evidence on epidurals:

> *"Women need to be accurately and completely informed of their choices for pain relief in labour before they can provide their true consent. No matter how well intended, epidural analgesia increases the likelihood that women will have a variety of other interventions, especially if the epidural is given without specific medical indications ... When used routinely as a first line agent, epidural analgesia can create problems that could have been avoided."*

Epidurals increase the risk of requiring a C-section, especially when given too early. According to Dr. Kelly Brogan's brilliant analysis of the research, there's been a 60% rise in C-sections since 1996. A study has shown that a prolonged second stage of labor is the main reason for the most cesareans. This prolongation can be directly linked to the use of epidurals, for many reasons, including a mom's decreased ability to push effectively and her needing to be in a supine position that makes birthing more difficult, as it goes against gravity and pelvic capacity is at its smaller dimensions.

What happens after this prolonged stage? A myriad of interventions to "help" to induce the birth: from restricting food, drink, and mobility, IV fluids, bladder catheter, medications to augment labor, more frequent internal exams and procedures like artificially rupturing the membranes of protective amniotic fluid around baby, and continuous monitoring that has not improved outcomes in babies, but has led to dramatically increased rates of cesareans. All of these will only encourage the need for even more interventions, like vacuums, forceps, episiotomy, increased probability of more severe perineal tearing into the anal sphincter and rectum, or major abdominal surgery. All medications, invasive interventions, and operative deliveries risk birth trauma and injury to the baby as well as the mother.

Epidurals can prolong all stages of labor, combined with the associated procedures that increase the risk of infection. Epidurals also increase the incidence of non-infectious fever for moms, which leads to IV antibiotics in case of infection that, most likely, is non-existent. Antibiotics disrupt the microbiome and lead to all the associated health risks of interfering with the healthy balance of bacteria within the body for both the mom and baby. It can also lead to signs of fetal distress, which then lead to other interventions from needing oxygen to emergency surgical delivery.

This drug administration upsets the normal hormonal balance during labor. While the very nature of an epidural is to alleviate at least some of the pain and so easing a good chunk of stress, some stress during labor is actually quite good for both mother and baby. Cortisol, the stress hormone, for example, lessens a mom's exhaustion. It gives the mother energy to push and heightens her euphoria and sense of excitement—a big part of the natural birth experience—and this euphoria actually increases bonding with the baby. For the baby, the healthy "stress" of being born turns many biological processes on during the whole birthing process, like the baby's breathing instinct at birth, which eases transition to adjusting to life outside the womb. No surprise that babies may need more assistance to breathe when epidurals are administered, and tend to be too sleepy to nurse well initially.

There are so many effects that also take place in the aftermath of the birth since an epidural is a narcotic that will pass from the mother's circulation through the placenta into the baby's bloodstream.

Evidence supports risks to the baby from epidurals that include reduced muscle tone, poor feeding, jaundice, withdrawal, and sensorimotor impairment. Epidurals have been linked to failure to establish breastfeeding, and this is not to be taken lightly, as breastfed babies have much healthier outcomes and less health risks than formula-fed babies.

Newborns also can get a fever and increased heart rate from the epidural, without having an infection, but separation from mom and extensive work-up in the neonatal intensive care unit ensues for evaluation, including blood tests, spinal tap, and precautionary IV antibiotics.

Renowned physical therapist, labor expert and childbirth educator Penny Simkin highlights:

> *"Epidurals can result in short-term subtle neurobehavioral effects, such as irritability and inconsolability and decreased ability to track an object visually or to shut out noise, bright light. There are no data on potential long-term effects ... Decreased infant responsiveness may lead to long-term consequences for the parent-infant relationship ... [risking] labels of 'difficult child' or 'incompetent mother' [self-imposed or by others]."*

The mother can experience some annoying but distressing side effects, mostly from the medications entering her bloodstream and/or administration error, like itching, nausea, shivering, spinal headache, residual numbness, tingling and weakness, backache, as well as alarming side effects, like difficulty swallowing and breathing, rare permanent nerve damage, convulsions, respiratory paralysis, cardiac arrest, and even death. Evidence-based care expert Henci Goer points out in her ongoing evaluation of risks and benefits of maternity care that epidurals cause "somewhere between 1 in 1,400 and 1 in 4,400 women to experience a life-threatening complication."

This is some very scary stuff! And yet, epidurals aren't so much the problem as are our society's tendencies to consider them a benign and advised common practice for the majority of healthy laboring women.

Epidurals necessitate hospital birth and eliminate the homebirth and birth center option, which are associated with better health outcomes physically and emotionally for a mom and baby, when it comes to low-risk healthy childbirth. Neonatologist, pediatrician, family physician, and medical researcher Dr. Michael Klein poignantly elaborates on the concerns that epidurals have medicalized birth so much so that they increase the demand on the nurse to pay greater attention to the technology of all the resulting interventions, and consequently, they have less time, experience, and skill to provide needed hands-on and emotional support for the laboring woman.

Disruption of the normal hormones of labor with epidural use can cause the laboring mom to feel detached from her own childbirth process and to becomes more of an observer than a participant. Studies indicate that women who had an epidural may have had less pain, but were most dissatisfied with their experience even up to a year later. The provider and nurse can no longer assess labor progress by observing the mother and must rely on the monitor, which makes the experience more impersonal, and vaginal exams, which are invasive and increase risk of infection. The use of epidurals and the anesthesiologist alone raise the cost of care, which increases exponentially with the cascade of hospital interventions that result.

The Pros

One of my founding philosophies in helping women to have a safe, healthy, and transcendent birth experience is that a birth—of any kind, in all settings!—isn't a medical procedure. It's a natural and miraculous process of life. It is not, in and of itself, a dangerous crisis.

That being said, I'd like to affirm that an epidural has its place in childbirth.

When a labor isn't proceeding normally, when there's a prolonged or arrested labor or the mother is experiencing exhaustion, extreme pain, and/or anxiety, the compassionate use of an epidural could be the answer and can enable her to relax, rest, and progress to vaginal delivery. There could be a real medical need for medications to help induce or augment labor, which makes labor sensations much more painful. As a last resort, an epidural can help relieve the pain and stress from an emergency situation.

A woman suffering from preeclampsia, for example, who receives an epidural anesthetic, will likely not have a prolonged second stage of labor. Epidurals tend to lower blood pressure, which is a benefit in cases of hypertension.

An epidural could also be an advantage during a major operation like a cesarean; in most cases, it carries much less risk than general anesthesia and is a great alternative to being unconscious from the high doses of those medications.

An epidural or spinal anesthetic could relief or reduction of pain without seriously impacting a mother's mental state. Since birth by C-section is still a birth, an epidural or spinal anesthetic can help the mom stay fully alert and pain-free during this operation. She'll be involved and fully capable of holding and bonding with her baby even after a a cesarean birth, as opposed to being put out from a general anesthetic.

Keep in mind that I'm speaking of C-sections that are necessary because of endangering complications and serious issues. This is not the same as C-sections that are caused by epidurals themselves like we spoke about before. Cesareans, in and of themselves, are supposed to be the last resort and indicated for serious life-threatening health problems. The fact that we have them more and more often in America and that they are treated as a normal procedure during a labor is a sore reflection of our society's ideas of pregnancy and birth.

How to Prepare for an Epidural-Free Birth

The women who come to me want to have their pregnancy and labor their own way, and they don't want to numb themselves to the healthy and normal sensations of giving birth. It is, in fact, your own birthright as a woman to have this right of passage into motherhood. The women I work with want to feel that empowerment and the high of successfully bringing their child into the world on their own. Here are some reasons why, that go beyond commitment to avoiding risky unnecessary interventions.

The physicality and courageous mindset of overcoming challenges that are required to give birth has been compared to the performance of an endurance athlete! There's an inherent strength in every woman to go beyond what she knows herself to be capable of. And when she does that, she is darn proud of herself; she has discovered her strength and capacity she can draw on for the rest of her life.

As Dr. Sarah Buckley pointed out:

> *"In labor, such high-levels [of beta-endorphins] are released and help the laboring woman to transcend pain, as she enters the altered state of consciousness that characterizes an undisturbed birth. In the hours after birth, elevated beta-endorphin levels reward and reinforce mother-baby interactions, including physical contact and breastfeeding as well as contributing to intensely pleasurable, even ecstatic, feelings for both."*

Kelly Brogan, MD regards fully feeling and experiencing natural birth as an "empowering life journey, an opportunity for psycho-spiritual transcendence ... to behold a glimpse of what we are capable of as mammals and most importantly, as a human female ... As most women who have experienced natural birth would attest – just when you think you can't do it and your mind demands surrender–you meet your baby, and the world stands still in a moment of unparalleled beauty and wonder."

Understanding what your body is capable of can begin to give you the confidence you need to begin planning your natural birth. My Love Your Birth course can help you prepare for the entire process from beginning to end. You'll equally learn how to cope with and handle labor pains, so much so that you can love your experience no matter how challenging. The right preparation really begins with a shift in mindset, not just about labor but in what your body is capable of doing. The pride and joy that a woman experiences after giving birth naturally is overwhelming. So many mamas are empowered and overcome by their own capability to bring their child into the world.

My rate of successful women having natural births is 93%. The other 7% of cases had complications that required medical attention or surgical intervention. But, in over two decades of practice as a homebirth midwife, I've never once had to transfer a mother to the hospital for an epidural or any other pain medication because she couldn't cope with sensations of normal labor. Not once! It is not that women who come to me have different bodies. It has more to do with how well they prepare themselves in advance, their attitudes and mindsets, and how they are cared for and supported during birth.

Women have been giving birth naturally around the world since the beginning of time. Today, we interfere more with it, and sometimes we get in our own way. Have faith that your body and nature both have your back—they were divinely designed to know what to do! We just need to step aside. That takes advance preparation in the modern world, as well as choosing care providers and settings that have the philosophy and expertise to support normal healthy physiologic birth without unnecessary disturbance.

Don't deprive yourself of these sensations and this transcendent experience. You are able and you are supported!

VBAC—Vaginal Birth After Cesarean

If a woman has had a cesarean and wants to plan a vaginal birth for her next, it would be considered a VBAC, which stands for vaginal birth after cesarean.

A cesarean section is major abdominal surgery that involves serious potential risks for both a mother and her baby. Unfortunately, a cesarean can lead to trauma to the internal organs or reproductive tract, risk of hemorrhage, complications with scar tissue, long-term postoperative pain, wound infection, blood clots, stroke, and possible respiratory problems for the baby. High rates of cesarean section contribute to high rates of morbidity and mortality as well.

When medically necessary, a cesarean can be life-saving. I am very grateful for this. And it is still, of course, a birth to celebrate. However, cesareans have become so routine. Statistically, the United States ranks among the highest in the world for cesarean rates. It's approximately 30% and rising. It's as high as 40%-50% in some areas near to where I live, and this is absolutely unacceptable.

I believe women are not given the opportunity to explore all their options and are not offered education and empowerment to have a vaginal delivery after a previous cesarean, other than a repeat cesarean birth, if that is their choice. This is why I want to educate pregnant women on the possibility of VBAC.

Benefits of a VBAC

There are many benefits to a VBAC—physical, emotional, mental, and spiritual. These are only a few important benefits on the long list:

- The mother and baby do not face the risks associated with c-sections. This is enormous.
- There is an easier postpartum healing and recovery for the mother.
- The baby receives necessary bacteria for optimal health from the mother when passing through the vaginal birth canal.
- Breastfeeding may be more successful.
- There is no potential harm to the woman's future fertility.
- The woman tends to feel more positive about the birth experience.
- She has an increased sense of empowerment.
- VBAC allows for more involvement of family and support people.
- There is less risk of postpartum depression and emotional birth trauma.

Most major healthcare regulators and advisory organizations like the World Health Organization encourage VBACs:

> *"The World Health Organization recommends that the caesarean section rate should not be higher than 10% to 15%. According to the Society of Obstetricians and Gynecologists of Canada (SOGC), vaginal delivery represents the safest route for the fetus and newborn in the first and subsequent pregnancies."*

The WHO's recommended c-section rate is actually quite generous. When the cesarean section was originally implemented, it was intended to serve 5% of the birthing population–those with serious complications who really needed life-saving surgical intervention.

The National Guideline Clearinghouse Agency for Healthcare Research and Quality, and the American College of Nurse Midwives provide a lot of information on this topic as well, as does the International Cesarean Awareness Network (ICAN). The American Academy of Family Physicians stated the following:

"The AAFP strongly recommends that clinicians inform women who have had a prior vaginal birth, either before or after a prior cesarean birth, that they have a high likelihood of VBAC. Unless there are specific contraindications to a vaginal birth, these women should be encouraged to plan a labor and VBAC and should be offered referral to clinicians and facilities capable of providing this service, if it is not available locally."

I share the opinion of many concerned with improving maternity care and reducing our rising rates of maternal and newborn death and serious health consequences from the interventions in normal childbirth; that a woman should not be forced to have a major surgery against her will, rather she should be provided with the current evidence and empowered to make her own decision, considering she is having a healthy pregnancy.

The American College of Obstetricians and Gynecologists removed the previous unreasonable restriction requiring immediate availability of a surgical staff for an emergency cesarean, as most hospitals around the country, let alone free-standing birth centers and home settings, do not meet this criterion. Most hospitals are not able to have a surgical staff at all times and cannot perform an emergency cesarean in under 30 minutes.

Despite this, research is showing that far too many obstetricians do not offer VBACs. They routinely recommend repeat cesareans because they may fear lawsuits, have scheduling stresses, work in a restrictive hospital, have to abide by malpractice insurance policies, and/or feel pressured to uphold certain standards among their colleagues not supportive of VBAC. The hands of a midwife whose collaborative obstetrician and hospital do not support VBAC can often be unnecessarily tied as well for these reasons. Most repeat cesareans are not actually medically necessary and are commonly recommended due to various non-medical reasons. This is very concerning.

What also concerns me is that the risks of a VBAC are magnified in conversation with women while the risks of a repeat cesarean are downplayed, so women may feel forced, afraid, and powerless.

I want women to feel like they have a voice.

Some women who want to have a VBAC have limited options, and local doctors in the area are only offering cesareans. Some feel they have no option other than having an unattended homebirth, laboring alone at home until the last minute without any monitoring, or not being truthful with their providers about their previous cesarean birth—all of which can increase the risks for her and her baby.

A trained and experienced midwife who is continuously with the woman in active labor can detect concerning signs and symptoms before they can become a crisis, so that the mama is transferred and treated in time to save her and her baby's life and health. A midwife wears many hats, one of which is protecting the space, so the natural process of birth can proceed with ease and grace, and another is as a lifeguard to know when and how to intervene to prevent problems or manage emergencies. There are many wonderful obstetricians supportive of VBAC who have this training and style of practice as well; they are just harder to find.

Who Is a Good Candidate for a VBAC? What Are the Chances of Having a Successful VBAC?

The stats range from 60-80% of women, who have had previous cesareans, are candidates for a successful VBAC. In actuality, most healthy pregnant women carrying healthy babies are candidates.

The chances of a successful VBAC are higher if a woman is using a midwife, even higher in free-standing birthing centers and home settings. Going to a hospital and working with an OB/GYN with high cesarean rates will increase the likelihood that a woman will have another cesarean.

In some hospitals, there are a lot of restrictive procedures, like continuous electronic fetal monitoring, confining a laboring woman to lie in bed, not allowing her to eat or drink, and routine IVs and time limits, which increase the risk of another cesarean.

As a midwife, I fully support a mama's choice to have a VBAC. But, there are many important reasons why you could find yourself in a condition to have either a scheduled or an unplanned repeat C-section birth. For example, you have had multiple cesareans, a classical incision or prior uterine surgery called a myomectomy to remove fibroids, your baby may be in a transverse position (lying in the uterus across your abdomen), or you may be nearing term and have placenta previa—especially if the placenta is completely or partially covering your cervix. Read up on these situations to further understand what truly are indications for undergoing a C-section.

Once you've learned and weighed the pros and cons of both a VBAC and a C-section, complement your research with the knowledge and experience of your trusted doctor and/or midwife.

What Is the Main Risk of a VBAC?

The risk of separation of the prior uterine scar is approximately 2 in 1,000 VBACs, but often it is a mild superficial dehiscence (slight separation of some layers of the surgical wound) that has no clinical significance and does not impact the health of the mom or baby. The risk of a severe life-threatening emergency from a partial or complete uterine rupture of all the scar layers is significantly lower–a highly unlikely occurrence, significantly less than 1%. The main risk of a VBAC is this rare total rupture of the previous uterine incision that risks both the mother and her baby, and can lead to catastrophic outcomes. It cannot be ignored and must be monitored for appropriately. It also cannot be exaggerated or make the risk of repeat cesarean less alarming.

Although every decision has risks, a VBAC is a reasonable, appropriate, and safe option. If a woman planning a VBAC decides to give birth at home, I highly recommend working with a well-trained and experienced midwife and considering the distance to a hospital (thirty minutes or less driving time is ideal).

There are also risks of some vaginal pain or tearing that takes a few weeks or few months to fully heal (a much shorter time than it takes for the cesarean wound to heal), a slight increase in urinary and rarely anal incontinence, and birth injury to the baby from the uncommon complication of shoulder dystocia.

There are risks and benefits to every kind of birth and in every setting. I provide women with evidence-based information. I encourage each family to dig deep and look at the pros and cons of having a VBAC in a hospital setting, free-standing birthing center, or home versus a scheduled repeat cesarean. I make sure to have informed consent for her birth.

Are There Benefits to a Cesarean?

A planned cesarean is in a controlled environment, and some women find great comfort in knowing that. Perhaps a woman has a history of sexual abuse or had a previous traumatic, long labor the first time, and she just doesn't want to go through that experience again. Some women are very anxious about that, and they just feel safer knowing they will have another cesarean.

I take that seriously because she won't labor well if she doesn't feel safe.

As I have mentioned, the serious risks for a VBAC can often be prevented, treated, or transferred to surgical care in time, with a skilled midwife or obstetrician who is attending to the laboring woman and who is aware and mindful of the symptoms that lead up to any issues.

Thankfully, some hospitals are now at least allowing more time for the baby to get the cord blood from the placenta, skin-to-skin bonding, and the mother's partner or main support person in the operating room. Some providers are performing "gentle cesareans"–cesareans that are family- and woman-centered where they try to provide the environment of a natural birth as much as possible. This is a wonderful attempt to restore humanity to birthing in the operating room.

Dealing with Emotional Trauma from Previous Cesarean

A woman should get the support she needs. Many women who have had a prior cesarean have issues they need to discuss and process, especially if unplanned. There are therapists who specialize in this. Visit ICAN, a nonprofit organization that educates and supports women through their cesarean recovery. They also support families in their communities advocating for VBAC. One of my passions and areas of expertise is creating space, so a mom can debrief, process, and heal from her previous upsetting or traumatic birth experience. That is what I do for the women in my local practice and online for the global community. I work with them not only to heal, but also to help them to approach their next childbirth experience with positivity, confidence, and joy. Also, that is a main focus of my comprehensive online course, Love Your Birth.

I have personally found the most effective form of trauma healing to be Clarity Breathwork, which is explained in the chapter on breathwork. It is so much more powerful than almost any other modality, including talk therapy alone. I had such profound healing myself using this form of breathwork that I became a Clarity Breathwork practitioner to help others experience the huge healing and transformation I did and witnessed in so many others.

VBAC or Cesarean and You

A woman's childbirth is her own, and she should have the freedom to experience the full power of what she is capable of. If you know you want to have another baby, I would start with research and education, and digging deep to determine what you really want: VBAC or cesarean. Know what you want and why you want it. Find healthcare providers as well as other women who support you in your decisions and who can help you on your journey. Hire a doula, especially if you are planning a VBAC and you do not have that kind of calm mothering support for the big day.

This is a time to work closely with your provider(s) on bringing to life the successful birth you've envisioned for yourself. Make your needs and goals very clear to them, so that all you have to focus on is delivering your baby when the time comes.

A glowing vaginal birth after cesarean is possible for every mama who is a candidate, which is most of you. If you decide on planning a VBAC, you need to work extra hard to surround yourself with positivity and supportive encouragement in your local community and online. Look for positive VBAC stories of healing, beauty, and empowerment to encourage you. Fill your mind with positive birth stories, and what's possible for you instead of what you fear might happen. Draw, journal, meditate, visualize, play sensual music, and let yourself freestyle dance to it—these things help you to heighten and easily tap into the intuitive, feminine self. This is your heart and gut, your truth, your wisdom, the part of you that knows what you most deeply desire, and the part of you that knows exactly how to give birth. With easier access to this huge part of your being, you will more easily determine what it is that you want and need. This creates more confidence and assuredness in the decisions that you make, no matter what the rest of the world might be telling you.

Now that you know where to begin, take responsibility for your pregnancy and childbirth. This is the most empowering thing you can do for yourself and your baby. It is also the healthiest and will bring you a deep sense of inner peace and joy. You'll find that there are actually many resources and communities that can help you to have the kind of birth that you envision for yourself.

Watch my video on VBAC : *https://homesweethomebirth.com/ nbsbookbonus*

KIDS AT BIRTH

When you gave birth to your first, there was no one else to worry about–just you, your baby, and your partner. And if you have pets like a cat or dog, you likely made sure that they, too, would be looked after while you were in the throes of labor. So, yes, you made sure you had what you needed and that everybody else had what they needed. But all of that was a piece of cake compared to the plans you have to make when you have other kids on this side of your belly.

Should your children witness the birth of the newest family member? Should they not be present? For some, this is a no-brainer. For others, the answer isn't quite so clear. There are no absolutes when it comes to making this decision, except for one: you'll need to secure the services of a designated child person (DCP) who can help you change gears if necessary. A DCP could be a trusted relative, friend, or caregiver. Let me explain.

Scenario 1–you want your children there. A DCP can help the kids exit stage left if you do a 180 and need them out of the room. Why might that happen? A quick refresher, everyone–how you feel in labor can change super quickly from one moment to the next. You can't possibly know now all of what you'll need then. On the one hand, it might do you a world of good to see those angelic faces when you are between contractions. But you also might be anxious about how your kids are processing everything. Or they may become fearful, disruptive, or needy. Knowing someone is there to lead them out if necessary will help you all feel safe and secure.

Scenario 2–you don't want your children there. The process begins, and your kids aren't with you. Suddenly, you decide that you can't possibly do this without them! Well, your DCP will be just a text or call away, so they are able to bring your kids to your side quickly. Or keep them well cared for until you are ready for them to come meet the baby after birth.

No matter how you envision all of this going, secure your DCP coverage now. When you know your kids will be cared for, you will feel more relaxed. And that will serve you and your upcoming labor wildly well.

Also, make sure to prepare your kids about birth and what to expect. Some birthing centers, doulas, and childbirth educators teach a sibling class. There are many wonderful books and videos for them as well - I list my favorites in my online course. Bring your kids to prenatal visits when you can and encourage them to be involved in your care - some love to "help" the midwife measure your belly, check the baby's heart beat, feel the baby's body parts. Some love to be little doulas and help you in labor, some do not. So be flexible and respect not only their choices but also your needs - all of which may change in labor.

For more information, check out my videos about kids at birth and my other video on family and friends at birth: *https://homesweethomebirth. com/nbsbookbonus.*

LOVED ONES AGAINST HOMEBIRTH

Thanks to documentaries like *The Business of Being Born and Orgasmic Birth*, as well as celebrities like Alanis Morissette and Gisele Bundchen sharing their testimonies of ecstatic births at home, modern women all over the world are stepping into a positive experience of birthing their babies in out-of-hospital settings and sharing it all over the media; and more are returning to giving birth at home, where women have birthed their babies since the beginning of time. Home is still globally the most common setting to have a baby.

I believe many women and their families are not informed of homebirth or a midwifery model of care, and this is where much of the uncertainty and discomfort comes from when it is discussed among partners and family members. Despite the latest statistics showing that a homebirth with a qualified midwife is just as safe as birthing a baby at the hospital–if not safer–many are still apprehensive about the perceived risks involved.

Even so, women continue to birth at home because they feel the calling within their bodies, within their hearts, within their souls. Many women have shared with me that they desire greatly to have a homebirth experience and know that it's what they feel is best for them and for their babies. Many very educated professionals of all careers are making well-researched and informed decisions to have homebirths with a midwife.

Although I am optimistic about healthcare moving in the direction of the more prevalent homebirth midwifery model of care, our modern society still expresses an opinion that babies are to be born in hospitals.

Or at the very least, in birth centers.

What to Do When Your Partner or Family Is Not Supportive of a Homebirth?

I have worked with women who gather as much information as possible and share it with their partner in hopes of helping their partner understand where they are coming from. Sometimes these are the pregnant moms. I have also had partners feel very passionate about having a homebirth, although the mom wasn't completely sure.

In my experience, when partners feel heard and validated, they oftentimes come around. This is through meeting with me as the months go by and having the opportunity to ask questions, get answers, and receive support through the pregnancy process. But a woman who is unsure must dig deep, as she will labor best where she feels safe–and that may be the hospital. If her spouse is zealous, and she agrees only intellectually, I am wary of her being able to relax and give birth at home.

While some of your extended family may have had homebirths themselves or are very supportive, some could be very against the idea, especially if it's a situation they don't fully understand, like going to a midwife or having a homebirth. They may be very vocal about their opinions. If family members don't have the knowledge or direct experience with home or even natural birth, it understandably may not sit well with them, and they may have safety concerns.

I have dealt with these situations often as well. Every situation is different. It is not a time for the pregnant mama to get into debates defending her position. I help empower her to set boundaries and maintain a fortress of positivity around herself. In some more challenging situations, after discussion, we agree that the couple does not need to tell their family they are planning a homebirth at all or until after the birth. They can just say they are seeing a midwife, mention the backup hospital if asked, and that's the end of the conversation.

In most cases, I encourage expectant couples to bring their anti-homebirth family members to prenatal visits to ask me their questions and discuss with me their concerns. When this happens, those family members see the licenses on the wall and medical equipment–like for labs, checking blood pressure and fetal heart rate–even if tucked away in the homey office setting, and they relax a bit. Most significantly, the more time we can spend together, the more answers they receive and feel lovingly validated, they come around to at least stop resisting. Many times I am amazed by how they transform to offer support and even excitement around the upcoming homebirth. Some do tell me they won't relax until it's over and everyone is healthy–but then, after the birth, they become big homebirth supporters, telling everyone how wonderful the experience was.

Watch my video on this topic:
https://homesweethomebirth.com/nbsbookbonus

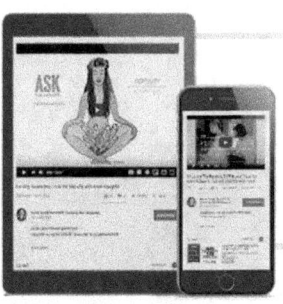

Want to learn more or have more questions?

Grab your free Book Bonuses below:
https://homesweethomebirth.com/nbsbookbonus

Expect the Unexpected

When it comes to birth, oftentimes things don't go as planned. Sometimes this means a woman never makes it to the birthing tub she prepared and dreamt about birthing in because, in the moment of giving birth, she found her groove and prefers to stay on the squatting stool or her labor progresses quickly, and she needs to push before the tub is filled with water. Sometimes this means certain family members or friends aren't present for the birth like originally intended because, for example, a mama is not laboring well with her kids present, they want to leave, or her best friend is sick and could not come to help.

Other times, when things don't go as planned, this means a woman might need IV fluids or other treatments that can be done at home, or medical or surgical interventions that only can be done in hospital. A common example: a mama is experiencing a hard-back labor at home or at a freestanding birth center, her baby persists in the posterior position, she is not progressing for hours despite trying everything and is exhausted; she is transferred to the hospital for Pitocin to augment her labor and the compassionate use of an epidural. A less common example: a baby is not tolerating the labor and is showing signs of worsening distress in any birth setting, and a cesarean is needed to save the baby's life.

Overall, we must surrender to the process of labor and birth, and know that we are being guided and well-cared for. To avoid needless suffering, we must embrace what comes our way that is not in our control, as what is meant to happen–because it is happening or did happen. We can rise to the level of being grateful that we were given exactly what we needed for our growth and benefit, what we each needed on our own journey as a soul temporarily living in a body, even if we do not understand the reasons.

I am not apologetic about my spiritual perspective and my firm belief that the infinite all-powerful being, Spirit, or G-d of our own understanding is beneficent and has pure love for each and everyone one of us.

Want to learn more about this topic? Watch my video *https://homesweethomebirth.com/nbsbookbonus*.

What Do You Do if there is an Emergency in Out-Of-Hospital Birth Settings?

In general, healthy mamas with healthy pregnancies have healthy births. The stats on homebirth and free-standing birth center outcomes are excellent when there is a trained, experienced midwife in attendance.

My transfer rate from home to hospital in labor is 7%, and that is comparable to those of my colleagues. The vast majority of transfers are non-urgent. In most cases, it's usually first-time vaginal birthers whose labor stops progressing with exhaustion despite us trying every one of our "tricks" to remedy the situation. The need to call 911 and have an urgent ambulance transfer has happened a handful of times in over 20 years.

The midwife is, of course, there as a lifeguard, as rarely, emergencies do occur. I bring the same emergency equipment and medications that any free-standing birth center has. Most of the time, I don't use it and all is well. But when I need it, I have saved lives, as any seasoned midwife can say.

I saw much more catastrophic events when I was an OB nurse in the hospital. I have never lost a mother, but our country's high maternal mortality rate is largely from risky hospital interventions, which are not happening at home.

I have had to resuscitate significantly less babies at home–we have a screened healthy low-risk population and are watching closely and WITH the mama in active labor. We do not intervene unless medically necessary and do not cut the umbilical cord until it stops pulsing or the placenta is birthed, unless there is a problem or a request for lotus birth.

In over two decades of homebirth midwifery practice, I have had to transfer three babies to the hospital who did not respond to resuscitation and needed intensive care due to unrelated complications. This is significantly less than our country's high newborn morbidity and mortality rates.

Yes, we need to be prepared for and be able to manage a rare shoulder dystocia (stuck shoulders), but it happens less as our mamas are laboring and birthing in positions that use gravity and maximize the diameter of the pelvis. Yes, we have had to treat postpartum hemorrhage not responsive to natural remedies with medication and IV fluids. That's a big reason we are there.

Why Mention Cesareans?

Cesareans can be both planned and unplanned for serious complications or illness. In both cases, they are indeed a birth, for baby, for mom, for dad/partner, and of a new family.

I want all women to feel lovingly supported and cared for however they give birth, and that includes a cesarean. I like to talk about a gentle cesarean. It's still using a homebirth model of care, with the principle of restoring humanity to maternity and newborn care–especially in the operating room. A gentle cesarean can include pulling the curtain down, allowing the baby to birth itself gently through the incision, encouraging mom to receive her baby directly from the surgeon and to hold her baby skin to skin, delayed cord clamping, and early breastfeeding. It can also include allowing her partner, doula, and anyone else she needs in the OR by her side.

I want to offer support to all women, and especially women who feel their birth did not go as planned and needed a c-section. Although it's rare for normal healthy births to lead to complications or emergencies requiring lifesaving medical and surgical interventions, it can happen and those mamas, babies, and families need extra love and supportive care.

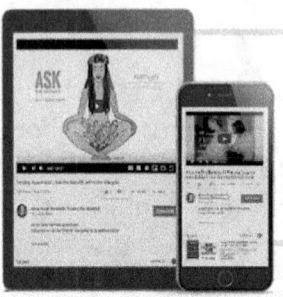

Want to learn more or have more questions?

Grab your free Book Bonuses below:
https://homesweethomebirth.com/nbsbookbonus

Precipitous or Rapid Birth

Precipitous birth is medically defined as a birth that occurs in three hours or less—from the onset of the regular labor pattern to the baby being born. Sometimes, though, it can happen much more quickly than that—two hours, one hour, or even 15 minutes! It tends to happen more often in second and subsequent births, but it can happen to a first-time mama too! A mama can also be in earlier stages of labor but rapidly progress to later stages and pushing.

Is It dangerous?

There are some potential risks, which is why it is important to get help, but in the vast majority of cases, the outcome for mom and baby is good. Normal, natural births are not considered emergencies. Precipitous birth is a variation of normal and natural—it's just crunched into a smaller timeframe than usual!

What If It Happens to You?

First and foremost, stay calm! There is no need to panic. Take a deep breath and feel yourself grounded on the surface you are on. Remember, your body knew how to grow your baby, so it knows how to give birth, and your baby knows how to be born. Connect to the divine, to the spirit of your own understanding, and know you and your baby are guided and protected. It never hurts to say a prayer for the wellbeing of you both.

You can act more effectively when you are calm, and it is ideal to bring your baby into an environment that is peaceful and gentle. If you were planning to go to a hospital or birth center, but you are feeling like you're ready to push, don't get in the car. It is safer to have the baby at home than on the side of the road. Instead, find a comfortable spot to labor in. Your partner can call 911 and then call your care provider. Ask your provider to stay on the phone with your provider until help arrives. If you were planning a homebirth but haven't called the midwife yet, call your midwife and keep her on the phone or ideally FaceTime until she arrives.

Next, find a comfortable spot and ask your partner to put waterproof padding under you, such as a flannel-backed tablecloth with the more comfortable flannel-side up, or even a shower curtain with Chux pads (or cloth versions of them) on top. Remove your pants and underwear. Your care provider will hopefully stay on the phone with you and guide you as you birth your baby. Have your partner gather clean blankets and towels for the baby.

Are Precipitous Labor Sensations Much Different Than Those of a Longer Labor?

This is subjective. Some mamas love their fast birth and are grateful for the surprise and that they were not in labor for a long number of hours. Some mamas can find themselves overwhelmed by a labor that ramps up quickly with little warning.

It might seem harder to cope when she hasn't had time to process what's happening. It is helpful for the partner to remind her that things are progressing quickly because everything is going right.

Helping mama into a side-lying position or hands and knees can help slow things down slightly and give her a better sense of control. Help her tap into her slow, deep breathing to keep her relaxed, and when pushing, pant through pursed lips to not only help slow things down but prevent tearing as the baby is emerging.

Tension and fear not only don't help anyone, they make things worse. It is important to stay relaxed inside, take some deep, slow releasing breaths, and feel yourself on the ground or whatever is beneath you. Find your center. And remember, birth works the vast majority of times, or we would not have survived as humans. It really is an instinctual process. Mamas' bodies know how to give birth and babies know how to be born. We just need to get our minds out of the way. As renowned midwife Ina May Gaskin says, "Let your monkey do it."

Can You Predict a Precipitous Birth?

There is no real way to know if you will have a very fast labor, although it is more common in mamas who have given birth vaginally before. If you had a fast labor with previous babies, it is more likely you'll have another fast labor, and you should prepare for one. If labor begins and contractions are quickly close together (i.e., every few minutes for a first-time mom or approximately every five minutes for a subsequent vaginal birth), lasting 45 seconds or longer, and they feel intense enough that you cannot talk through them, make sure you don't wait to contact your care provider.

Also, keep your provider updated with changes in a "normal" or fairly typically progressing labor, and definitely if your main bag of water breaks and the amniotic fluid releases.

Watch my video about this topic for more details:
https://homesweethomebirth.com/nbsbookbonus

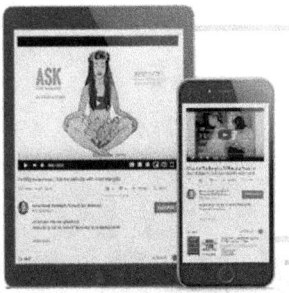

Want to learn more or have more questions?

Grab your free Book Bonuses below:
https://homesweethomebirth.com/nbsbookbonus

Anatomy and Physiology of Birth

A woman, miraculously made is a perfectly designed vessel to bring a baby into the world. Each body part is created for a purpose and specifically placed, so babies can be born. It's a dance between feminine bodies and their babies … each knowing exactly what they are supposed to do. I empower women to get their minds out of the way and learn to work with the brilliant natural process.

When given the opportunity to flourish and to rise up to the moment, a woman's body has the capacity to deliver almost every time.

What Is Your Body Doing During Childbirth?

During pregnancy, you're looking at what your appearance is on the outside. You see your skin stretching, meeting the physical space of encasing a growing being. Most of the conversation is external, comments of size, possible stretch marks.

Just behind this wall of protection lives a breathing, vibrant, and meticulous ecosystem. Swimming in a double-wrapped membranous bag of amniotic fluid lives your baby. The baby is encased in the womb, which is surrounded by the uterus. The placenta connects to the baby through the umbilical cord. All of the baby's nutrients are delivered to them through this cord, which also removes waste.

Five of Many Things That Change with Pregnancy and Labor

1. Through pregnancy, your uterus grows as your baby grows.

2. Moving into labor, your cervix changes. It is firm, thick, long, and closed during pregnancy, and during labor, it softens, thins, shortens, and opens.

3. As your cervix dilates and its tiny vessels break, you may release a mucus plug. This could, but not always, allow for some blood to show.

4. Your vaginal canal of muscles is stretched, holding space for your baby's head and body to come through.

5. Your pelvis, which is three bones connected by ligaments, can stretch. It can get smaller or larger, depending on your position. When we talk about "station," it's in reference to whether the baby's head is engaged in the mid-pelvis or how many centimeters it is above or below it.

Movement and Position During Labor Is Important

Lying down gives the pelvis less room to allow for the baby's head. Squatting, kneeling, hands and knees, lunging, standing, walking, or dancing works with the force of gravity and opens up the pelvis to help the baby to navigate their way down.

What Does It Mean for Your Water to Break?

Because your baby is double-wrapped in two bags of amniotic fluid, the first bag can break, sometimes in early labor, which releases no more than a few tablespoons of fluid that can make up to a pancake-sized stain in your underwear. This could prompt thoughts and concerns about "ruptured membranes"–your main bag of fluid breaking–and may lead to unnecessary interventions to prevent infection, especially when there is a prolonged period of time between this and birth–when in actuality your water did not break.

On the contrary, this tiny gush of fluid is usually a sign that labor is beginning, and only the first bag has broken. As long as there is no continual flow of fluid and no signs on evaluation, the main bag is often still intact and will break during later stages of labor. It's imperative to wear a pad for monitoring and check with your healthcare provider if you have concerns over any flow of fluid to confirm what is going on.

What Is Happening to Your Body Before You Go into Labor?

Everybody is different, but there are some general signals. Pre-labor could last a few weeks. Here are some signs labor could be approaching:

- A dropping sensation as the baby descends lower in the pelvis
- More pelvic pressure
- More frequent bathroom trips
- Loose bowel movements
- Easier breathing
- Less heartburn
- More uterine tightening sensations as the uterine muscles warm up and ripen the cervix
- Excited surge of energy
- "Nesting"–feeling the urge to clean, organize, and prepare.

I am humbled by the many various and unique ways women start labor! Just as women come in so many different shapes, sizes, and forms, so do their labors.

Physical and Emotional Sensations

Generally, when you start to feel a regular pattern of sensations of uterine tightening, we would consider that the onset of labor. These regular sensations are commonly referred to as contractions, but that is a limited term and can create a sense of tension.

The top of the uterus does contract, so the bottom shortens, thins, and expands. Similar to waves, the sensations come and go, build to a peak, then gradually lessen with no such sensation in between, like the calm waters between the waves. Because of this, let's use the word "wave" instead of "contraction"–some mamas prefer "surges" or make up their own affirmative positive term, like "hugs" to the baby.

Labor waves are different than Braxton Hicks' "false" labor waves. Labor waves tend to be felt low in the pelvis and go around the back of the body. They come in a pattern. This means they keep coming. Maybe one comes in five minutes, another in ten, then another in seven, and then another in 20 … It becomes a pattern when they persist. Just like they can range in interval, they range in duration, lasting in the early stages from 20-60 seconds on average. And they feel different.

How Will You feel at the Onset of Labor?

Early waves can feel like menstrual cramping. As they progress, the sensations become more intense, last longer, and come more frequently. They can feel like a tightening with pressure down low in your belly and sometimes low back. You'll be able to have a conversation and go about your day. You'll be coping well and feel sociable and excited.

How Do You Know When You Are Progressing in Labor By How You Are Feeling?

Waves of the cramping will come more frequently, lasting a little bit longer. They tend to come more consistently, like every 4-6 minutes, and last anywhere from 45-75 seconds.

These feel more intense, and you'll generally not be able to speak through them. Some women will begin to moan, breathe, and need to become inwardly focused. When not disturbed, laboring women make natural opiates that lessen sensations of pain and enable them to enter a trance-like state.

Midwife Pam England calls this "labor land." This trance-like state is important because it takes us out of our thinking brain and more into an instinctual, primal, and sensual space that allows our bodies to do their job of birthing.

As labor progresses, the main bag of amniotic fluid may break. This could result in a big gush of fluid releasing at once or periodically–either making a large puddle on the floor, soaking through your clothes and the surface beneath you, or making a large maxi-pad heavy like a baby's full diaper after a night's sleep. There can also be a small amount of normal bleeding from a few streaks or spotting, to no more than a light period.

Moving into active labor, a woman needs more support. Some women in transition will vomit, get sweats, or feel shaky and restless.

Emotions to Consider

When the first stage of labor reaches the final stages, "transition" labor feels most intense–but it also means the progression to pushing out and meeting your baby is coming soon. Labor sensations are coming every few minutes, lasting an average of 60-90 seconds. They are still coming in waves, which rise and fall, with a delicious rest in between.

I encourage women to stay present and know what is common, so they can embrace, rather than fear it.

I like everyone at the birth to know that our birthing mom will experience intense emotions towards the end of labor and that this is normal. So no one will be scared, I reinforce to everyone that she is working hard and she is internally focused.

It's important for everyone at the birth, including the birthing mom, to know and understand the signs during this period, as it may help relieve concern, doubt and fear that arise.

A woman in transition may:

- Lose her ability to cope and feel overwhelmed
- Doubt her decision to birth in the way she wanted to
- Want to give up
- Ask for drugs
- Curse
- Panic
- Think she is dying or that something is really wrong.

These are all signs that even more support is required.

At this point, we bring her back to the present, let her know she is not alone, reassure her all is well, she is doing it, and remind her that we are moving closer to meeting her baby!

This intensity is normal and it's healthy. It is just part of the process, necessary for the huge transformation that is about to occur. And in the scheme of things, it does not last that long. To the mama experiencing it, it feels long, but the earlier part of labor, although easier, is usually much longer–up to several days. And in transition we are talking no more than several hours in the course of a lifespan–around one minute plus, at a time. You can take normal healthy labor sensations for 60-90 seconds with rests in between.

How Is a Baby's Head Able to Make It Through Such a Small Area?

The miraculous design of it all: a baby's skull is not yet fused. The soft spots ("fontanels" located between certain suture lines) on it are there because these bones are not yet closed together, so your baby's head can mold to accommodate the pelvis. And a woman's birth canal can stretch and expand to accommodate her baby.

So Should You Actually NOT Push When Fully Dilated?

This is something I feel very strongly about. The medical model of care defines active labor when a woman is at least six centimeters dilated and the pushing or second stage when a woman is fully dilated. Fully dilated means there is no longer any cervix in front of and encircling the baby's head.

This time is not to be spent trying to push before the natural urge is felt but honored as a resting phase. Often the waves naturally slow down, and there is a sense of calm. Some women sleep to recharge and wake up to a surge of increased energy needed for pushing. I believe we are to honor this time and allow our body and baby to do the work they were perfectly designed to do–the vast majority of times. When the natural physiologic process of birth is allowed to progress on its own, the baby will soon lower into the pelvis on its own, and then you may feel a strong instinctual urge to push. That is the actual start of pushing, the second stage of labor, not when your cervix is examined to be fully dilated.

When a woman is told to push as soon as she is fully dilated, especially for her first vaginal birth, she will exhaust herself, as the baby is not low enough in the pelvis to create the urge to push. She can become swollen and increase the risk of tears. She will have to work longer and harder, as her baby is higher, she is working against her body, not with it. It's like pushing out a bowel movement when you don't feel the urge to. Once the stool lowers in the colon to the point that you feel you have to poop, you poop easily. When the baby naturally lowers and mom has new energy from having the chance to rest, her body creates a natural, strong urge to push. It is much easier to wait and use that internal force to do much of the work for you.

I like to respect the resting phase when all is well. It typically lasts several minutes to an hour or more.

The baby will lower down, and a woman will feel pressure and a powerful urge to push. Like having a bowel movement, you will know when you have to push your baby out.

Although contractions are not as frequent as they were in the last part of labor, many women feel a renewed excitement and determination, becoming hyper-focused on what is happening and getting the job done. Now they can do something to work WITH their body and the intense sensations.

The baby starts the descent and glimpses of their head may be seen that come and go, as it makes a few steps forward and a few back, before it begins to actually come out. The birth canal opens to accommodate. In a healthy childbirth, the baby's head emerges, then the shoulders and rest of the body follow more easily.

What About the Cord and When Should It Be Cut?

During birth, a third of baby's blood supply backs up into the placenta and is essential to return to the baby after birth for the baby to transition to life outside the womb. After the birth of your baby, the cord is still pulsing strong, returning to the baby a substantial amount of their own blood volume, blood which is crucial for the baby's health. One of the most dangerous routine interventions is immediate cutting of the umbilical cord. Immediate clamping deprives the baby of this large amount of blood, equivalent to a hemorrhage that no one sees, creating the need to resuscitate more babies and a whole variety of other short- and long-term health problems.

A critical addition to your birth plan: leave your baby's cord intact at least until it stops pulsing. Or keeping the cord intact until it empties and stops significantly pulsing or after the placenta emerges. That is part of a physiologic undisturbed birth—the immensely wise natural process that has sustained the human species since the beginning of time. Delayed, lately termed "optimal cord clamping" should be the norm, and a must to add to your birth preferences in any setting.

Pediatrician Dr. Alan Green eloquently describes why:

> *"There's something important parents need to know about that moment when the umbilical cord is clamped the moment a baby's born—a third of their blood, the blood that's been going through them for all of pregnancy, is still outside their body. What happened for all of human history is that after the baby is born, the cord would pump, pulse, push blood into the baby. They'd get 30% more blood, 60% more blood cells. They get iron to last them through their first year, white blood cells to fight infection. They would get antibodies. They would get stem cells to help repair their body. What happened in the 20th century is we got the idea to immediately put a clamp on the cord. To clamp it, cut it, and lock out the oxygen, lock out the iron, lock out all those wonderful things ... At the moment of birth, about 2/3 of the baby's blood is in the baby. The remaining third is still in the umbilical cord and placenta. During the third stage of labor, from the delivery of the baby to the delivery of the placenta, the cord actively pumps iron-rich, oxygen-rich, stem-cell-rich blood into the baby ... Wait until the cord stops actively pumping fetal blood into the baby, unless there is a strong reason otherwise. This has been studied in countries such as Argentina, Australia, Bangladesh, Canada,*

India, Libya, Mexico, Pakistan, United Kingdom, USA, and Zambia. Optimal cord clamping (a more accurate term than the more frequent 'delayed' cord clamping) has been shown to be both safe and effective at significantly reducing the risk of iron deficiency. Other benefits include reducing birth asphyxia (inadequate oxygen to the brain) and cerebral palsy. The health benefits from receiving the cord's stem cells may be the most significant impact, but has yet to be understood. Immediate cord clamping is a (harmful) medical intervention with unproven benefit. The WHO no longer recommends immediate cord clamping."

Not clamping the cord immediately, even waiting at least 60-90 seconds per ACOG recommendations, can be done during cesarean birth, and more providers are practicing this as more compelling research is coming out in its favor. Time limits are more crucial for the mom during major abdominal surgery. Watch Dr. Green's more elaborate TedXBrussels presentation on the subject. See the link to it in references.

When Does the Placenta Come Out?

The third stage of labor is between the birth of the baby and the birth of the placenta. When left undisturbed, this stage can last anywhere from five minutes to an hour. This is a sacred time between parents and their baby. Everyone is meeting for the first time.

Physically, you'll know when the placenta needs to come out. Cramping will occur. It's not like in labor, but cramping increases and is accompanied by a gush of blood. It's common to lose up to a half-liter of blood or a bit more at a vaginal birth.

The uterus clamps down and pushes out the placenta. It contains no bones, like a slab of raw meat, so it doesn't hurt to push it out.

In the meantime, the baby takes time to adjust to life outside the womb. They become very alert, and an unfolding is happening. They are looking around, moving their arms and legs, and eventually start rooting, sucking, and doing other breastfeeding reflexes.

For more information on this topic, check out my video on this topic
https://homesweethomebirth.com/nbsbookbonus.

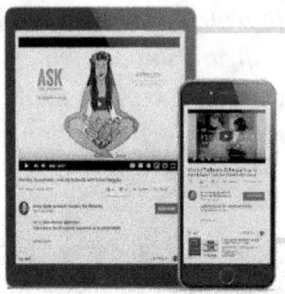

**Want to learn more or
have more questions?**

Grab your free Book Bonuses below:
https://homesweethomebirth.com/nbsbookbonus

Managing Pain During Labor

As written in Dr. Sarah Buckley's book Gentle Birth, Gentle Mothering:

"Undisturbed birth does not imply that birth will be pain-free. The stress hormones released in birth are equivalent to those of an endurance athlete, which reflects the magnitude of this event, and explains some of the sensations of birth. And like a marathon runner, a woman's task in birth is not so much to avoid the pain-which usually makes it worse-but to realize that birth is a peak bodily performance, for which our bodies are superbly designed. Undisturbed birth gives us the space to follow our instincts and to find our own rhythm in an atmosphere of support and trust, which will also help to optimize our birth hormones, aiding us further in transmuting pain."

You may have had a similar experience to the one I share: being given Pitocin to make my labor progress more quickly, then an epidural-as I could not take the pain of the stronger sensations from the medication, lying on my back, attached to continuous monitors and intravenous fluids, without any labor support or doula. I was in my early twenties back then. I didn't ask many questions and assumed this was standard procedure when giving birth. And I was an obstetric nurse on the unit where I was laboring! This was what I saw and thought was routine.

Also, statistically, these are very common practices. However, no one shared with me the opportunity to have a natural, undisturbed, well-supported childbirth. There was no online information or many books about it available to me back then. Because I didn't have anyone in my life talking to me about intuitive natural pregnancy and birth as a normal physiologic process, I thought I was covering all my bases when I was eating healthy, exercising, attending all my check-ups, doing all the required tests, and taking Lamaze.

They say that when the student is ready, the teacher appears ... and perhaps I was not yet ready to dive into myself ... and let go ... I was so young and scared by what I saw in the hospital and heard from others.

This chapter focuses on the mindset around "pain" during labor and childbirth, as well as my perspective on managing it in an out-of-hospital birth setting.

In all my years as a homebirth midwife, I have never had to transfer a mama to the hospital for an epidural or pain meds because she could not cope with the sensations of normal labor. It is not because women who have homebirths have different bodies and no intensive sensations. It is largely the mindset, the language we use, the attitude, the preparation in advance, and how the mamas are cared for and supported in labor.

I was always terribly frightened about pain after my experience giving birth to my first two babies on the obstetric unit where I worked as a nurse. They were similarly handled second birth were among my most traumatic experiences ever. I will cover birth trauma in an upcoming chapter.

When I woke up, went to midwifery school, and began to heal from my own birth traumas, I was still petrified of the pain and wanted to see if the wimp I considered myself to be could do it without an epidural. I wanted midwifery and natural birth to work for ME, to be authentic about providing that kind of care.

I told my fears to my midwife, and she validated me. She also reassured me she was confident I could do it naturally as I was now with a midwife and my care would be very different. I would be eating and drinking, upright, moving, vocalizing freely, and would be more empowered, supported, and encouraged to trust my body's ability to give birth. She was sure I would surprise myself.

She was so right. I felt so healed and like a superstar after my next two babies were born without epidurals or any pain meds; just loving, excellent midwifery care and encouragement to tap into my own capacities and strength as a woman.

Being in the water helped. Movement and moaning helped. But a complete shift in mindset and perspective was key, as was my preparation. I learned to use different language for the sensations of labor–instead of "pain," which implies illness and something that needs to be remedied–and to see them for what they were. I learned to use other words for "contraction," which implies tension and negativity, thus a word that is not empowering, and does not fully explain what is happening. Yes, the top of the uterus contracts so the birth canal can open and expand, as well as push out my baby. So, "expansions" are also happening in labor. That is really the goal of what I am doing–expanding so my baby can emerge from my womb to the outside world, and we can both be birthed as a new mother and baby.

Suffering is a choice. And I chose to embrace my intense sensations for what they were; as healthy signs, what was needed to birth, and what my baby needed to transition earth-side. They came in waves with a delicious rest in between, and I kept staying in the now. My yoga, breathwork, and mindfulness helped me calm myself, witness, and get curious about the sensations, to release and dive right into them without fighting them, and to notice that most of my body actually felt fine. I also noticed that when I was more relaxed, the labor was easier, and the sensations were less intense and easier to deal with.

I could do anything for 60-90 seconds, every few minutes at the maximum. I also felt confident with the support I had. The peak intensity was only at the peak of the wave in later stages of labor, when the waves are at their most intense, closest intervals, and longest duration. Prior to that, they were shorter, less frequent, and not as strong–so even more manageable. I knew that the hardest part, the end of labor was a relatively short period of time and indicated that my baby would be born soon.

So, that's the kind of care I provide and encourage others to provide, and that's the level of preparation I encourage to maximize success.

Natural Hormones for Management of Labor Sensations

Dr. Sarah Buckley in her book *Gentle Birth, Gentle Mothering* explains:

> *"In labor, such high levels [of beta-endorphins] are released and help the laboring woman to transcend pain, as she enters the altered state of consciousness that characterizes an undisturbed birth. In the hours after birth, elevated beta-endorphin levels reward and reinforce mother-baby interactions, including physical contact and breastfeeding, as well as contributing to intensely pleasurable, even ecstatic, feelings for both."*

These natural pain-killers are programmed perfectly to release and work with a woman's body and her baby as she progresses through pregnancy, labor, and after birth. Beta-endorphins work with another hormone produced naturally, oxytocin, the love hormone, to contract the uterus before and after the baby is born. A woman's body is a divine machine that was designed with miraculous and purposeful intent.

Although epidurals and other interventions have their place and are beneficial when necessary, their routine use interferes with the natural tendencies and process of labor, birth, and early postpartum, where breastfeeding and bonding between mother and baby are so important.

Can Labor and Birth Actually Be Pleasurable?

Many women who I have cared for in my practice have used the word "ecstasy" to describe it! I have helped mamas dance, laugh, sing, breathe, and sensually release their babies out.

I liken some of the experience of labor and birth to that of a marathon runner, with the feelings of ecstasy compared to something similar to a runner's high. Although birthing your baby is a much more powerful, peak-life experience, this is an experience a woman may only have once or a few times in her life, so why not LOVE it? Why not aim for ecstasy?

Here's what Christine B. said about it, as given in Elizabeth Davis and Debra Pascali-Bonaro's book, *Orgasmic Birth: Your Guide to a Safe, Satisfying, and Pleasurable Birth Experience:*

"I never thought I would see the day that anyone other than me would describe childbirth as total ecstasy! I know exactly what orgasmic birth is–I have experienced it myself. There is absolutely nothing else on earth like it. There is no moment in a woman's life when she feels stronger, more capable, more an embodiment of the Divine than when she pushes her child into this world."

Oxytocin is released both during love-making and during labor. There is a deep connection between the love that put a baby there and the love that helps the baby come out. It's the same sensual energy that is needed, in an atmosphere and mindset conducive to it flowing organically ... as in making love, as in giving birth. A woman's relationship with her body, both sexually and sensually, can be an integral part of experiencing labor. The contractions and expansions that occur during labor and childbirth are comparable to those of orgasm.

Most of us have grown up with a belief about childbirth, one in which it has to be painful. We hold a vision in our mind of a pregnant woman, screaming in pain, wearing a hospital gown, with her legs up in the air, an obstetrician and nurses taking over and doing all sorts of emergency care on the laboring mother. That is what we are told by many others who have given birth in standard hospital settings for the last few generations.

Even if it's just something we've seen in the movies, it would lead anyone to sign up for an epidural without question. No wonder there is a prevalent fear and lack of self-confidence. However, it is possible to embrace and lean into the sensations of labor, rather than fear them or try to escape them. It is possible to birth with joy and even sensual pleasure. Think of all of your senses and bring to your birth setting what pleases them. That includes the nourishing foods and hydrating fluids you like to taste, the essential oils or scented lotion and flowers you like to smell, the clothing, bedding, and towels you like to feel on your skin and how you like to be touched (firmly/softly, deeply/lightly steady pressure, or massage), the sounds you like to listen to (nature or sound machine of running water, rain, jungle or forest, a playlist of your favorite songs), and what inspiring things you like to see (from string lights or electric candles, birth art, affirmations, pictures of family)—all of which creates an ambiance of sensual pleasure.

When a woman prepares for this process, she can feel the momentum that labor provides. She can be guided by her own intuition and the trust of a supportive team around her. Her mindset can shift to a positive perspective about the sensations of birth, and it's fully possible to have a birth that leaves a woman feeling empowered, strengthened, and deeply satisfied. It is possible for her to feel a sense of bliss like no other, despite the intensity and challenges she may face.

Watch my video about labor coping techniques and another video on managing pain of labor at home:
https://homesweethomebirth.com/nbsbookbonus.

Optimal Labor Positions

Modern-day medicine and common hospital birth experiences lead many women to believe that birthing on the back is standard and optimal. But it was never standard before birth was moved to the hospitals in some localities in the early 1900s, nor is it a naturally assumed birthing position around the globe today.

The reclining position may be optimal for the attending care provider to control the delivery, but it is not at all optimal for the healthy mom or baby whose birth does not need to be controlled. Using gravity, a woman can assume positions that are more comfortable, help the baby navigate its way down and out, prevent tearing, lower the risk of complications, and optimize her birth experience.

When it comes to optimal labor positions, the most important component is for a woman to listen to her body. Unless directed otherwise because of a problem, intuitive instinct and what feels best will align a woman with her best laboring and birthing positions. In general, activity alternated with rest is best.

- Rest
- Move
- Repeat.

Changing positions is important to keep the good energy and flow going while gradually encouraging the baby to move downwards.

Positions and Movements That Can Help

The Side–if a woman feels like taking a rest, she can lie on her side, rather than her back, which causes the pelvis to have a smaller diameter. She can use pillows and receive help from a partner or doula to get most comfortable. I suggest alternating between sides periodically while raising the bent leg at different intervals and resting it on a pillow.

Wide Child's Pose–this is one of my favorites, as mamas tend to assume a form of it naturally and find it most comforting! It's a resting pose used in yoga. I especially love the restorative, supportive child's pose, where a woman's knees are open, she rests her buttocks on her heels and her forehead on a bolster, stacked pillows, or sofa cushion. Periodically, a woman can take a knee up and rest on her hands on the floor, rocking back and forth.

Hands and Knees–in this position, a woman can also rock back and forth, circle her pelvis, and move it side-to-side. Her knees can be on padding like a pillow, a folded yoga mat, and blankets, for more comfort. This allows her to move around and get into the music. She can rotate her hips, move side to side, and raise her leg up on each side intermittently, lunging in and out to cope and make more space for baby.

Kneeling–some prefer to kneel on their knees, with their torso more upright, with knees on padding on the floor, leaning forward on a chair, birth ball, or into a partner who is sitting on a chair. She can also kneel on a sofa or bed and can lean forward with her hands resting on the wall, the furniture's back, or a birthing tub. There are many ways to kneel comfortably.

Sitting--on a birth ball and bouncing, circling or swaying; cross legged or with knees bent leaning into or back to back with her partner or doula; on yoga blocks against the wall in a supported squat. Towards the end, many women want to sit on the toilet. This is where they feel most comfortable and private and in a position to push and birth.

Standing–many women feel best standing and leaning forward on a wall, high dresser, or partner's shoulders. It helps to periodically alternate one leg up in a lunge, with a foot resting on a stool or chair. Her hips can sway from side-to-side. Hips in motion to the music can be a great way to labor, and a woman can do this while kneeling or standing.

Dancing Styles

I always suggest to my families to make a few playlists. They can include those that are:

- Spa-like – soothing and relaxing
- Slow dancing like R & B with a sensual feel
- Funky, Hip hop or free flow primal to drumming

Many of the mamas I have worked with have danced their way through labor! Dancing styles vary according to preferences, how you feel, and what is needed at different stages of labor. They can encompass:

- Slow and sensual dancing with a partner, either facing each other, side-to-side, or back to back, rocking back and forth with one another
- Sexy and sassy
- Tribal
- Belly dancing
- Upbeat and enlivening
- Anything that gets you to shake your booty and move your hips like no-one is watching.

To learn more, watch my video:
https://homesweethomebirth.com/nbsbookbonus

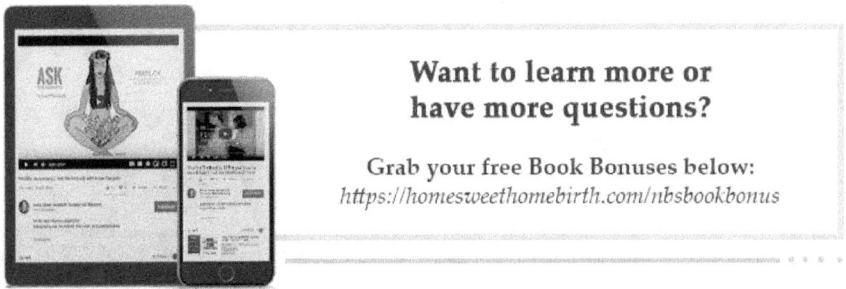

Want to learn more or have more questions?

Grab your free Book Bonuses below:
https://homesweethomebirth.com/nbsbookbonus

PLACENTA

The placenta is an essential organ that forms during the womb in pregnancy and attaches to the baby via the umbilical cord. It belongs to the baby. It is the only organ critical for fetal survival but is not needed by the baby post-birth after the baby receives the cord blood, which is one-third of the baby's blood supply that backed up into the placenta during birth. The placenta is the organ that gives a baby life. It provides oxygen and nutrients, and also filters waste products. It makes hormones that support the pregnancy, helps the baby grow and develop, and provides protection against bacteria and infection. Toward the end of pregnancy, the placenta passes antibodies from the mother to the baby, which can provide immunity for up to three months after birth.

But what happens to the placenta after pregnancy is over? Many people simply allow the placenta to go to medical waste in the hospital or want it to be discarded after birth. However, for those who want to keep or use the placenta, there are several options.

Ingestion

Placentophagia is the act of mammals eating the placenta of their young after childbirth. Most mammals, left to birth undisturbed in nature, will eat the placenta, even herbivores. It is theorized that this is done instinctually to avoid predators, but also because the placenta contains high levels of prostaglandin, which stimulates the uterus to shrink back to its normal size. It also contains small amounts of oxytocin, which can ease emotions after the birth and contract the uterus to prevent hemorrhage, as well as facilitate breastfeeding and increase milk production.

It is said to restore iron levels in the blood, increase levels of stress-reducing hormones, and for women, decrease the incidence of postpartum depression.

In humans, placenta ingestion is practiced most often in Chinese medicine, and the tradition is centuries old. Most often, it is dried, steamed, ground, and encapsulated although some eat it raw in a smoothie or cooked into other foods. It can also be made into a tincture.

There have only been a few scientific studies on the benefits of placenta encapsulation, and they have not conclusively supported or dispelled the proposed benefits. Most information about placenta encapsulation is mostly from a holistic understanding of health and wellbeing, science, intuitive traditional wisdom, and anecdotal reports. In over 24 years of being a midwife, all women in my practice who chose to ingest their placentas have reported positive results without complications (except one who felt it made her more agitated). I do not claim this to be scientific evidence, but I do like to listen and validate their experiences, as well as provide the information I currently know and options so each can make their own informed decision. I am eager to learn the results of research as natural approaches to health, including placenta ingestion are increasing in popularity and are being studied more scientifically.

If you are interested in encapsulating your placenta, you can look for a certified encapsulation specialist in your area, who has completed encapsulation training to make sure it is done properly. Be sure to research the techniques used to make sure safety and hygiene standards are upheld. It is wise not to encapsulate if there is any maternal or newborn infection, or testing positive in pregnancy for group B strep. More and more childbirth professionals are offering this service, and Dr. Aviva Romm, in her book *Natural Health After Birth*, has instructions on how to do this yourself.

Lotus Birth

Lotus birth takes delayed cord clamping up a level. It is the practice of leaving the umbilical cord attached to the baby after birth until it naturally separates, which can take approximately three to ten days. It is not as essential as refraining from immediate clamping of the umbilical cord at birth but does have some perks, but can be cumbersome, you can't do placental encapsulation and does risk serious infection from decaying tissue that can breed bacteria and spread to the baby. It is not supported by most medical organizations.

In addition to the benefits from delayed optimal cord clamping to allow the baby to get back essential blood volume, oxygen, nutrients, and stem cells for healthiest transition at birth and long-term survival earth-side, lotus birth honors the third stage of labor and allows for a more gentle transition from fetus within the womb, to a baby outside in the world. It encourages the baby and mom to stay in extremely close contact and discourages others from unnecessarily moving the baby. It also encourages the mom to stay still and quiet in the days following birth.

The placenta does require some extra care for a lotus birth. Immediately after birth it should be alongside or slightly above baby so their blood does not flow out of them, back into it before cord vessels completely close. It should be gently rinsed with water and patted dry, then placed in a sieve or colander for 24 hours to drain. It is ideal to place the placenta in a shallow bowel filled with sea salt and sprinkled with sea salt daily to preserve it and prevent bacterial overgrowth. It can be wrapped in an absorbent material, such as a clean dishtowel or cloth diaper, and placed in a placenta bag. There are many different crafty options for these that can be purchased on etsy.com. The wrapping should be changed every day. The placenta and baby should be monitored for signs of infection; of course the practice needs to be discontinued and baby should be immediately evaluated and treated by their healthcare provider if infected. As common sense dictates, do not do a lotus birth if you tested positive for GBS while pregnant, either of you had an infection during or soon after childbirth.

Ceremonial Burial

Many cultures honor the placenta by burying it. Some believe this will give the child a strong connection with the land. Others bury the placenta under a new tree, as a symbol for the placenta acting like the "tree of life" for the baby and believing the organ will bring richness to the soil to help the tree grow. The tree can then be looked upon in remembrance of all the placenta accomplished and the life of the child it nourished.

Placenta Art

You can also make a placenta print keepsake. Take the fresh placenta and press the side with all the blood vessels branching out like a tree against a white canvas or art paper. This can then be framed when dried or placed in a scrapbook along with a dried part of the umbilical cord shaped in a heart or spelling out LOVE.

For more information, watch my placenta video: *https://homesweethomebirth.com/nbsbookbonus*

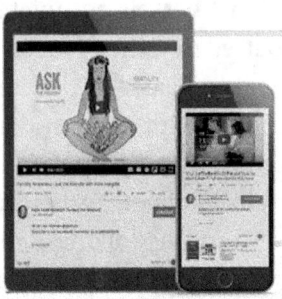

Want to learn more or have more questions?

Grab your free Book Bonuses below:
https://homesweethomebirth.com/nbsbookbonus

POSTPARTUM BLEEDING: HOLISTIC PREVENTION STRATEGIES

It is normal to have light bleeding in labor as your cervix dilates and breaks its tiny blood vessels. And as the baby emerges from the birth canal, there can some local tearing that can cause bleeding. Expect to experience the most bleeding at delivery and postpartum. Most of this bleeding is from where the placenta was located in your uterus.

With a normal vaginal birth and immediate postpartum, it is common to lose up to a half-liter of blood. After a cesarean birth, one liter of blood loss is the average. After birth, your uterus needs to contract around the major blood vessels that supplied the placenta to close them off and prevent excessive bleeding.

The first few days, bleeding can be like a heavy period. Then, it tapers to a moderate period, after which it becomes lighter and changes color over several weeks from shades of red, then pink to brown. The body is healing the former placental site, shedding the internal scab there (which explains a day of increased bleeding around 2 weeks postpartum) and the extra tissue and blood that was lining your uterus during pregnancy.

Postpartum hemorrhage usually occurs immediately, or up to the first 24 hours post-birth, and remains a major cause of maternal death in the US and around the world. It must be taken seriously. Currently, there is substantial evidence in support of what is termed "active management of the third stage of labor," to reduce the risk of severe excess postpartum bleeding. It includes the use of:

- The synthetic hormone oxytocin (referred to as Pitocin in the US) via intravenous or intramuscular injection
- Early cord clamping with waiting one to three minutes until the baby gets at least most of the cord blood
- Controlled traction on the cord along with counter pressure on the uterus to effect placenta delivery within the first 5-30 minutes after birth
- Uterine massage to make sure it is firmly contracted
- Assessments every 15 minutes for the first 2 hours

The above process, or a similar version, is done routinely in most hospitals, and can certainly be done in out-of-hospital birth settings. However, the studies that determined these procedures were based on hospital births in mostly resource-poor but also well-developed countries. Like all studies, they have their limitations and flaws; some were even considered to be of poor quality according to the esteemed Cochrane Review. Also, these interventions are not without side effects and concerns. The American College of Nurse-Midwives supports the use of active management of the third stage of labor in low-resource settings, according to their position statement, although they do admit its benefits are not as clear in the low-risk healthy population and encourage the provider to have a risk-benefit discussion with each pregnant family, so they can make an informed decision about it.

Most homebirth and birth center moms and their providers are passionate about physiologic birthing, minimal interventions, and holistic modalities, so they do not routinely want an injection of medication and are more interested in natural alternatives. They trust the incredible wisdom of the normal birthing process, which has worked for thousands of years (or we would not have survived as a species). They share a common belief that if it is not broken, don't fix it, so they are wary of medication and interventions unless absolutely necessary and the benefits outweigh risks. They tend to like the alternative "expectant management" approach, which also entails close observation by the provider, but tends to take longer, allowing for the normal physiologic process to take its course, and for interventions only if needed in select cases.

After birth, a mom and baby are, of course, carefully assessed, but encouraged to bond skin-to-skin. There is no rush. Cord clamping is delayed until pulsation has ceased or after the placenta is birthed. Mom and baby are assisted to breastfeed, which helps release mama's own natural oxytocin.

The provider waits and watches for signs that the placenta is naturally separating and then assists the mom into an optimal position, usually using gravity, and encourages her to use her own bearing-down efforts to birth her placenta. The provider may sometimes guide the birthing placenta with gentle traction on the cord, while supporting the uterus, then massage the uterus to make sure it is firm, assess the bleeding until stable, and assess for and repair tearing as needed.

Certainly, if there are certain concerns or risk factors, you may truly benefit from medical prevention and active management.

If there is an actual hemorrhage, make sure your provider is skilled, experienced, and fully equipped to deal with it with at least the commonly-used effective medications, IV fluids, suturing material for lacerations needing repair, and hands-on care that are usually sufficient to control it successfully.

However, you can build up a strong blood supply and reduce excess bleeding and its risks with the following suggestions for natural support, both in your pregnancy and postpartum.

Prenatal Support

Make sure you get checked and treated for anemia common in pregnancy and that your iron stores (ferritin) are sufficient.

Eat three large servings of wild greens or dark green leafy vegetables every day. They can be made into a salad, lightly sautéed, or steamed. Good options are parsley, dandelion, alfalfa, kale, collard greens, comfrey and turnip greens. For additional support, you can try the following:

Nettle and Raspberry Tea

Starting in the third trimester, drink one cup of this nourishing herbal infusion several times per day:

1. Combine a handful each of the dried herbs of nettle and red raspberry leaf with one quart of boiling water.
2. Steep for at least four hours.
3. Strain to a glass canning jar.
4. You can add fresh mint leaves, lemon juice, or honey to taste.

Green Drinks

Drink one ounce of fresh, frozen, or powdered wheatgrass juice, one to two times daily, to enrich and build your blood.

Or, try one scoop daily of powdered greens in your smoothie, one to three tablespoons of bottled chlorophyll, or tablets or powders of spirulina and chlorella.

Postpartum

You need to rest in bed, on the couch, or an outdoor lounge chair as much as possible for the first two weeks to recover. Make sure you arrange for help in the home during this special time. Limiting activity and increasing rest helps the area of open uterine blood vessels where the placenta detached to heal.

Check the top of your uterus regularly for firmness, and massage it if it feels soft, until it hardens. Postpartum bleeding can be minimized when mothers are taught regular postpartum self-massage of the uterus so that it stays firm and contracted around the blood vessels that supplied the placenta.

Start breastfeeding right away, and every 1.5-3 hours thereafter, especially taking advantage of the times when your baby is awake and alert and eager to suck. Nursing frequently causes the body to secrete its own natural hormone oxytocin to keep the uterus firm and decrease bleeding.

Urinate frequently to keep the bladder empty, so the uterus can contract more easily.

You can also take homeopathic caulophyllum 30 or 200 C immediately after delivery, then three to four pellets of arnica 30 C under your tongue every two to three hours. And try herbal shepherd's purse, one dropperful of the tincture, three times daily, for the first three to five days after birth. If you need additional herbal support for heavier or persistent bleeding, you can try a dropperful of angelica tincture a few times daily.

If bleeding becomes heavier than a heavy period, and you are soaking through two maxi pads an hour, for two hours, empty your bladder, make sure the top of your uterus is firm, and massage it if it is soft until it becomes hard. If this gives no relief, take one teaspoon of shepherd's purse herbal tincture under your tongue. You can repeat the dose a few times. See the section on bleeding in the "Postpartum Care at Home" chapter for more details and when to call your provider.

Following Childbirth

Preparing for Postpartum

I remember sitting at my kitchen table holding my newborn, staring bleary-eyed at the glass of water Cindy placed before me. Cindy was an angel sent from heaven. Her wings may not have been visible, but I know they were there. Cindy was my postpartum doula, and my husband and I don't know how we would have survived those early days without her. When she observed on our first day together just how sleep-deprived, hormonal, besotted, and bewildered I was, she asked, "How can we better prepare new mothers for this?"

I carefully considered her seemingly simple question. I mean, I had taken a really good childbirth class, and I had devoured the words and opinions of as many pregnancy books as I could possibly digest in 41 weeks. I had enjoyed many heart-to-hearts with my mom and friends who had babies. But there was nothing–absolutely nothing–that could have prepared me for motherhood. I was exhausted, fragile, clueless, and sore. I was a mess, oddly sad, but madly in love, and I was not ... the ... same. I felt changed forever. How does someone gear up for that, exactly?

I looked up at Cindy, through my fog and fatigue and utter cobwebiness, and gave it to her straight: "You can't," I told her. "Not today." Parenthood, I have come to tell moms, is like an exclusive club that you join as soon as your baby is born. You can ask other members about it, research it, get a glimpse of what it might be like in advance. But it's not until that baby is in your arms that you really, truly, on a visceral level, become a card-carrying member of the Whoa!!-I'm-Wholly-Responsible-for-Another-Human-Being Association.

Therefore, think about whatever it is you can do now to give yourself and your family the best shot out of the gate. Shore up your relatives, your friends, your co-workers, your community. Explore the myriad of ways you can procure professional support: postpartum doula, baby nurse, meal delivery, housekeeping, etc. If resources are limited, any of those options make an invaluable gift. Have your best friend spread the word when she sends out your baby shower or mother blessing invites. Most postpartum doulas offer payment plans and some provide services on a sliding scale.

Do You Want to Play a Game?

Close your eyes, imagine you are more bone-tired than you have ever been in your entire life. You are recovering from a marathon, and your hormones have left you to deal with the aftermath. Now, walk yourself through a day with a newborn who depends on you for literally everything, and remember, keep your expectations low.

Nope, lower than that. Now, go even lower. Awwwww–it's super cute that you see yourself getting dressed! Keep going …

If you all you pictured was, maybe, just maybe, brushing your teeth and squeezing a shower in between feedings, then you are a WINNER!

Why does accomplishing next to nothing except nourishing your baby and yourself, sleeping, and perhaps getting in some personal hygiene activities before you collapse into bed equal success? Because if you do much more than that, you'll be pushing yourself too hard, that's why. I know–this all sounds ridiculous now. It certainly did to me when friends warned me about taking it easy. But if you don't heed this advice and if you don't secure some kind of support before you give birth, you will only set yourself back. And if you go down, who's going to be there for your little one?

Don't panic. Of course, you'll achieve a new normal once the baby grows a little and you begin to feel stronger and get the hang of things. But the adjustment period is big. Respect it as such, and your whole family will benefit.

You have so much to think about when you are pregnant, and at this point, you are likely even making lists of your lists. But building a strong postpartum support system before your baby arrives will help ease your initiation into this pretty awesome club we call parenting. Preparing for postpartum in pregnancy is so critical, I have devoted an entire section of my online Love Your Birth course just for doing exactly that.

For more information about postpartum and how to prepare for it, watch my video: *https://homesweethomebirth.com/nbsbookbonus.*

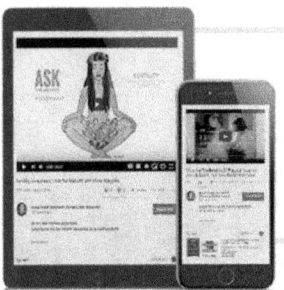

Want to learn more or have more questions?

Grab your free Book Bonuses below:
https://homesweethomebirth.com/nbsbookbonus

BREASTFEEDING TIPS AND DISPELLING THE MYTHS

"The newborn baby has only three (main) demands: warmth in the arms of their mother, food from her breasts, and security in the knowledge of her presence. Breastfeeding satisfies all three."

–Grantly Dick-Read

Breastfeeding is a magical experience for the entire family, and it's one I am proud to support wholeheartedly, especially as it's so incredibly beneficial for mamas and babies. I am determined to help mamas and babies get the support they need so their breastfeeding journey is a successful one. I have helped thousands of mamas on their breastfeeding journeys, and I am happy to share the wisdom from my education and those experiences to help you too.

Breastfeeding is a natural process that healthy mamas and babies know how to do. But it's not always straightforward and uncomplicated. "Natural" unfortunately doesn't necessarily equal "easy," especially in the beginning and for first-timers! It is a learned instinct, but once you and your baby get it, it can be so easy, even pleasurable, and incredibly worth it. While many do get it right away, for others, there is a learning curve, and it can take a few weeks to get into the groove. In this chapter, I give five tips to help you get started.

#1–Advance Education

Prepare in advance with education and learn all you can about breastfeeding. Whether you are expecting one baby, multiples, or plan to tandem nurse, the best way to prepare to breastfeed is the same as the best way to have the most positive birth outcome: through education during pregnancy, especially when you do not know about it!

My online Love Your Birth course goes into great detail about breastfeeding and preparing yourself in advance with knowledge and support, the hows, whys, and what you can do to prevent potential common breastfeeding obstacles and set yourself up for optimal success.

#2–Support

Sometimes extra lactation support is needed–especially if it's your first experience and you are not surrounded by other mamas breastfeeding, as women were throughout history and still are in many parts of the world. It is the way all mammals naturally feed their babies. Animals just know what to do. In unusual cases, if a baby animal was having difficulty in the wild, they did not survive. And that is simply part of wildlife reality. If an animal is owned by a person, they usually help the rare little one that is having trouble. Humans who want to breastfeed but are facing challenges are fortunate to have all sorts of lactation support options available. Absolutely take advantage of them and get that support. More and more mamas today approach their birth full of information, which is great! But many mamas do little to prepare themselves for breastfeeding their precious little ones before they are faced with it postpartum. It is much easier to breastfeed when you are determined and surrounded by breastfeeding mamas and support, which you can seek out while pregnant. Lactation support throughout history included wet nurses; we now have regulated donor milk banks, and pumping, storage, and alternative feeding methods to get babies breastmilk. Again, seek out this support while you are pregnant and before your baby is born so that you are prepared, come time to breastfeed.

It is crucial to have breastfeeding support available before and as soon as possible postpartum. Often guidance from your midwife is all you need. Sometimes some shared wisdom from other seasoned breastfeeding moms or your local La Leche leader does the trick. If not, and more extensive assistance is needed, contact your local lactation consultant with IBCLC training and credentials. Make sure to ask for that help right away, as the earlier breastfeeding is established, the better for both you and your baby. It does take a village of wisdom, love, and support. We must bring back that village.

#3–The First Hour

Start breastfeeding within the first hour of postpartum, or as early as possible. Unmedicated babies are most alert that first hour after birth with active breastfeeding reflexes.

#4–The Breast Crawl

Place your baby skin-to-skin on your abdomen or chest, and allow for the breast crawl. The first hour after birth is an ideal time to start breastfeeding as babies are naturally wide awake, and have strong suck, root, and crawl reflexes from the hormones of an undisturbed childbirth. Make sure the lights are dim and the room is quiet. Healthy babies have reflexes to actually crawl up and find their way to the breast and nipple, and start sucking on their own. It takes patience, but there is no rush, and it's truly amazing to watch. Check out movies like The Breast Crawl and others on YouTube.

Healthy postpartum mamas have a huge maternal instinct to love and care for their babies, enhanced by the hormonal cocktail circulating in the body after an undisturbed birth. Their breasts are filled with colostrum, commonly referred to as "liquid gold," that transitions in a few days to breast milk, which completely meets your baby's needs at least for the first six months and beyond.

#5–Assistance

There are times when some assistance is needed. But don't give up. Make sure your baby's latch is wide. If your baby is falling asleep and your efforts to wake them have not worked, or your baby seems frustrated and is starting to get fussy trying to find your nipple, there are things you can do to help. You will have an easier time getting your baby to breastfeed before the crying starts. Sit up and get yourself comfortable with pillow support as needed, cradle your baby in one bent arm, so their face is directly in front of your breast a tad below your nipple, leaving your other arm free.

When your baby is held close, facing your nipple, wait for them to open their mouth wide enough to get a good latch to breastfeed. A good latch includes as much of your areola as possible, meaning the darker circular area surrounding your nipple where the breastmilk is contained, as well as your nipple, where the milk is released into the baby's mouth. Your baby needs to compress and squeeze the milk out of your milk sinuses in the areola prior to sucking, which is all part of the breastfeeding process.

Sometimes the baby's latches are occasionally shallow in the early learning stages, which usually means the baby is sucking mostly on the nipple. This not only feels painful, but the baby is also not getting the proper amount of milk needed. If that happens, press down on the nipple with your finger to release the baby's strong latch and try again for a wider latch. Until you both get the hang of it, you may need to hold your breast and slide the nipple up and down against your baby's lips. This will stimulate your baby to open wide and then you bring them to your breast to feed. Practice and patience do make perfect and are well worth it.

Busting Some Breastfeeding Myths

Let's dispel a few myths that inevitably pepper nursing conversations whenever they pop up:

MYTH: It's a fact–breastfeeding is hard, especially in the beginning and for first-timers.

Yes, it might be. But it might not be at all. Some babies have a little difficulty in the beginning, some nurse like champs from the get-go. We've done such a good job of warning women about potential issues that now everyone expects challenges. But you and your baby are likely to be just fine, either immediately or very shortly thereafter. Professional support is critical, so don't be shy about asking for some!

MYTH: Women need to prime the skin on their nipples prenatally for nursing.

When moms-to-be ask me about this, they don't gently inquire about creams and salves. No–they want to know about *sandpapering* their nipples. I reply, "Don't even think about engaging in such suffering." It's wildly unnecessary, and, um, ouch! However, you might consider getting your nipples analyzed (yes, seriously) by your midwife, or an International Board Certified Lactation Consultant (IBCLC). She will be able to tell you if your nipples are flat or inverted, which could be predictors of early nursing concerns. The good news is–if your nipples meet the criteria, you can actually do something about it! The "something" comes in the form of suction cups made just for this purpose (fun fact–these "Supple Cups" were actually initially developed for porn industry actors).

MYTH: Breastfeeding shouldn't hurt.

Well, ultimately, when the baby has established a good, solid latch, it's true, nursing shouldn't make you want crawl out of your skin and actually should be quite pleasurable. However, it's not unusual that until you get the hang of it (remember, this a learned art for both parties), you might experience some discomfort. Pain upon the initial latch, slightly cracked and/or bleeding nipples are not uncommon, as the nipples are being sucked frequently, strongly, and for some duration each day. If any of these things persist or become excruciating, please make sure you contact an IBCLC specialist right away for help. It may be related to something like an issue with baby's latch or a tongue tie that can be remedied.

MYTH: No one will be able to help me.

Wrong! There is so much help out there! Midwives know about breastfeeding, and so do postpartum doulas. Some pediatric practices have lactation professionals on staff. Support groups like La Leche League have chapters all over the world. Optimally, IBCLCs are specialists who can help you tackle any issue you may be having. Web resources can be invaluable, but make sure to be selective and choose only reputable sites.

MYTH: Breastfeeding = Birth Control.

Please take this one to heart: nursing exclusively might offer protection for some women, but not for all. Don't fall for this rumor unless you are ready to have another bun in the oven, like, now. Your care provider should discuss birth control options with you at your six-week postpartum visit, but if you want to discuss it sooner, then, by all means, pick up that phone!

MYTH: I will be totally exposed if I nurse in public.

This is, of course, a natural concern, and our culture can be so confusing. After all, we seem to have no trouble exploiting women in mainstream media for entertainment and advertising purposes, but post a photo of a mother breastfeeding her baby? Well, stop right there and contact the Breast Police! Babies can eat anywhere, and there are laws that protect the rights of breastfeeding. Walk into a midwife's office or a La Leche League meeting, and you'll see that nursing is as normal as drinking from your water bottle.

Unless you are already completely topless when you leave the house, you won't be exposed at all. Think about it. If you lift up your shirt, and if you have a nursing bra on, your upper breast is covered by your shirt, your baby's head covers the rest of your breast, and their body covers your belly. It's really that simple. If you still have modesty concerns, just drape yourself with a jacket, blanket, or one of those nifty nursing covers.

MYTH: Those who had breast surgery, are adopting their babies, are having babies through surrogacy, or who are experiencing severe nursing issues don't have any options.

Happily, there are indeed options for these awesome mamas! I advise women to consult with providers who specialize in the above, so they can gather the facts and make the feeding decisions that are right for them and their babies.

I hope that has cleared the air a bit and that you enjoy this nursing knowledge as you go forth in feeding!

Learn more by watching my video:
https://homesweethomebirth.com/nbsbookbonus.

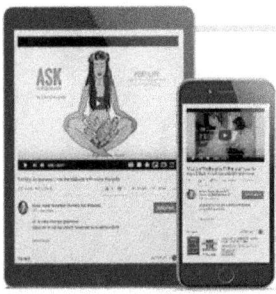

Want to learn more or have more questions?

Grab your free Book Bonuses below:
https://homesweethomebirth.com/nbsbookbonus

Postpartum Care at Home: Your Comprehensive Guide

Congratulations to you and your family on the birth of your baby! You did it! You are a rockstar, a superhero, however and wherever you birthed. Now it is time for some postpartum care. Through it all, do what you can to go with the flow. Tune into your body and your baby's natural rhythms. Embrace it all as a normal, healthy phase of your life as a new mama, shared with mamas around the world since the beginning of time. Try to have fun with it and keep your sense of humor.

Welcome to the postpartum period, the fourth trimester, a period of healing and huge adjustment, of getting to know and comfort your baby and mastering breastfeeding. All your baby needs now is love and breast milk. If you are unable or choose not to breastfeed, consider feeding your baby pumped breast milk or donor breast milk from registered milk banks. Breast milk is the ideal food for your baby, although organic goat milk formula is most similar to human milk and if necessary, you can discuss the best alternative options with your pediatrician.

The rest will follow naturally as you learn on the job, take guidance from wise, experienced others, and let your baby be your teacher. As in pregnancy and birth, trust your instincts and your heart. But do not hesitate to ask for help and support as needed. Hopefully, you prepared in your pregnancy so that you are well-supported during this sensitive time, as it has always taken a village to raise a baby as well as new parents. A postpartum doula is a must if you do not have family and friends to help you.

After the first week or so, but before your memory of details fades, it is recommended that you reflect on your pregnancy and birth with heartfelt honesty and write your pregnancy memories and childbirth story down in a journal. This is something special to share with your child one day, and it is also a wonderful gift to yourself. It can be especially helpful for healing if things were difficult or your labor and birth did not go as planned or as you hoped. Journaling will help you express, later process, understand, come to terms with, and make peace with any painful feelings that come up more deeply.

Below are some helpful hints to make the next few weeks easier and more comfortable, so you are more able to heal, enjoy, and reflect upon your extraordinary new miracle. The most important advice is to slow down, stay in the moment, try to resist the temptation to do, do, do ... and just be, be, be. Trust that you will heal, as you are perfectly designed to do, given the proper care and support.

Nutrition for Postpartum Care

Maintain at least the same healthy nutrition as you did in pregnancy, especially now for recovery after birth and during breastfeeding. This will help you to make good quality milk and nourish your baby as well as yourself. Make sure to eat at least three whole-food, varied, healthy meals and snacks, and even a little bit more than you would normally consume. And keep well-hydrated.

Traditional foods for the early postpartum weeks across cultures typically include soups and stews with a lot of vegetables, with the starchy ones, like sweet potatoes and winter squash, stewed meat or chicken, and whole grains (ideally gluten-free). Also, do eat plenty of seasonal fruits and vegetables. Much nourishment can be added to fruit/veggie smoothies, soufflés, whole-grain hot cereals, and breads/muffins, like zucchini-apple, banana-date, or carrot-raisin, enhanced with almond flour or chopped nuts and seeds, nut milk, and eggs.

Herbs and Supplements

Make sure to supplement your diet as in pregnancy, with herbs, vitamins, minerals, omega threes, and probiotics to complete nourishment not supplied by diet alone. This will aid in your recovery and help supply all of your and your baby's nutritional needs. Refer to the chapter on nutrition for more details on the ideal diet and supplements. Do increase iron-rich foods and take an herbal iron, especially if you were anemic in pregnancy, have low iron stores, lost a lot of blood at birth, gave birth by cesarean, and/or are still anemic. Follow the recommendations in the chapter on anemia.

Do continue your nourishing pregnancy herbal infusion of red raspberry and nettles, but add alfalfa and red clover. You can have a support person make this:

1. Blend a handful of dried nettle leaf, a handful of dried red raspberry leaf, a pinch of alfalfa, a large pinch of red clover, and several rose hips.
2. Add a pinch of comfrey to help with healing (optional).
3. Brew it in a quart glass canning jar of boiling water for one to four hours. The longer the brew, the stronger the taste and effect.
4. Strain, and drink plain or lightly sweetened with rose hip-infused honey and/or a splash of fresh-squeezed lemon or lime juice.
5. Enjoy hot or cold, up to four cups per day.

You can make it in larger quantities and store it in the fridge.

Other herbal tonics for new moms to promote general physical and emotional postpartum recovery and healing include ashwagandha, gotu kola (a half to one teaspoon each, twice daily), and milky oats (a half to one teaspoon, one to three times daily), in addition to herbs mentioned below as appropriate for each specific issue.

To promote healing after birth, take three to four pellets of homeopathic arnica 30c under your tongue every few hours for the first three days, then three times daily for a week. You can also dissolve the pellets in a clean, unused bottle of water, shake vigorously a few times, then gargle a mouthful before swallowing, which increases the strength of the remedy.

There are some nice herbal breastfeeding teas like those made by Earth Mama Organics and Traditional Medicinals. Use two bags per cup of tea to get the benefits. You can have your special someone make your own delicious, nourishing combination of herbs, which helps with breastfeeding and enhances the nutritional content of your breast milk:

1. Mix a handful each of dried chamomile blossoms, catnip, and blessed thistle, a pinch each of fennel seeds and fenugreek powder or seeds, and a few dried lavender flowers.
2. Put one tablespoon of the mix in a cup, fill with boiling water, and steep for ten to 15 minutes.
3. Strain in a glass jar, and drink plain or lightly sweetened with rose hip-infused honey and a dash of anise.
4. Drink one to three cups daily.

Breastfeeding

You will find in the chapter "Breastfeeding Tips and Dispelling Myths" ways to prepare for breastfeeding and common myths to be busted, as well as five essential tips to get the breastfeeding going.

Your newborn baby's stomach is tiny, like the size of a cherry, the first few days, a small apricot at one week, and a large egg at one month of age. Only tiny amounts of milk are tolerated initially. Expect your baby to drink about one to 1.5 teaspoons per feed on the first day, 1.5-2 ounces by one week, and 2.5-5 ounces per feed by one month of age. This is just what you have to give.

The liquid gold colostrum that your breast produces makes no more than a few teaspoons per feed, but when your full breast milk comes in, you will have more than enough to accommodate. Often women have a misconception that they do not have enough milk when they have exactly what the baby needs, and they get into a tension and supplemental feeding cycle that actually decreases supply. Frequent nursing on-demand, without giving baby any supplements prevents this problem for the vast majority of healthy newborns.

If you had labor or birth complications, needed epidural or spinal anesthesia, your baby was birthed by cesarean or had to be in the intensive care unit, then establishing breastfeeding can be more challenging at first, but you can do it. Get help from a certified lactation consultant (IBCLC) as soon as possible if there is any difficulty. Baby-friendly hospitals should all have them on staff, or you can ask your midwife, pediatrician, or local La Leche leader for recommendations. If you need additional guidance to boost a low milk supply, first follow these steps: www.kellymom.com/hot-topics/low-supply/. All you may need to do is keep nice and calm with your baby skin-to-skin and nurse more frequently, avoid formula and glucose water, and not use pacifiers until your breastfeeding is well established.

You can increase emptying if needed, which boosts your supply, by using a double electric breast pump every 2-2.5 hours for 15-20 minutes, but know that a healthy baby is the best breast pump. If you do pump, freeze the milk for later use, like when you need to go out or want a break from a nightly feed. Take herbal combinations like More Milk Special Blend oor a similar lactation supplement and drink non-alcoholic beer or hops tea and several cups sesame milk daily. You may need to add increased amounts of individual herbs like goats rue, blessed thistle, and fenugreek, two to three capsules each, up to three times per day, or add the tincture of More Milk Special Blend, 2ml, four times per day, to increase your supply.

Treatment for Afterpains

Periodic cramping, known as afterpains, commonly occurs as your uterus muscle fibers contract around the blood vessels that supplied the placenta. This is your body's natural defense in order to minimize excessive bleeding and return to its nonpregnant size. They can be quite painful and can occur with increasing intensity after each subsequent baby.

Breastfeeding can temporarily increase the severity of these pains, which is actually helping your body heal and prevent excess blood loss. Afterpains should gradually subside over the next week and lessen significantly over the first three days after birth.

Below are some suggestions to lessen the discomfort.

- Frequently empty your bladder, even though you don't feel like you need to pee, as is common from the swelling after childbirth.
- Especially during the first 24 hours, check the top of your uterus several times per hour to make sure it is nice and firm like a hard nectarine or knuckle. Massage the top of your uterus gently when it begins to soften or feels boggy.
- Lie on your stomach with a pillow under your lower abdomen.
- Apply warm moist towel compresses, hot water bottles, hot herbal packs, rice packs heated with a few drops of essential oil of lavender, or a heating pad to your lower abdomen.
- Practice your breathwork, deep breathing, and conscious relaxation exercises during the afterpains, dropping your focus right down into them, relaxing with surrendering to the intense sensations as you did in labor.
- Try soaking in a well-cleaned, warm bath with drops of lavender or chamomile.
- For an effective herbal infusion:
    - Mix a large pinch of chamomile blossoms and/or catnip in one cup of boiling water.
    - Brew, covered for 10-20 minutes.
    - Strain in a glass canning jar.
    - Add honey to taste (optional).
    - Drink very warm, one to four cups daily.
- Take a dropperful of motherwort herbal tincture, up to four times daily. If without relief, try cramp bark herbal tincture, one dropperful, every 30 minutes to 2 hours, then two to three times daily. You can add a dropperful of black haw tincture, three times per day. You can make your own cramp bark infusion by steeping a handful of cramp bark and black haw

with a pinch of hops and generous pinch of blue cohosh root in a quart glass jar overnight.

- Take Wish Garden AfterEase herbal tincture as directed.
- Take three to four pellets homeopathic chamomilla, arnica, or caulophyllum 30c. Try a few pellets of one remedy under your tongue. If no relief, try the other. If the remedy works, repeat several times daily as needed.
- Get Moxibustion treatments by an acupuncturist.
- Try additional suggestions and remedies mentioned already in a previous chapter on pain in pregnancy. They work!
- If the pain is too much for you and interfering with your ability to breastfeed, rest, and sleep, you can take ibuprofen (up to 800 mg, every six hours) OR acetaminophen (up to 650 mg, every four hours) 30 minutes before nursing for the first several days only, as needed. But before reaching for these medications, try 1-2 grams of curcumin (turmeric), a natural herb studied to be as effective for pain relief as most over-the-counter synthetic analgesics without their associated potential risk of toxicity.

Consult your practitioner for severe cramping or cramping that lasts longer than one to two weeks, or if the cramping is accompanied by uterine tenderness, fever, or foul-smelling discharge.

Home Remedies for Bleeding

During the first two to five days, bleeding is no more than a heavy period with an occasional clot the size of a 50-cent piece or egg, dark red in color with a fleshy smell. It tends to be less after a cesarean birth. Clots are simply congealed blood mostly that pools in the vagina when you are reclining and can occasionally be as long as the vaginal canal. Sometimes bleeding increases with nursing, strenuous activity, heavy lifting and pushing motions, a full bladder, and as you rise from a lying-down position.

During the next week or so, the bleeding becomes paler pink or brownish, and it lessens in amount so that you only need to change sanitary pads several times per day. Over the following two to four weeks, discharge becomes creamy white or yellow and even less in amount, but usually returns to red bleeding or spotting for a day or two around the second postpartum week.

Some women occasionally spot on and off for longer periods of time or throughout breastfeeding. Suggestions for keeping clean, healthy and comfortable are:

- Take a daily bath in a well-cleaned tub (add calendula tincture and lavender oil to water if desired) or shower.
- Change disposable organic sanitary pads or herbal-infused natural pads every four to six hours and after going to the bathroom. Do not use tampons, menstrual sponges, or menstrual cups. The first day or two, especially at night, consider wearing adult diaper-type pads simply because it is easier, as bleeding can be heavier than common postpartum maxi pads can accommodate and can leak onto your clothes and sheets. Use them with a smile.
- Wash hands before and after changing pads.
- Remove pad from front to back, squeeze a peri-bottle of warm water over your perineum. If you had tearing with or without repair, you can also add one teaspoon of calendula tincture and lavender oil to the water. Pat dry.
- Do not douche.
- Check the top of your uterus for firmness several times per hour when awake for the first 24 hours, then several times per day for three days. It should feel as firm as a hard nectarine. If it feels soft, massage it firmly so it re-contracts.
- To prevent excessive bleeding, take homeopathic arnica 30c as described in the previous herbs and supplements section.
- Take herbal shepherd's purse, one dropperful of the tincture, three times daily, for the first three to five days.
- Wear an abdominal binder or Bellefit's postpartum support girdle. You get a $20 off with the code ANNE20 at checkout at www.bellefit.com/a/12/.

- Continue your herbal iron dose until your bleeding stops in four to six weeks, which may need to be increased per your practitioner if there was hemorrhage. Eat foods high in iron, mentioned in the chapter on anemia.
- If bleeding becomes heavy (you are saturating more than a large maxi pad every half-hour):
  ○ Try herbal shepherd's purse tincture (one dropperful under your tongue), repeat every few minutes as needed).
  ○ Add three dropperfuls of the tincture of cotton root, two dropperfuls each of lady's mantle, witch hazel, and blue cohosh, and one dropperful of yarrow. Take them every 10 minutes under your tongue until the heavy bleeding resolves, but only up to an hour.
  ○ If heavy bleeding persists, take two dropperfuls of HerbPharm's tincture erigeron/cinnamon under your tongue every 20 minutes for no more than 2 hours, and add one dropperful of angelica if without relief.

Report to your practitioner immediately if you are saturating more than one pad an hour for over 2 hours (or > 2 cups) and/or passing large clots (like a tennis ball or bigger), not relieved by the above suggestions - especially if you feel lightheaded, dizzy or faint or oddly unwell; are unusually pale, weak, drowsy, spaced out or disoriented or anxious; and you feel cold and clammy with rapid, shallow breathing and pounding heart. Contact them also if you have foul smelling vaginal discharge, severe pain, a temperature over 100.4 after the first few days, and any other deviation from the described normal pattern of bleeding.

Treating Breast Engorgement

Your breasts will begin filling with milk and can become engorged by the third or fourth postpartum day, whether or not you are breastfeeding. Initially, you may notice that your breasts become larger, fuller, heavy, lumpy, slightly tender, and warm. They may leak milk and you may notice a short-lived low-grade fever. The skin of the breasts may be pulled tight and become shiny, hard, painful, and throbbing, and the baby might be less able to grasp the nipple.

Suggestions to minimize discomfort with breastfeeding include:

- Practice early, frequent breastfeeding (on-demand or every 1.5-3 hours) without supplemental bottles for at least the first month. The breasts will learn to replace only what the baby takes. (This is a good reason not to pump significantly in addition to nursing initially, as your breasts will replace that too). Allow the milk to run freely into a bottle from one breast as the baby nurses on the other side. The bottled milk can be frozen for a later nighttime feed your partner can give to your baby to give you some much-needed sleep once engorgement resolves.
- If your baby is having a hard time latching, try manually hand expressing a small amount of milk before nursing. You can also do so afterwards if still uncomfortably full after each feeding.
- Rub arnica oil gently over breasts, except nipples, then apply a comfortably hot washcloth/compress or stand under a warm shower 5-10 minutes before nursing.
- Gently massage your breasts downward while nursing using arnica massage oil or lotion.
- If you are uncomfortable between feedings, you can let comfortably hot shower water run over your breasts and massage them downwards using a fine-tooth comb dipped in soap, or gently hand express just a small amount, or soak your breasts into a sink full of comfortably hot water. If engorgement is severe, add 1-2 ounces of marshmallow root tincture to the water.
- For severe engorgement, apply cold packs just during the short-term period of extreme discomfort. Ideally, make these by defrosting frozen cabbage leaves rolled over with a rolling pin.
- Apply cold compresses of comfrey (soak washcloths with the tincture and store in the fridge). You can try comfortably hot comfrey compresses and add parsley tincture.
- If you are not nursing and need help drying up your breastmilk, drink lots of sage tea and do not pump.

Report to your provider any areas of increased heat, redness, swelling, and severe pain; a fever over 100.4 after the first few days; and chills, headache, and generalized aches like you have the flu.

Sore Nipples

Your nipples may be tender or downright sore during the first two weeks or so of getting accustomed to breastfeeding your baby, whether you are a first-time mom or have nursed successfully before. You may also feel some pain, usually lasting no longer than 1 minute each time the baby latches onto the breast in these early weeks, which lessens as the baby nurses. If your baby is improperly sucking or incorrectly positioned, your nipples can become very sore and the pain is intense the entire feed.

Suggestions to minimize nipple soreness are:

- Remember this pain is temporary as your nipples adjust to normal, healthy breastfeeding, and use your tools from labor and breathwork to breathe and relax into the sensations rather than to fight them. This actually helps tremendously.
- Have an experienced person observe for proper positioning, latching, and sucking during breastfeeding from the beginning, especially if you have severe nipple pain during the entire feed and your nipples are very sore.
- Release the baby's suction with your finger before removing the nipple from the baby's mouth any time you need to stop the sucking, especially when the latch is shallow or only on the nipple. It needs to be wide, over as much of the areola as possible.
- Soak nipples in a cup of 0.9% physiologic saline solution, then expose the breasts to fresh air 20 minutes after each feeding, ideally in the sun, in front of a 60-Watt light bulb, or a blow dryer. Yes, spend some time topless.
- Apply some breast milk to the nipple.
- Avoid synthetic breast creams and nipple shields.
- If mild, massage plain organic cocoa butter, almond oil, or vitamin E onto the nipples after each feeding. If without relief,

apply homeopathic calendula cream or herbal salve made with calendula, marshmallow, aloe vera, and chamomile, or lanolin designed for sore nipples after each feed, and gently remove any residue before nursing. Apply pure aloe vera gel to the cracks and cuts, as well as comfrey, but wipe off before nursing so the baby does not ingest it. Try several remedies or combinations and see what feels best for you.

- Nurse more frequently for shorter periods of time.
- Alternate positions of nursing each feeding to vary pressure points on the nipple.
- Initiate nursing on the least sore side. You can nurse only one breast a day to allow the other to heal, pumping the sore breast to relieve engorgement during each nursing session. Then nurse the alternate breast the next day (pumping the other), and continue this until your nipples have recovered.
- Take a daily bath or shower, washing nipples with water only (no soap).
- Wear all-cotton bras, avoid tight bras, and minimize the use of breast pads. If breast pads are occasionally needed, use organic bamboo or cotton washables or nontoxic, disposable breast pads without plastic, changing when wet to keep nipples dry.

Report to your practitioner if your soreness lasts longer than a week or is getting worse, if your nipples are cracked and bleeding, or severe nipple pain persists during the entire feed, indicating a latch issue that needs to be addressed as soon as possible.

Perineal and Vaginal Discomfort

After delivery, your perineum and vaginal area may feel sore, swollen, and uncomfortable. Any pain or tenderness should gradually lessen over the next several weeks, or longer if you had a large tear.

Suggestions are:

- Practice good perineal hygiene as previously described in the section on bleeding.

- Don't forget to take the homeopathic remedy arnica 30c, as directed above, in the first few weeks, to support healing after giving birth, which definitely helps your perineal and vaginal areas.
- For a small tear that did not need stitches, using a peri-bottle, squeeze warm water with several drops of calendula tincture and lavender oil over the area as you urinate to reduce stinging. Squirt vitamin E oil a few times daily on the tear to promote healing. Motherlove and Earth Mama make wonderfully soothing and healing herbal combination perineal sprays.
- Apply a perineal ice pack or frozen maxi pads saturated with witch hazel for the first 24 hours (with a 30-minute respite each hour) or as long as you feel it is soothing.
- Periodically sit in a cool sitz bath during the first 24 hours or as long as you feel it is comforting.
- After the first 24 hours, take a warm sitz bath or warm shallow bath, two to three times per day. You can also add tea tree oil, tincture of calendula, garlic, ginger, and/or lavender, or try herbal sitz bath combinations with uva ursi, comfrey, sage calendula, oatmeal witch hazel, yarrow and/or plantain. You can also try herbs with Epsom and Dead Sea salt or herbal salt soaks and see which feels best for you. You can use any leftover, unused liquid for compresses or your peri bottle rinse.
- Apply warm wet compresses. You can soak a washcloth with any of the above herbal liquids or add any combination of comfrey, witch hazel, aloe vera, St. John's wort, and/or calendula tinctures to the compresses and apply them warm (or cold) to the perineum. You can apply pure aloe vera gel directly as it is very soothing and pain-relieving. After the third or fourth day postpartum, apply evening primrose oil and/or vitamin E oil to minimize scarring, and you can use the oil to make a paste with slippery elm, comfrey, and a little water to relieve pain, strengthen the tissues as they bind together, and enhance their healing.
- Apply hot or cold packs as needed throughout the day and night.
- Place a therapeutic red heat lamp a foot away from your bottom for 20 minutes, three times per day.

- Lie on an organic absorbent washable pad or disposable underpad without panties for air exposure, as much as possible (at least an hour daily).
- Use a pillow or cushion when you need to sit.
- Contract your pelvic muscles (kegels) or even better, engage your mula bandha (all of your pelvic floor muscles) when changing positions.

Report to your provider pain that worsens or does not improve over time or you notice an increased area of redness, swelling, or pus-like discharge.

If You Have Difficulty Urinating

During the first four hours after birth, many women have trouble urinating such that they feel no urge, feel the urge but cannot urinate, or feel burning after the urine comes out. It is essential that you urinate within four to eight hours after birth (sooner if you had IV fluids) as difficult as it may be, to prevent infection and excess uterine bleeding.

Suggestions to help you urinate are:

- Listen to running sink water.
- Squeeze warm water with your peri-bottle, infused with a few drops of peppermint, on your vulva, letting it flow down over your urinary opening towards your perineum
- Dabble your fingers in water.
- Apply light pressure to the area above your pubic bone.
- Put oil of peppermint in the toilet.
- Sit in a sitz bath with several drops of the oil of peppermint.
- Take a bath or shower.
- Blow your thumb.
- Concentrate on relaxing and opening your pelvic floor muscles while imagining the urine flowing out.
- Drink eight glasses of water per day.
- Try homeopathic arsenicum or causticum, both at the 30c dose.

Report to your practitioner an inability to urinate more than eight hours after the birth, burning pain before or as the urine is coming out, feeling the urge to urinate frequently but little urine comes out, fever, chills or back flank pain.

Cesarean Birth

If you birthed your baby by c-section, it will take more time to heal physically and psychologically—especially if unexpected and unplanned, or traumatic. Trust that you will get back to your new mama self. The scar will be there but will eventually fade. Allow for at least three months recovery for your body from major abdominal surgery and possibly longer to heal the mind and heart. Homeopathic remedies help tremendously and definitely speed and enhance your recovery safely and naturally. If your cesarean is planned, start arnica 200c, three times daily, the day before and continue through, three to four days postpartum.

Other remedies helpful to have on hand are aconite 30c for intense fear and panic before surgery; bellis perennis 200c post-cesarean to boost healing after you finish the arnica; staphysagria 200c for incisional pain and healing; and hypericum 200c for shooting nerve-type pain from the spinal anesthesia (only if needed). Use one remedy at a time, and take it three times daily until you feel improvement. Consult your classical homeopath for more personal guidance.

The first week is the hardest in terms of postoperative pain, so take analgesics prescribed in the hospital, and once home if absolutely needed; then switch to more natural pain-relief and anti-inflammatory remedies that are safe for you and your breastfeeding baby, but still effective. Samples include curcumin (500 mg four times daily), and ginger (500-1000 mg once or twice per day).

Use the skills from breathwork and mindfulness to center and ground yourself, stay present one breath at a time, surrender, lean into and embrace the temporary painful sensations you feel, without the story but with love and compassion towards yourself. Whenever you feel overwhelmed or stressed, take a few minutes to simply breathe, keeping your focus softly on a distant nonmoving object (*drishti*) or close your eyes and internally gaze between your eyebrows, relaxing deeper with each exhale. Send your love and breath (divine life force) and imagined light to areas of pain. Use visualization to support you as you desire. This is powerfully healing.

While in the hospital, it is important to take deep abdominal breaths also to keep your lungs fully expanding (use the incentive spirometer many hospitals give you) and to get up and walk within 12-24 hours after birth for 10 minutes each waking hour, especially to prevent serious blood clots and painful abdominal gas buildup. The more you walk, the sooner you pass gas and get your bowels moving, and you keep your blood flowing rather than stagnating from immobility.

Ask to be progressed from a clear to a regular diet within this time, and choose healthy foods and bottled spring water from the hospital menu (if that even exists!) or have your family and friends bring you more wholesome, real-food meals and snacks. For gas and bloating, limit:

- Gluten-containing foods found in wheat, spelt, rye, barley, and some oats
- Certain fresh fruits and veggies
- Cow dairy if lactose intolerant
- Carbonated liquids
- Chewing gum.

Eat slowly, chew thoroughly and mindfully. Natural remedies for gas and bloating include chewing fennel seeds, drinking fennel tea, or taking 2-4 ml of the tincture, three times per day, taking slippery elm lozenges, three to four three times daily, and taking a high-quality multi-species probiotic twice daily on an empty stomach. Eat and drink fermented foods like kefir and kombucha. For bad gas and abdominal pain, take one dropperful each of chamomile and passionflower, half of a dropperful each of hops and lemon balm, and ¼ of a dropperful lavender tinctures, every four hours.

The dressing over your incision should be removed within 12-24 hours so your incision is kept clean and dry to prevent infection. You can apply a clean maxi pad over the incision if your belly is folding over it so that it does not stay warm and moist, inviting bacterial growth. You have been sewn back together in many layers, and the skin is brought together by a glue-like substance, absorbable stitches or staples, or removable metal staples. While it takes time to heal, when all is proceeding normally, it is unlikely to open as commonly feared.

Sometimes they use steristrips over the incision, which will come off eventually, or you can remove them in a few days. You can definitely shower, but do not use soap initially on the incision. Dry the area gently. A little oozing of blood is common to see on the dressing, as is a tiny amount of clear, white, or yellowish fluid, as long as it is not pus-like discharge. Look at your incision so you can monitor its healing as well as work on acceptance and appreciation for the journey you and your baby needed, made especially for you both. Once you go home, you can apply herbs for perineal and vaginal tears mentioned above to soothe and enhance healing. Earth Mama makes a lovely herbal balm specific to healing a cesarean scar, and there are other organic balms that also help the scar fade.

Make sure to keep your baby skin-to-skin in dim quiet as much as you can, bonding and soothing your baby with your love, telling them all is well, that they are safe, and acknowledge that it was a tough journey for both of you. Get help with breastfeeding as soon as possible. Your baby may be sleepy from the medications, and it takes longer for the full breast milk to come in, but you will get the breastfeeding going with excellent support and patient perseverance.

I encourage you to love and be proud and grateful for your cesarean scar. This may take time to cultivate, but is a worthwhile goal. Do not be shy to ask for extra needed help and get support processing and healing emotionally. For online and local group support and advocacy, there are many wonderful resources like ICAN and Childbirth Connection, but you may want to consider breathwork to release the strong stuck emotions and trauma energy in your body if it is interfering with your wellbeing.

If you are suffering from birth trauma or you suspect your baby has it as well—as is common after cesarean birth—there are resources for healing for you and for your baby. Refer to my chapter on birth trauma.

Consult your practitioner if you find yourself enduring any of the following:

- A fever over 100.6 with general muscle aches and chills
- Persistent or worsening pain
- Area of tenderness, foul smell, pus, redness, and/or swelling by your incision
- Area of leg swelling, redness, warmth, and pain that worsens when you flex your foot
- Unusually frequent, urgent, or painful urination
- Heavy or foul-smelling vaginal bleeding
- Vision changes, nausea, vomiting, chest pain, and/or headache, especially if you had high blood pressure
- Anything unusual you are concerned about.

Obviously, if you have problems breathing, feel weak, disoriented, and faint, call 911.

Constipation and Your First Bowel Movement

It is normal to go a few days after delivery without having a bowel movement. Many have loose stools before labor and pooped during pushing, and those who birthed in hospitals who don't allow eating in active labor probably did not eat much, if at all, in labor, unless they (hopefully!) respectfully challenged that outdated policy, or simply sneaked in some food. So you have a few days leeway. Some mothers are afraid that a bowel movement will be painful or open their tear more or stitches if they had them. Other women are too busy and preoccupied with all that is involved postpartum to even think about taking the time. Do rest assured that although the first few bowel movements may be uncomfortable, they will not open your tear or affect the stitches. Even if you had a large tear, it's extremely rare for it to be torn by a bowel movement.

Suggestions to limit your discomfort and prevent constipation are similar to remedies in pregnancy as given in the chapter "Constipation During Pregnancy: Relief Measures and Natural Remedies" with some additions:

- Eat organic, clean, whole foods and stay away from the highly processed ones.
- Drink lots of water.
- Do kegels and abdominal muscle-toning exercises.
- Drink warm prune juice or a cup of tea or coffee on an empty stomach.
- Drink Smooth Move Tea, which tastes yummy and works like a charm.
- Mix two to three tablespoons of oat or wheat bran or ground flaxseed in your hot cereal or applesauce. Or, mix it with stewed prunes or dried figs.
- Try raisin bran muffins with black strap molasses (ask someone to make you a batch, with whole grains or Paleo, i.e, gluten-, sugar-, and dairy-free).
- You can take these remedies in these doses for preventing and treating constipation, which include Magnesium glycinate, citrate or the powdered liquid equivalent in Natural Calm, triphala, psyllium seed husks, or a homemade dandelion and yellow dock root infusion.
- Use Colace (stool softener) as directed if your bowel movements are getting hard despite these above suggestions and you are on opioid pain medication after a cesarean birth.
- If you are taking iron, use alternative sources of iron other than ferrous sulfate, such as ferrous fumarate, ferrous gluconate, or herbal iron (review the chapter on anemia).
- Do not ignore the urge to have a bowel movement, which usually occurs a half-hour after breakfast.
- Take an interesting book or magazine into the bathroom with you to enjoy some relaxing time on the toilet.
- While on the toilet, rest your feet on a low stool and avoid straining. Support your perineum by applying counter pressure with a folded tissue if needed.

- If it hurts while having the first few bowel movements, do some relaxation and deep breathing exercises, relax into the discomfort instead of fighting it and tensing up, or try splinting the perineum with your hands to provide extra give to the area.
- Avoid relying on enemas and laxatives on a regular basis.
- Ask your classical homeopath or refer to a reference book for a homeopathic remedy specific to your unique symptoms.

Consult your practitioner if there is no bowel movement by the end of the fourth postpartum day, or you experience unusual pain or bleeding.

Treating Hemorrhoids

Hemorrhoids, varicose veins of the rectum, are a common postpartum occurrence. They resemble a pile of red grapes or marbles just outside the anal area, but they can be internal as well. They can itch, bleed, and be quite painful during the first two to three days before gradually becoming smaller. Refer to the suggestions in the chapter on natural remedies for varicose veins and hemorrhoids in pregnancy as many still apply now.
Suggestions for relief are:

- Herbal sitz baths as mentioned above for your perineum, with Epsom salts, witch hazel, and/or comfrey.
- Use a pillow or special round donut cushion when you need to sit on a chair.
- Sleep on your side.
- Lie down several times each day with your hips and legs elevated with pillows.
- Try gently placing the hemorrhoids back inside your rectum with a lubricated finger and then tightening your rectal muscles around them for two minutes.
- There are effective natural remedies for internal and topical use, and include applications of already-made witch hazel compresses (known as Tucks in the pharmacy). Or you can make your own by pouring witch hazel onto round cotton pads, adding plantain, pure aloe vera gel, clove of garlic insert, and homeopathic

Hamamelis.You can also use herbal combinations in an herbal salve or ointment.

- Shine a red heat lamp on the affected area.
- Avoid constipation and straining. See above.

Report to your provider if pain, swelling, or bleeding worsens or becomes severe.

Postpartum Dizziness or Faintness

It is very common to feel dizzy, light-headed, or faint the first few times that you get up from a lying or sitting position, especially after a long, hard, exhausting labor with a large amount of blood loss.
Suggestions are:

- Make sure you are eating well and drinking enough water as described in the nutrition chapter, and refer to the chapter on dizziness for additional suggestions.
- Have someone assist you the first couple of times that you have to rise.
- Rise from lying down gradually. First sit, then stand slowly.
- If feeling lightheaded or woozy while standing, lie down with your feet elevated up the wall or bed headboard or sit down with your head between your knees. Ask for someone to bring you a few large glasses of juice, as well as a high-quality whole carbohydrate, fat, and protein meal. For example, a nut butter and jelly sandwich on sprouted multigrain bread, or yogurt with fruit and granola.
- If you feel faint or do faint, sniff ammonia or smelling salts. This is an important first aid item to have, especially if birthing at home.
- Open windows to get fresh air.
- Splash water on your face.

Contact your practitioner with dizziness that lasts longer than the first few days or any actual fainting.

Dealing with Postpartum Exhaustion

Welcome to motherhood! Caring for a newborn and recovering from childbirth is no small task. Fatigue can easily lead to exhaustion, infection, irritability, and depression if you do not listen to your body's signals for increased rest during this time.

The best way to minimize fatigue is to spend the first two to four weeks after birth (longer after cesarean) caring only for yourself and your baby, while someone else (like your partner, a close relative, or friend) tends to the other needs of the household. Try to plan so that for the next two, ideally four weeks, someone else other than you is doing errands, cleaning, preparing meals, and tending to the older siblings. There is no need to feel guilty for doing nothing other than resting and taking care of yourself and your baby during this time. This is your sole job right now, with nothing else on your plate.

Many of the suggestions for fatigue in pregnancy still apply—see chapter "Managing Fatigue During Pregnancy"—but other suggestions specific for postpartum to prevent exhaustion include:

- As discussed at length in the nutrition chapter, eat well, at least three whole-food, varied, healthy meals and snacks without skipping them, drink lots of water, and take recommended supplements to ensure you are getting all the nourishment you need for yourself and your baby while you recover and breastfeed.
- If you are anemic or had excessive blood loss after birth, be sure to take an herbal iron supplement at least for the first six to eight weeks postpartum, until you feel back to yourself and your labs, including iron stores, are normal. See the chapter on anemia for more details.
- Consider hired help (such as a mother's helper or postpartum doula, a cleaning lady, and even a personal chef or healthy meal delivery like www.daily-harvest.com) if you do not feel you have enough support or after your support leaves. This can be put on your online baby gift registry and is much more essential than stuffed animals, toys, and an oversupply of newborn clothes your baby will soon grow out of.

- Be honest and direct about communicating your needs. Don't be afraid to delegate responsibilities to others.
- Gratefully accept offers to help. Remember this is not just a much-needed time to heal from the birth, but it is also a sacred time to get to know your baby and learn to breastfeed. As long as you are well-supported, allow yourself to enjoy this special time and bask in the loving support of others.
- Rest, sleep, and lounge as much as possible during at least the first month postpartum. Nap when your baby naps and ask a friend or relative to take the older kids for even an hour or two each day so you can do this. When you have a choice between folding the laundry, doing the dishes, and napping, choose napping. Do not give in to the temptation to do any housework, errands, childcare, or cooking, as these tasks can be delegated to others during this time while you are recuperating. This is not a time to be supermom. Allowing yourself this extra time to rest now will help you stay well physically and emotionally for you and your family, and will help you feel back to yourself sooner.
- Be strict with visitors. Don't be shy about suggesting when it's best for them to visit or excusing yourself if you feel tired. Ideally, put a sign on your front door saying something like,

"New parents and babies need lots of rest and help. We are resting now, please do not disturb us. But, we would love a short quiet visit between [insert baby's most awake hours]. If you would like to stay longer, please bring or cook a meal, play with our older children, or do some housework like the dishes or laundry."

- Ask your partner to tend to the baby at night after you breastfeed for burping, diaper changing, settling, or holding skin to skin. Once breastfeeding is well-established, your partner can also give the baby a bottle of expressed breast milk for one or two of the night feedings.
- Keep night feedings dark, quiet, and boring so that baby will eventually learn to sleep longer periods of time during the night.

- If you can't fall asleep at night, try the suggestions for insomnia in that chapter, and make sure to take one to two daily naps or rest periods when the baby sleeps. Remember to silence your phone. Better yet, keep it out of the bedroom.
- Limit caffeine and avoid it after 4:00pm.
- Limit time on the computer and phone, and avoid it after dark.
- Get daily fresh air and sun exposure during the non-peak hours.
- Treat yourself to a nice deep tissue massage focused especially on areas of aching muscles, or ask your partner to do it. A soothing simple combination for massage oil includes 3.5 ounces of almond oil, a half an ounce of arnica oil, 15-30 drops of your favorite uplifting essential oils like rosemary, evergreen (pine) peppermint, spearmint, rose, geranium, ylang ylang, orange, lemon, citrus blend, lavender, or jasmine. Shake well before each use, and store in a cool, dark place in a glass bottle. A few drops of vitamin E oil can be added to preserve it.
- After the first few weeks, an occasional weekend in a nice hotel with your partner and baby can be a really nice restorative rest and treat. And so worth the expense, as the hotel staff will clean your room and cook your meals!
- Practice regular gentle yoga and light stretching when you feel ready. There are many ways to do it with your baby, or you may benefit more from having some space to do it alone, leaving your baby with pumped breast milk and a trusted sitter. Gradually get back into exercise in the morning or early afternoon after the first several weeks, and increase as tolerated after your bleeding stops and you feel up to it.
- Do daily 10-20 minutes of conscious connected breathwork that provides you with natural energy and increases vitality.
- Heed signs of not getting enough rest, which include:
    - Ongoing exhaustion
    - Feeling run down and achy
    - Excess or prolonged bleeding
    - Inflamed clogged milk ducts
    - Frequent infections and colds
    - Excess emotional irritability.

Report to your practitioner if you cannot sleep, are too exhausted to cope, or your fatigue worsens or does not ease up by six weeks after your baby is born.

Excessive Sweating, Peeing, and Shaking

A normal increase in perspiration and trips to the bathroom are common as your body rids itself of additional fluids that developed during pregnancy, and of IV fluids if given during labor. Intense shaking right after birth is also common due to the hormonal fluctuations and temperature and body changes after the huge work your body just did to give birth. This is a normal stress response to release the intense energy that was involved.

Suggestions are:

- Ask your partner to hold you when shaking, but do encourage and embrace the shakes without trying to stop your body from doing what it needs to do in order to reset.
- Take Rescue Remedy to support your normal stress response, if you feel you need it.
- If you are cold, wear absorbent, all-cotton clothing and warm socks, dress in layers, and cover yourself with warm blankets.
- For sweating and chills not related to infection:
  - Sleep on a large towel or terry-cloth sheets.
  - Drink ginger tea alternating with cinnamon tea. It is best homemade by adding a pinch of freshly ground ginger or a stick of cinnamon to one cup of boiling water and brewing it, covered, for 15-20 minutes. Or steep a stick of cinnamon in the water for a few minutes. Strain into a glass jar, and add honey and or pure nut milk to taste.
  - For severe sweating, get an acupuncture treatment to balance your Chi and promote healing.

Report to your practitioner any persistent sweating that lasts several weeks, chills, muscle aches, and temperature over 100.4 after the first few days.

Dealing with Feeling Fat

This is one of the most common postpartum complaints. Women often struggle with body image issues postpartum and feel fat. Typically, only about 12 pounds are lost with delivery, another 5 pounds are lost during the first week, and an additional few pounds are lost by the six-week check-up. It can take several months for the fat stored around your hips and buttocks for breastfeeding and nourishing you during the pregnancy and postpartum to be used up. It is good to remember that the calories used for breastfeeding will help you lose this extra pregnancy weight.
The rest of the weight gained during pregnancy you will have to lose through a healthful diet and exercise program. Also, it takes at least six weeks for the uterus to return to a non-pregnant size, and it takes time and abdominal exercises to tone up the muscles and overlying skin that were stretched. It takes at least several months to return to your pre-pregnant size.

Remember, breast milk production requires even greater caloric intake than pregnancy, as you are the primary provider of nourishment to your rapidly growing baby. So, this is definitely not an appropriate time to diet, as it deprives you and your baby of essential nutrients. If you gained excessive weight in pregnancy or were overweight before pregnancy, eat varied whole food of high quality and avoid processed foods high in unhealthy fats, refined carbohydrates, and sugars, and engage in regular exercise when you are ready. This should be sufficient in most cases. If you need extra help consult a holistic nutritionist.

To summarize:

- Drink well and eat a clean, wholesome, real-food diet as discussed in the chapter on nutrition.
- Avoid the junk foods that are heavily processed and loaded with chemicals and unhealthy ingredients.
- Begin regular exercise like brisk walking or dancing as soon as you are able and the bleeding stops. Aim for 30 minutes, four to five times per week. Pilates is a great way to strengthen your

muscles and especially to tone up your core. Yoga will tone your core as well, in addition to increasing your total body flexibility and strength, while helping you to calm and ground you. Ideally, take a local class like "mommy and me" yoga or postpartum yoga and Pilates. There are also plenty of online classes until you can manage to get out to an actual class. Light walking, gentle yoga stretching, side-lying leg lifts, pelvic floor muscle strengthening, and gentle abdominal toning exercises can be done after the first few weeks. Gradually increase the time and intensity as you are able. Listen to your body, though. There is no need to rush or push yourself during this time of needed rest, healing, and recovery.

- Historically and in plenty of cultures around the world, a fuller figure is more glorified, respected, and honored, and being too thin is not considered healthy or attractive. While obesity is unhealthy and it is important to have a healthy weight and body image, there are many variations in normal weight and body characteristics. Ditch the pervasive media pictures of thin models. They are not realistic, they wreak havoc with body image, and they often result in you feeling unnecessarily bad about yourself. If you need to, look at the #BodyPositive images of mothers on social media. Be mindful of unhealthy thoughts from modern, Western cultural stereotypes that imply "Thin is most beautiful" and "Looking fat is ugly." Try to replace them with more true affirmations of pride and gratitude for your body having just grown and birthed your baby. Maintain acceptance and love for your unique body type which is forever changing. Know that you are more than just a body, but a beautiful eternal soul with your own special gifts, attributes, and purpose far bigger than that of your body. Even though you are a postpartum woman who has just birthed her baby, you are also physically radiant, lovely, magnificent, and have a deeper sort of beauty and wisdom.

Postpartum Blues, Depression and Anxiety

Intense emotions, mild depression, anxiety, and mood swings are common in the first few weeks after having a baby, as are postpartum struggles, overwhelm, increased sensitivity and reactivity - and are labeled postpartum blues. Symptoms are especially worse if you are overtired and exhausted, without help or support from others, and/or have other stresses, personal issues, or other problems. You may find that you are at times down, irritable, easily upset, extremely sensitive, cry without apparent reason, overwhelmed, tense, anxious, and unable to concentrate or remember things.

Natural remedies to lessen the emotional ups and downs, and help you cope include many that are mentioned in the chapters on Emotions and Natural Stress Alleviation.
Suggestions specific for postpartum include:

- Minimize fatigue with the tips from the exhaustion section above. Adequate sleep is crucial.
- Eat a healthy well-balanced diet as described in the nutrition chapter, but many feel best completely off gluten, dairy, soy, and all forms of cane sugar. Consider eating an organic Paleo diet. Try it for a month. You will be amazed by how much better you feel physically and emotionally.
- For general health and physical and emotional wellbeing, make sure to take the supplements recommended in the nutrition chapter that include a whole food multivitamin, omega threes, probiotics, vitamin D, plus those specific for symptoms of anxiety and depression:
   - Calcium, 250-500 mg, two to three times daily
   - Magnesium, 200-400 mg, two to three times daily
   - Vitamin B complex, 20-50 mg, once daily with methylated folate and
   - Vitamin B12 sublingual (under the tongue) in the form of methyl, hydroxo, or adenosyl cobalamin, 1,000-5,000 mcg daily to two to three times weekly, depending on symptom severity and blood levels

- ○ Curumin (tumeric), 500 mg, one to three times daily to reduce inflammation linked to depression, anxiety, and other mental health challenges
  - ○ Evening primrose oil, 500-1,300 mg daily
  - ○ Continue your iron supplement if prescribed during pregnancy until you stop bleeding.
- Spend extra time breastfeeding and cuddling with your baby, skin-to-skin.
- Share your feelings with a close friend, relative, transformational life coach, or integrative health professional. An occasional good cry does wonders, as does a good hug, a good laugh and a good dance - to move the emotions through your body.
- Write and feel free to share your birth story. Include the details, the lessons you learned about yourself and others, your strengths you have discovered, how you and your partner have grown, and qualities you found that exceeded your expectations.
- Commiserate with other mothers by taking a postpartum yoga or exercise class, or joining a mothering, breastfeeding, or parenting class or support group.
- Every day, remember to protect your emotional wellbeing by doing things that cheer you up and avoiding things that upset you.
- Each morning, shower, brush your hair and get dressed, even if it is just changing PJs or sweat pants and shirt. After the first two weeks, get dressed in clothes and put on your usual make-up.
- As soon as you are able and the bleeding stops, begin a regular exercise program such as brisk walking, hiking, low-impact aerobics, more active yoga, dancing, or swimming for 30 minutes, four to five times per week.
- Get out of the house and get some fresh air at least once daily, even for just a little walk in the park, a trip to the farmer's market, or enjoying a cup of tea with a friend.
- Plan some leisure time away from the baby at least twice a week in the early weeks and more frequently later postpartum, even if just an hour each day.

- Avoid drugs, alcohol, and caffeine.
- Before attempting medication, try the recommended lifestyle changes, natural remedies, and herbs for stress and emotions first (mentioned in those chapters), as they are non-toxic, effective, and address the root causes, unless symptoms are too severe. If you are already on medication, the natural modalities and suggestions here can be used in adjunct, and can ultimately support you when you one day taper down to lower doses and choose to stop taking them.
- For persistent symptoms, make sure to have your provider check a comprehensive thyroid panel with thyroid antibodies, your vitamin D and B12 levels, fasting glucose and hemoglobin A1C, and address issues accordingly. Do what you can to prevent postpartum depression and anxiety and minimize underlying possible causes.
- In Chinese medicine and many other ancient traditions, the dried placenta powder is recommended postpartum for its powerful healing properties, especially helpful for balancing emotions to prevent or lessen postpartum depression if there is a risk or history. Many doulas and birth professionals encapsulate placentas. If you encapsulated your placenta, take as directed by the provider who encapsulated it.

Report to a healthcare professional if your symptoms of depression or anxiety worsen or last more than the first few weeks, if they interfere with your ability to carry out your daily tasks, if you notice significant changes in your eating and sleeping habits, if you feel desperate, hopeless, afraid, unable to cope, scared of how you are thinking, or have thoughts of harming yourself or your baby.

Siblings

Postpartum is always a time of adjustment for siblings. It's healthy and normal, and they each handle it differently. The youngest tends to have the hardest time, but not always. Some temporarily regress a bit. Some show upset towards mom, dad, or the new baby. Others become more needy and try to get negative attention and act out if they cannot get enough attention in a positive way.

Although your heart doubles with each new baby, meeting the needs of the older children and balancing that with your own healing and newborn care can be challenging. Having a strong network of family, friends, mothers with similar-aged children, or hired help is essential in the early weeks. This support system can help with the siblings' care and give you time to heal, rest, and focus on the baby and mastering breastfeeding. Extra support is especially important if the sibling is a toddler or young child, as they usually need the most tending to.

Take a deep breath and let compassion run through you, and imagine how you would feel if your partner just brought home a new girlfriend everyone's all excited about and loving towards, and encouraged you to love her too. Reassure them they are loved, give them a lot of approval, and include them in age-appropriate ways if they are interested in helping to encourage them to feel involved and important. Try to spend some quality time with each of them alone regularly, so your attention can be focused on them completely without interruption, ideally after the baby has been fed and can be held by someone else.

It is important to avoid expressing criticism or anger towards them when they are seeming to be acting out or trying to help, and do not suppress the expression of their feelings. A wonderful book written in easy-to-read comic strip form, with great suggestions on helping older children adjust healthfully is *Siblings Without Rivalry* by Adele Faber and Elaine Mazlish.

Relationship Issues

Having a baby, while associated with immense joy and euphoria, is a major life change for both you and your partner, and can affect you both individually and as a couple. Although it can bring couples much closer than before, postpartum can be challenging for your relationship with your partner, even if it was wonderful before and during pregnancy. And all the more so if there are ongoing difficulties and unresolved issues between you.

Your partner may be going through a variety of personal emotions, such as:

- Recovering from the intensity of labor and birth
- Questioning their performance and ability to provide sufficient support for you and the new baby
- Fatigue from lack of sleep and doing a lot of extra work around the house
- Struggling with an increased sense of responsibility and finances
- Anxiety over you and your baby's wellbeing
- Balancing outside pressures from work
- Taking care of their own health needs
- Conflict regarding their new role as a parent, especially if they had issues with their own parents
- Guilt about not being able to completely fulfill professional responsibilities or meet your physical and emotional needs.

It is a time for healing and integration for your partner as well, and they may also feel overwhelmed, stressed, and exhausted. Although you need lots of care and support, your partner may also. Tensions can escalate, so be mindful of doing what it takes to minimize or diffuse them. It is important each day to spend even just a few minutes alone to talk, laugh, hug, have a good cry if needed, and let each other know you appreciate and love each other. Individual or couples counseling by a holistic qualified therapist or life coach may be needed down the road, and it has helped many adjust to this major life change in healthy transformative ways.

Postpartum Sex

It is normal to have a decreased interest in sex for several months after having a baby, but once you are ready there are ways to navigate the journey and reclaim your sensual sexual relationship, which we explore in the upcoming chapter "Sex After Postpartum." For now, it is safe to resume sexual intercourse when the vaginal bleeding has stopped, after the perineal area has healed, and after your 5-7 week postpartum checkup is normal.

Suggestions to make your postpartum sex life better are to:

Communicate your temporary limitations to your partner. Be honest and tell them how you are feeling. Include your partner in the postpartum experience since they often feel left out.

Until you feel comfortable having intercourse, just cuddle, kiss, and spend some sensual, affectionate time together doing recreational activities you enjoy. Focus on the pleasure of being together.

Practice mula bandha exercises several times per day to strengthen your pelvic floor. For a thorough explanation of these exercises, you'll find it the chapter "Varicose Veins and Hemorrhoids in Pregnancy: Natural Remedies and Relief."

When ready to try intercourse, plan a date together with your partner when you expect the baby to be sleeping. Be prepared for occasional interruptions and keep your sense of humor. Remind them to be gentle as it may still be tender inside. Use extra lubricant. Explore the various natural scented and unscented sensual massage oils and see which one you like best. Experiment with different positions. Try being on top, or a pillow under your buttocks with you on the bottom for comfort.

Add maca powder to your smoothies or baked goods, or take it in capsule form to support a healthy stress response, balance hormones, and enhance your sex drive.

Seek help if the sexual problems between you and your spouse run deeper than this, if you have worsening pain during sex, or if your discomfort or lack of sexual desire or feelings do not resolve over the next few months.

Remember that if you are interested in preventing another pregnancy at this time, or if you feel that you cannot handle having another baby so soon after this one, do not resume intercourse until you have discussed contraceptive options with your practitioner. Whether or not you are breastfeeding, you can become pregnant as early as five weeks postpartum.

If you haven't already done so, get the wonderful book written by herbalist, midwife, and doctor Aviva Romm, *Natural Health After Birth*, for a more complete, holistic, and heartfelt guide to postpartum healing and wellness.

Natural Newborn Care

Congratulations! Having a new baby in the house is such an exciting and wonderful blessing. But it can also be overwhelming, especially if this is your first or if you're trying new things with this baby. Below are some tips to help guide you through this special time.

Feeding

Breastmilk is best for you and your baby, but it is a learning process. Allow a few weeks for the both of you to become pros. Get help from your midwife or lactation consultant as soon as possible if you are having difficulty.

General suggestions to ease the process include:

- Nurse your baby on demand or every 1.5-3 hours while you are awake. If the baby is healthy and is a normal weight for their age, and has a 4-6 hour stretch in the middle of the night, let the baby sleep.
- If the baby is too sleepy to nurse—this often happens in the beginning—try to rouse them by unswaddling and undressing, a diaper change, a gentle back rub, or applying a cool washcloth on the baby's forehead.
- Nurse one side each feeding. Start the next session on the other breast.
- Alternate feeding positions between side-lying, cradling, and football holding.
- Burp your baby as needed if they appear gassy during and after feeding.

- Do not give your baby glucose water or common formula, especially while you are trying to get the breastfeeding going. Breastmilk alone, including colostrum—the "liquid gold" initial breast milk—is adequate nutrition and hydration for at least the first six months when all is well. The water or formula fills up their tiny stomach, so they nurse less, which makes you produce less milk, and the bottle's teat confuses them and can impair their ability to suck on your nipple. If there are issues and you do need to supplement, pumped or donor breast milk from certified milk banks is the choice method of feeding. If you must give formula, go for organic goat milk brands that most closely resemble breast milk. Use a dropper to the side of the baby's mouth, supplemental nursing system, or slow flow nipples that are more similar to the breast.
- Avoid smoking, alcohol, and drugs while breastfeeding. Always consult your practitioner before taking any medications or herbal preparations.
- Limit caffeinated beverages to no more than one to two cups per day.
- To calm a screaming baby that is too upset to nurse, try:
    - Changing their diaper
    - Burping the baby
    - Swaddling the baby in a blanket
    - Giving the baby a warm bath
    - Cradling or cuddling the baby close to your chest
    - Rocking
    - Singing
    - Swinging
    - Talking softly and lovingly to the baby
    - Giving the baby a gentle back massage
    - Taking the baby for a walk or car ride
    - Holding the baby in a position that allows the application of slight pressure on their abdomen
    - A homeopathic remedy like chamomilla 30 c if they seem gassy and hard to console (place one pellet in the side of their mouth)
    - If all else fails, give the baby to your partner, take 30 minutes, and try again.

Some excellent breastfeeding and milk bank resources are:

- *www.kellymom.com*
- *www.breastfeedingonline.com*
- *www.ibconline.ca*
- *www.breastfeedinginc.ca*
- *www.llli.org a*
- *www.askdrsears.com*
- *www.milkbank.org*
- *www.hmbana.org*

Sleeping

Newborns sleep about 18 hours per day. Place your baby on their back or side to sleep, with the baby's back supported by a rolled receiving blanket.

Bowel Movements and Voiding

Newborn babies have a greenish-black, sticky stool for the first few days. This is called meconium. Breastfed babies' stools will then become golden-yellow, soft, and seedy-looking. Once your full milk comes in and replaces colostrum, your baby will have one to four plus stools and six to eight wet diapers in a 24 hour period; sometimes that is combined together in one diaper after a longer stretch. Change the baby before each feeding to prevent diaper rash. For a reddened diaper area, use homeopathic calendula, zinc oxide, or an herbal diaper cream, A & D ointment, Desitin cream, plain or with zinc oxide.

French green clay is excellent for diaper rashes. Use talcum-free baby powder. Place your baby on an absorbent pad and allow periods for them to be diaper-free, or read up on elimination communication—training a baby to poop and pee on the potty!

Cord Care

Keep the cord stump dry by folding the front of the baby's diaper down.

Squeeze a saturated cotton ball of alcohol or hydrogen peroxide to the cord stump, three times per day, to keep it clean. Open a capsule and apply powdered goldenseal herb or herbal combination cord powder around the base. The cord stump should fall off by itself within 8-12 days after the birth.

General Care

Wash your hands before handling the baby.

Bathe the baby with mild natural soap and water (ideally every day–they love it), and wash the baby's hair with a gentle, tear-free natural shampoo several times per week.

After the first 24 hours and the baby's body temperature stabilizes, dress them according to the temperature as you would dress.

It is best to file then cut long nails with scissors, so your baby does not scratch themself.

Take the baby for a daily outing, but keep the baby away from crowds and people with contagious illnesses.

Wear your baby. Experiment with a few safe baby carriers and see which one you and the baby like the best.

Add to your collection *The Baby Book* by Dr. William and Martha Sears, as it is a wonderful "must-have" comprehensive reference and guidebook to the baby's first two years of life and virtually every aspect of care.

If you had antibiotics or the baby was born by cesarean, take extra precautions to restore the baby's microbiome.

Safety

It is state law in America and a safe practice that babies ride in carseats every time that they travel in a vehicle.

Always make sure that the baby is not unattended on changing tables, beds, or other high places.

If the baby sleeps in bed with you, make sure the baby is in a sleeping pod or safe baby lounger, and that the bed has a guardrail. Do not keep pillows, stuffed animals, or extra blankets in the baby's sleeping area.

Danger Signs

Contact your pediatrician immediately if:

- The baby becomes listless, will not nurse, is inconsolable, has high-pitched screaming, or behaves in an unusual way.
- The baby does not urinate within the first 24 hours or voids less than six diapers per day after your milk is in.
- The baby has no bowel movement for 48 hours or has more than ten watery-green, foul-smelling diarrhea diapers per day.
- The cord starts to smell bad or has pus oozing from it, and the area around it becomes red and swollen.
- The baby's temperature is below 97 degrees or above 99 degrees when taken under the baby's arm.
- The whites of the baby's eyes become yellow, or the skin color becomes a progressively yellow or tan tinge, moving from face downward to abdomen and extremities.
- The baby's skin turns blue or white, especially the trunk or around the mouth.
- The baby has projectile vomiting.

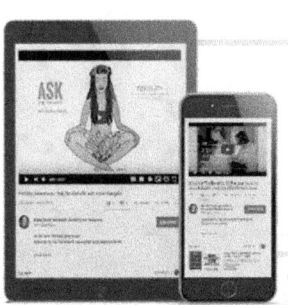

Want to learn more or have more questions?

Grab your free Book Bonuses below:
https://homesweethomebirth.com/nbsbookbonus

Postpartum Sex After Birth

There are so many psychosocial pressures to maintaining a strong and healthy loving relationship these days. One of the most concerning and yet least talked about pressures is reviving your sex life after having a baby.

- How extensively will a baby affect our sex life?
- Will it ever be again like it was before?
- Will it hurt?
- Do I have to think about this now?
- I have little or no interest in sex, and I feel so unattractive and guilty—what to do?
- My partner wants to have sex again, but I can't even deal with the whole thing. I just need a hug. Is this normal? How do I get in the mood?

Please remember, if you have any of the above questions, you are not alone.

Not only is sex after birth and baby not often discussed, especially on a mental/emotional and relational level, but the so-called "fourth trimester" is practically completely forgotten and disregarded in many parts of today's world. Let's begin to shed some light on an important topic in an open manner.

Where to Begin?

Postpartum is indeed an extremely self-conscious time for the new mama and could be an equally insecure time for the partner as well.

Many partners feel excluded due to the new and acute bond between the mother and baby.

Communication is crucial at this stage between partners. If both partners know how vulnerable they each are, the pressure to "perform" or "satisfy the other's desires" would probably greatly diminish. And what you can learn is that if a woman knows her desires and her desires are satisfied, her cup is full, and she will naturally want to please her partner ... or not. If a woman is turned off and unsatisfied, you can forget about her interest in desiring to serve her partner. But no one really talks about it. This lack of communication isn't only within the couple itself but throughout society and even between client/patient and their midwife or doctor.

As stated in the *New York Times* article, "Sex and Intimacy": "Sexual problems are common among new parents but discussing them with doctors or close friends is not."

Are There Any Practical Steps?

While there's no one trick to get your sex life rocking and rolling again, much like the first time (fortunately or unfortunately!), you'll both have to rediscover yourselves and find your own groove.

Here is the big and empowering news. A critical ingredient to a wonderful life that includes awesome sex is largely dependent on the woman. Reclaim and own your feminine power, which defies logic. As a woman, it helps to dig deep to know what your desires are and what turns you on—using all of your senses—so that you can create what you want, stay in your pleasure, be turned on, and communicate your requests to your partner. Partners tend to really want to please and do not always know how or what their love is thinking. There's probably nothing easy or nonchalant about finding your desire again either, but know that it takes time and that it is doable.

Regina Thomashauer (Mama Gena), who has been advocating for women and studying the discipline of female pleasure for years and in all aspects of life, argues: "As a woman, you can actually design a life that will allow you to experience pleasure any time you wish, ongoingly. Pleasure is deliberate, not casual. She requires planning, she does not happen by default."

In her latest New York Times bestselling, provocative, and revolutionary book, *Pussy: A Reclamation*, she writes:

> *"You'll discover what no one taught you about the source of your feminine power and how to use it. It's no secret that women today are still undervalued at home, at work, and in a relationship. Too many of us are at war with our bodies and disconnected from our truth.*
>
> *See, we live in a culture that teaches us to turn off. To play small. To take care of everyone else first. To keep a lid on our dreams and a cork on our truth.*
>
> *This book is written to reacquaint a woman with her own power source—which is the part of herself she has been taught to ignore, push down, and despise ... It's a call for her to tune in, turn on, and not drop out—but live more richly, fully, and lusciously than she ever thought she could."*

Here's what else you'll learn—how to know and speak your truth, how to radically accept, love, and celebrate everything that is you and feel the rewards of this transformative practice, how to move from depletion, obligation, overwork, and resentment into embracing what life brings your way and all of what you feel, how to cultivate an attitude of immense gratitude, how to healthfully process your emotions, how to listen to and trust your sacred inner wisdom, all about creating sisterhood and passionately creating and loving your life. This will ultimately rock your sex life, but you will also learn practices on how to further enhance it. I am convinced this book is a must-read for all women.

Some other must-have sexual resources include the following:

- *Women's Anatomy of Arousal* by Sheri Winston, CNM
- *The New Art of Sexual Ecstasy: Following the Path of Sacred*

Sexuality by Margo Anand
- *Pure Sex: The Intimate Guide to Sexual Fulfillment* by Anne Cooper

But Let's Talk Basics First: When and How to Resume Sex After Birth

For most new mamas, sex after having a baby can be as intimidating as the very first time. While much of social convention will have you thinking that partners are more than ready to jump right back into bed, this is often not exactly the case. They can be exhausted too, doing what they can to help, keeping up with work, also getting broken and less sleep, while adjusting to their new role as parent to this baby.

At this stage in your relationship, open and honest, kind and sensitive "nonviolent" communication is the key.

On a practical level, as mentioned, most practitioners recommend waiting between four to six weeks before trying intercourse again in order to give the new mother time to recover—at least until the bleeding stops and any tearing has healed. But, this recommendation is based mostly on physical readiness. Many women after giving birth, report not being ready for sexual intercourse for much longer.

What about your psychological readiness? How do you work through the possibly daunting task of beginning sex again after birth, when you may feel some or all of the following: your breasts are full, tender, and leaking milk; the baby is nursing every few hours; you feel overtired and are not getting the sleep or help you need; you feel dry and still sore vaginally; you feel fat and less attractive than you used to; you are preoccupied with caring for your new baby and balancing all of your other responsibilities; you are afraid to get pregnant again; you can barely find the time to eat; you are feeling emotional and overwhelmed; you just need hugs and cuddling; you have very little, if any interest in sex, but feel guilty and pressured to do it for your partner when you really don't want to; and you are just madly in love ... with your baby.

A great way to begin is knowing that what you're feeling is totally normal and very common. Not only is it normal for your libido to be low during this time after birth, but many women have expressed how uncomfortable it is to have the sex conversation at the six-week mark. They don't even want to think about sex for another six months, sometimes even longer.

And, there are many reasons for not feeling ready or downright apprehensive. The key is to listen to and honor your feelings, talk your feelings through with your partner, and truly listen to your partner's feelings as well. You might be relieved at what your partner reveals. But do not have sex if you are feeling pressured into it, out of guilt or obligation, or if you really don't want to. That is not intimacy; it is actually nonconsensual sex, which can lead to an unhealthy sexual relationship, or worse, if it becomes ongoing, leading to deep psychic pain and sexual trauma.

Dealing with Discomforts After Birth

Social perception tends to emphasize birth as the predominant and climactic purpose of pregnancy. But, in uncovering this forgotten "fourth trimester," we'll find that the numerous discomforts and huge lifestyle adjustments a new mama has to make after giving birth can be just as strenuous, if not more so than labor and birth. Even though this is part of life, we have been birthing and mothering since the beginning of time, historically, we had a village, a community of support; but today, many women are alone. That is why I urge preparing for postpartum support during pregnancy and provide extensive planning guidance in my Love Your Birth online course, as I do with the mamas in my practice.

Here are just a couple of examples of prominent issues to deal with after birth—not to make you fear them, but for you to know what is normal, to prepare and find support for them. While these may be fairly obvious, I've paired them with some of the worries and concerns a partner might be feeling and not telling you.

Hopefully, this opens the door to more real and meaningful conversations that deepen your connection.

There are ways to prevent tearing when the baby emerges at birth; many women do not tear or tear a little but do not need stitches, yet the vaginal area feels raw and swollen from pushing a baby out through it. And sometimes, despite all of your and your attendant's efforts, tearing occurs and needs to be repaired with stitches. Tearing and swelling require time to recover. So, take it slow and cultivate patience and trust. The body has an incredible capacity to heal.

Episiotomy is another aspect of more severe tearing that has recently been deemed no longer medically necessary; it is actually one of the most harmful, unnecessary routine procedures that had become so widespread and remains despite the evidence that does not support its use in normal childbirth. Now, it's been found to actually cause more damage than any natural tearing would. It can, however, be needed in rare emergencies when a baby needs to be delivered immediately.

Many women who had tearing and stitches fear sex will worsen the tear or open the stitches after they are healed. You can be assured that this does not happen. Many women feel lingering discomfort and dryness, which some organic natural lubricant can relieve. Explore the various natural scented and unscented sensual massage oils and see which one is your favorite. Partners also may feel uneasy or nervous about penetration for these reasons. You might be thinking that the sex in your relationship will not be "the same" for a long time. But in time, if you do the work to cultivate and grow personally and deepen your intimate connection and sexual relationship ... It will get better and better. The possibilities are endless.

Don't be afraid to try something new and have fun with it. Invite the ambiance that is important to you—the scented candle or massage oil, the music, the feel of your lingerie or sheets, the lighting, anything in the environment that sets the mood. Experiment with doing something you enjoy together; games and role- playing, slowly and sensually breathing together, feeding each other strawberries or dark chocolate, reading erotica or romantic poetry together, looking into each other's eyes, placing your hands on each other's heart, caressing in a variety of ways. Expand the focus of intimacy way beyond sexual intercourse.

"Foreplay" is a huge part of arousal for a woman, but I am not crazy about the word. It implies less important activities that have value only in that they lead to sexual intercourse but do not really count as sex. It makes the end goal of the man's happy ending the main focus, when, in actuality, these "foreplay" activities enhance pleasure by themselves, build stronger intimacy, and are all part of the sexual experience. They are not separate from it. In addition, over half of all women do not reach orgasm from sexual intercourse alone; more women have an orgasm through oral and manual stimulation of their clitoris.

The clitoris has 8,000 nerve endings designed only for a woman's pleasure and ecstasy, so it's really essential for both of you to get to know her. It is very sensitive and honest, and takes its patient feminine time. It knows what it likes and what it does not like. It tends to like to be touched softly or stroked gently, especially around the left upper quadrant. Sensations can move. Experiment with your clitoris. Learn what feels really good, so you can help your partner touch you in ways that are deeply pleasurable.

A woman's sexual pleasure is just as important as a man's. So, bring on the whispered loving words, the soft touching, massaging, caressing, licking, kissing, and hugging—it is not only such fun for both of you, but it will also ease reintroducing sexual pleasure into your relationship and strengthen your connection.

Sexuality and Breastfeeding: What Do You Know? reports, "One study found manual genital stimulation to be a form of sexual activity considered most exciting and most pleasant by both genders postpartum" (221).

Don't expect your partner to read your mind. Gratitude and communication in loving honesty are key, as is a playful sense of humor!

Breastfeeding and Postpartum Sex

While breastfeeding is a very intimate and tender part of motherhood, it does cause hormonal changes that also contribute to vaginal dryness. Using a favorite natural organic lubricant will make all the difference. This is more commonly talked about in the literature and with providers.

What is less discussed are the feelings of jealousy and exclusion that the mother/baby dyad might create in the partner. While this may not be a concern readily brought up by your partner, it does create an opportunity to validate and embrace your partner's feelings as well as your own, discuss the importance of more partner/baby time, and spend quality time alone with just you and your partner.

A partner can feel quite out of the loop, especially if they don't have much or any parental leave at this time. So, how can they feel more involved and nurture their own special relationship with the baby?

Having this discussion with your partner can create a more unified and open relationship, making it easier for each partner to feel vulnerable with the other and so facilitate, maybe not a resumption of your sexual relationship itself, but at least the conversation. Also, as soon as you are able and feeling ready, ask a family member or hire a trusted babysitter, so you and your partner can go out—aim high—once a week, even if only for a few hours, leaving behind a supply of pumped breast milk. Do something you love and make it simple—especially in the beginning. It might be just to have a quiet cup of tea, eat at a lovely restaurant, go on a walk, play a game at a coffee shop or in the park. With time, you can expand out to going to a concert, sports game or show, doing a meditation or taking a tango class together. Imagination has no limits. You can play with taking turns planning and surprising each other with fun activities.

Contraception: Fear of Getting Pregnant Again, Before Feeling Ready or Wanting to Be

Full-time exclusive breastfeeding has been relied upon since the beginning of time to space children—at least for the first six months, as it causes a rise in hormones that suppresses ovulation. But not always. While there is no guarantee and much variability here, there are things you can do to enhance its reliability in preventing pregnancy.

It is called the lactational amenorrhea method (LAM), and it is as effective as the birth control pill. But I have women in my practice that are nursing a toddler a few times a day and have not yet returned to their menstrual cycling, and women who get their periods back within six to eight weeks after birth despite exclusively and frequently breastfeeding on demand, keeping their baby close, and not using pacifiers or bottles. It happened to me with all four of my kids. We did our best.

Once the first period comes, breastfeeding is not a reliable form of contraception; and those who get pregnant unexpectedly in the early months postpartum, doing all they can to exclusively nurse, get pregnant because ovulation occurs BEFORE the first period, meaning they were not aware they resumed fertility. The World Health Organization actually recommends waiting 24 months after birth before getting pregnant again to have the most optimally healthy outcome for you and baby. If you are sure you are not ready for another pregnancy, it is important to understand your fertility signs and to look into and discuss options for contraception with your provider. There are several effective ways to prevent pregnancy that are safe for breastfeeding, naturally or not. You will feel better and more relaxed about resuming intercourse knowing you have a good contraceptive plan that works for you.

How to Reclaim Your Sensual/Sexual Self After Birth

Sexuality is a part of self that cannot be ignored or glossed over, and, just over the last nine months, you, as a new mama, have become more of an expert on using the senses. All of them. You might have noticed a heightened sense of smell, taste, hearing, seeing, and feeling. But postpartum, you're probably all "touched-out", as we'd say—your baby has been growing and developing inside you. You gave birth to your baby, which took a HUGE amount of your energy and strength, is a HUGE transformational event in your life, and an incredible accomplishment! Now that baby is here, they constantly need you from a physical standpoint as well as a nurturing one. Your breasts are being nursed frequently. Your greatest desire right now is probably to shower, eat a delicious meal that someone else prepared, sleep, and for no one to even touch you! That being said, how do you nurture yourself without feeling like you're neglecting your sexual self and your partner, and equally somehow betraying your newfound mama-hood? How do you and your partner become intimate once again after a long while of focusing on the baby?

This is a great time to get to know yourself and your partner again. Honest nonviolent communication is crucial at every level of any kind of relationship, more so now than ever. Your relationship will probably never be the same. But, that doesn't mean your intimacy can't be as great as it was before ... or much deeper and closer. It really can be better! The conversation might not be easy. But this is an opportunity for you both to see who you are now that you've crossed over to this new phase of life. Don't be afraid to take things slow and do things in a new way. Read and discuss together the books I mentioned. Start in pregnancy if you can, but if you already gave birth, start now, even a few pages a day. You've probably only had a few hours of broken sleep; your baby could wake up at any minute for nursing; you feel fat, nothing fits, and you didn't have time to take a shower or put on any make-up.

Embrace the postpartum, beautiful self in all of its empowering, draining, frustrating, and glorious moments. Give yourself lots of self-care. A human being just came out of you--cut yourself some slack! In fact, I hope you've tuned into the empowering sense of motherhood and what it means to be a woman. This is why I really recommend reading Mama Gena's book *Pussy: A Reclamation*. Please don't be deterred by the title. This is a great work of writing encouraging women to come into their power and be fully tuned in and turned on in their life. To give you an idea of the book's content, Mama Gena shares a glimpse of what her work is all about in an interview with Dr. Kelly Brogan:

> *"A woman begins to plug into what it means to have the privilege of 8,000 nerve endings dedicated to pleasure, what it means to have her emotional truth embodied and considered important and righteous, and not try to be 'sugar and spice, and everything nice' but to actually feel free to express the full range of her passion, her grief, her rage, her devastation, her joy."*

Sex, despite being a big social topic, is the least talked about in an honest, caring, compassionate, and vulnerable way—sex after birth even less so.

The best way to figure out how to go about getting back into the mood is through talking openly with yourself and your partner, nurturing your relationship with yourself and your partner, and making sure you are living a turned-on life that you love—not simply turned on sexually, but turned on and excited about all aspects of living. Safeguard your own self-care and joy and consider them as important as eating and drinking healthfully. A happy, fulfilled mama takes everyone higher, including her family and relationships.

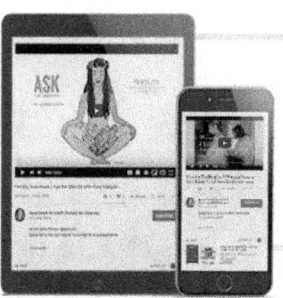

Want to learn more or have more questions?

Grab your free Book Bonuses below:
https://homesweethomebirth.com/nbsbookbonus

Postpartum Struggles Are Real

Statistics show that about 15% of new mamas experience postpartum depression. And 70-80% of us experience "baby blues," that two-week period after the baby is born when we can feel confused, overwhelmed, sensitive, and just not ourselves.

If this is you, you're obviously not alone. Here's what you need to know: **there is no failure in pregnancy, birth, and postpartum.**

You can move with grace through potential sadness, grief, fear, and anger to embrace and heal from your experience. When you are struggling with feeling overwhelmed and exhausted, depressed or anxious, unconfident and unsure, a holistic postpartum plan can give you back your joy and confidence. You've got this. But it takes a village to raise a baby and new parents. Sometimes we just need a little guidance and support—especially in modern times.

I know what it's like to experience birth trauma, and I struggled to put it behind me. Or to try to find balance when there's a new baby in the house—when the idea of "me time" seems like a cruel joke.

After My Own Last Birth, I Was Sick and Alone

Even as a nurse-midwife, I found myself in a postpartum situation that confused and scared me.

Several weeks after the baby was born, I began to feel like I was over-caffeinated. My thoughts were racing, I was extremely agitated, panicked, completely overwhelmed, and unable to function. Making decisions felt impossible, and I couldn't sleep. I felt faint and was losing weight.

I was ashamed and embarrassed. How could I, a professional in this field, find myself in such a state of confusion and intolerable symptoms of anxiety? I didn't want to ask for help. The people I did ask were unable to treat me, and my husband was confused and worried.

I started to have scary and repetitive thoughts. Noises seemed too loud. Faces seemed too big. What the hell was wrong with me?! I felt like I was drugged. Somehow, I suspected my thyroid was off, so I asked my colleague to draw my labs. Then I nearly passed out.

After a call to 911 and subsequent visits to a postpartum stress center, I learned that I had postpartum thyroiditis, an autoimmune condition in which the thyroid initially makes too much hormone, before not making enough.

The diagnosis gave me the confidence to finally accept help. I knew that I wasn't crazy. I knew I shouldn't be embarrassed ... but I was at the time. I stayed with my mother, who lived several hours away—near the center—for an entire month. And my husband and friends all worked together to care for my other kids at home.

I had to stop work for a whole year while recovering from my illness. And it took me a number of years to fully heal using a comprehensive holistic approach. My yoga and meditation practice were life-changing, but the complete healing happened after intensive Clarity Breathwork sessions. *It was the most delicious and miraculous feeling of relief I ever experienced.*

The Forgotten Fourth Trimester

Throughout history, children were raised in communities. When a woman labored, she was surrounded by friends and family. She was attended to by the community midwife, often the same person who was there for the births of all the other babies in the area and potentially even with her mama for her own birth. After birth, she was off-duty to rest, recover, and breastfeed while her tribe cooked, cleaned, took care of the other kids, and did the necessary errands.

Now, we live separated from our families and often experience pregnancy through postpartum more or less alone, and deliver our babies amongst strangers. A sister or mother-in-law might stay with us briefly after our babies are born, but then we're on our own.

In the US, women are sent home alone after a few days in the hospital, and maternity leave is shockingly brief. We're expected to pick up at work right where we left off after just a few short weeks at home with our new baby. Paternity leave is almost non-existent in this country, except for some more progressive family-friendly workplaces.

Of course so many of us experience depression, anxiety, worry, and a lack of confidence! This way of viewing motherhood is simply unnatural. You can't institutionalize the sacred.

But, thriving postpartum *is* possible. Especially when you go into it with a plan.

How to Thrive Postpartum

If you're currently struggling in your "fourth trimester," here are some tips you can implement right away to take the edge off.

Exercise. Try to make time for whatever type of movement feels good to you. Have someone take the baby while you go to a class. Put your baby in the stroller and go for a walk. Put on a workout video while they are napping. Turn on some music that reflects your mood and move your emotions with your body; then turn on something upbeat and dance like nobody is watching.

Connect with your community. Join a mommy support group, either online or in-person. Reach out to friends and family that tend to cheer you up or make you feel comforted. Ask a neighbor to join you for a walk. Take a postpartum "mommy and me" yoga class. Don't be afraid to open up about how you're feeling. You might be surprised by how many people can relate. And make sure to get daily soul-nurturing hugs.

Meditate. Taking time to center down can make a big difference in our energy and confidence. Spend quiet time in nature. If you're not accustomed to meditation, find a guided audio to listen to or just turn on some relaxing instrumental music, get comfortable, and focus on your breath. Review the relevant chapters on mindfulness, breathwork, visualization, and yoga, as well as stress and emotions.

Skip the sugar, cow dairy, and white gluten containing flours. Regularly eating sweets and simple carbs like breads and pastries puts us through a vicious cycle. Sugar crashes lead to low energy and low moods, which lead to carb cravings. Gluten and cow dairy are also inflammatory and have quite a negative impact on mental health. Stick to fresh organic, whole foods, and add more pastured animal protein and healthy fat for a balanced diet and a balanced mood. Refer to chapters related to healthy eating, stress reduction, and managing emotions in pregnancy for more details.

Do what you love. Each day, do things that bring you joy—even if it is for a few minutes at first. Think about what excites you and try to do more of it in your regular routine. Let it be easy and simple. That may be a quiet cup of tea, a visit with your friend, a stroll in the park, a flower or herbal bath in candlelight, watching comedy, getting a massage, doing some yoga. As your baby gets older, Make taking some time for yourself each day to do these things non-negotiable, in the same way as eating, drinking, and sleeping are.

Seek help. When your sadness or anxiety feels like more than "baby blues," seek a qualified professional to help you through it. If, like me, you have an undiagnosed medical condition, or a suffering from a serious mental illness, the suggestions above just won't be enough.

BIRTH TRAUMA IN MOMS AND BABIES

Women are so good at hiding their pain, especially when it comes to birth trauma. They hide deep emotional pain and feel disempowered, humiliated, and disregarded. They also feel they have no control or dignity, and the list goes on.

Did you know that over one-third of women characterize their birth experience as traumatic? Every year in the U.S. alone, nearly 4 million women give birth, so that is a lot of women. And many suffer silently—so how many go unreported? It certainly seems to me like much more than the reported one-third, as I help countless women to heal from it. The numbers of people and lives these impacts are staggering. Where is all of this birth trauma coming from?

What Is Birth Trauma and How Common Is It?

A trauma response is a normal set of reactions someone has after experiencing a life-threatening or dangerous, scary, intensely horrible, or overwhelming situation—the injured mind/body making sense of a traumatic experience. It is not a sign of weakness or inability to cope; it is not depression or anxiety, but it can lead to those feelings.

While most acknowledge that trauma is an expected occurrence after something like a war, serious accident, sudden death, grave assault, a mother's (or even a baby's) trauma following a birth is not widely discussed. Regardless of cause, trauma is trauma and may lead to post-traumatic stress disorder, known as PTSD, which can cause real and long-lasting symptoms of psychological distress. According to *Women's*

Health Today, "In at least one large study, the rates of full-criteria PTSD in the US following childbirth are now higher than those following a major terrorist attack."

The high rate of birth trauma is not acceptable, and we must do something about it by raising awareness and empowering childbearing women and their families to make choices that minimize the risk and speak up to their own providers. We can also get involved with organizations doing what they can to improve maternity and newborn care. In the US, there is Childbirth Connection, and there is the Coalition for Improving Maternity Services (CIMS), which recommend more humane, evidence-based care practices in the mother-friendly childbirth initiative, as well as certify hospitals as mother-baby-friendly based on adherence to these recommendations. In 2016, CIMS joined forces both with BirthNetwork National, a grassroots chapter organization, and Improving Birth, the nation's largest maternity care consumer advocacy organization. Fortunately, more and more hospitals are beginning the process and a number already have the designation, but it is not happening fast enough or on the large scale that is needed.

In countries like Holland and Sweden, where healthy childbirth is treated as normal, with minimal medical and surgical interventions, rates of birth trauma are significantly less, as are the rates of maternal and newborn morbidity and mortality. The United States is among the lowest-ranking countries when it comes to preventing fatality and sickness during birth. Despite being one of the most technologically advanced countries in the world, the USA loses more women and babies during childbirth than any other well-developed country. We're also known as being one of the countries that performs the most C-sections. The US cesarean rate is about twice that of Europe with significantly worse outcomes, and the majority of these C-sections are not medically justified according to maternal health experts.

As explained on the site BirthTraumaAssociation.org.uk:

> *"For most women, it is not always the sensational or dramatic events that trigger childbirth trauma but other factors such as loss of*

control, helplessness, loss of dignity, the hostile or difficult attitudes of the people around them, feelings of being invisible, not being heard or the absence of informed consent to medical procedures."

In a meta-analysis of multiple studies, women with PTSD from childbirth use words like "inhumane," "intrusive," "horrific," and "degrading" to express how they were treated by health care professionals during the experience. A woman can indeed feel traumatized in all birth settings, especially if there were unexpected serious complications or an emergency that required transfer of care or medical and surgical interventions. The most important determinant remains how she feels she was treated during all of it.

Characteristic symptoms of birth trauma can be mild to debilitating. They include persistent re-experiencing of the events with intrusive recurring memories or vivid flashbacks; nightmares; feeling triggered into extreme distress—pounding heart, faintness, nausea, shortness of breath, racing thoughts, and other symptoms of anxiety or panic when exposed to reminders or triggers; avoidance of anything that brings back recollection of the events or the need to talk about it repeatedly; feeling emotionally numb; difficulty bonding with baby or connecting with others, isolation, and loneliness; feeling hypersensitive and reactive, wound up, easily startled, hyper-alert, vigilant and on guard, on the lookout for signs of danger; trouble sleeping, concentrating, or remembering usual things; irritability or anger outbursts; feeling depressed, sad, and crying for no apparent reason; decreased motivation and interest in activities of daily life and absence of joy.

Psychological Impact of Birth Trauma

Sadly, the only goal of the medical world where birth is concerned is to have a breathing mother and baby with heartbeats who appear physically healthy. Not all birth attendants are trauma-informed. The psychological impact of giving birth is not really a concept a hospital or its staff can grasp on maternity wards. So, naturally, modern medicine does not necessarily take into account a woman's fears, emotional pain, or inner stress when managing their labor and birth, let alone the baby who is born fully conscious. In a culture that fails to recognize, understand, or validate the significance of the psychology of childbirth for the mother or baby, care is given without that sensitivity, leaving a birthing woman and her newborn baby's emotional wellness unchecked, which can make labor, birth, and postpartum all the more difficult, and increase the risk of her and her baby feeling traumatized.

With our quick and deep-rooted dependence on technology and modern medicine—the providers, institutions, and products—women have let go of their power and the inner knowledge that their bodies already have for giving birth. Unfortunately, in giving up our power to them, we've also forfeited our voice and our choice. Now, it has become part of routine procedure to use machines, tools, and drugs to monitor and "treat" normal, healthy birthing mothers when all is well; we are conditioned that they are actually necessary and beneficial, despite mounting evidence of their harm.

There are other causative factors—like the impersonal nature of busy, short-staffed, but costly hospital care. Hospitals need large volume and use of their services and products to keep them in business. We live in a litigious society and healthcare providers and their institutions are under a great deal of pressure to do all that they can to prevent litigation that entails millions of dollars, risk of licensure penalties or loss, and long years of extreme duress for them; perfection is expected when it can never be guaranteed.

Far too many women are experiencing some kind of trauma during or after their baby's birth, and many hospitals and their healthcare professionals are not paying attention, even if unintentionally. This type of care and trauma go hand-in-hand.

How Hospitals Typically View Birth

At the beginning of my career, I was a nurse working in a typical hospital. You'd think I'd have been prepared for the idea of labor and delivery when I found out that I was pregnant with my first child. In fact, working with mothers and their newborn babies as an OB nurse is where I developed my strong fear of birth in the first place!

I wish I could say that my own birth trauma story is an exception, but unfortunately, it's still a common experience today. I hear it from thousands of women. In most hospitals in the United States, labor is looked at as a very precarious and potentially problematic situation. A catastrophe or disaster could happen at any moment, resulting in a potential lawsuit. Labor, in the hospital in which I had worked, felt like an emergency or intensive care situation the majority of the time. I was actually in more operating rooms than delivery rooms, and I was assisting more cesarean births than I ever imagined I would be. I was then rescuing women and babies from complications caused by the routine medical interventions we claimed were called "standard procedures."

These highly volatile crisis situations scared me not just as a mother but even as a nurse. And, this is where birth trauma begins: chronic fear and inner stress are the enemies of healthy living without dis-ease and of giving birth. If a birthing mother is feeling stressed and afraid, she will not labor well, especially if her feelings go unheard or are completely disregarded. She will need interventions that lead to more problems and the cascade of more interventions.

What Did My Labor Look Like?

I had no sense that pregnancy and birth were normal and beautiful. As a nurse on the unit, the staff gave me the royal treatment. But it did not feel that way in my body. When I was in labor with my first baby, the treatment I received from my own doctor was very detached and impersonal (despite this doctor being my colleague). Even though I often told my doctor that I felt worried and afraid, my feelings were dismissed and overlooked, making me feel as though they were unimportant and irrelevant. I started to think something was wrong with me. My stress only inclined from there.

One of the first things to happen to me when I arrived at the hospital was having to take off my own clothes and put on a hospital gown. It seemed innocuous then. I look back on that now and know that this begins the disempowerment and depersonalization. A hospital gown creates a sense of increased vulnerability, a feeling of being sick and dependent, and of being an assembly line patient. It simply felt wrong: I wasn't a patient—I was a birthing mother; I wasn't sick—I was in labor. But I did not know any different and that there were options.

The second thing to happen was I was placed in a bed lying down even though I wanted to stand; my body needed to move around, which was discouraged because the nurse and doctor would be unable to read the monitors placed on me. When a mother is in labor, her body assumes a natural upright position. And, when you think about this, it only makes sense—it is not only more comfortable and helps her better cope with the intense sensations of labor, also, in the feat to get your baby to come down and out through your birth canal, gravity is your friend! The pelvic diameter is smaller when lying flat on your back. The baby is pressing on the cervix to dilate it during labor and needs to navigate through the pelvis, so your body will want to be up and move around, mimicking your baby's moves in order to facilitate the baby's travel.

I was also attached to an IV and told not to eat food and drink. As any athlete knows, without question, if you are about to embark on a long and arduous physical event like running the 26-mile marathon (or childbirth!), you do not go without oral fuel and hydration.

My doctor didn't talk to me much or explain things. He just kept giving me frequent internal exams without asking, then telling the results to the nurse outside my room: "She's still 4," and finally I heard, "Hang Pit." As a nurse, I knew what that was. I was familiar with the procedures. I knew they were going to give me medication that would intensify my labor, causing contractions to come more frequently and be much longer and harder than they naturally would.

When I said no, I did not want Pit, my nurse's well-meaning response was, "honey, you don't want a cesarean, do you?" It was either take the medication or be faced with the possibility of a C-section; to instill fear rather than provide knowledge and encouraging support (I now know that these weren't my only two options and that my body was capable).

Of course, I did not want a cesarean, major abdominal surgery, so I agreed. I was feared into it. Then my coping went out of the window. I couldn't deal with the agony brought on by the medication. The doctor came in and walked out again and said, "She's still at a 4. Give her an epidural." It seemed like forever, but then they were giving me an epidural anesthetic via a big needle in my back, into the area around my spinal cord. I was so young and afraid.

All of the things that come naturally are discouraged by most hospitals still today. I was uncomfortable, and I did not feel safe or secure. Not only were my feelings, worries, wants, and needs completely unheard and ignored, but I was also made to stay put when my body was screaming to do what comes naturally ... until it was numb. Then I did not know what was going on in me. I had no sense of control over my own body and my birth. I was in unnecessary pain and discomfort from the Pitocin that made me need an epidural.

The epidural caused a prolonged and severe drop in my baby's heart rate, so there was a frenzied panic around me. I was rushed to an operating room for an emergency cesarean—my biggest fear. As a nurse, I knew that if you don't operate within minutes of this happening, you could have a damaged or dead baby. I waited prepped and tied to the operating table in the OR for about an hour, watching the clock, waiting for the assistant surgeon who never came!

I was left completely alone all that time. My husband wasn't even allowed in the room. I ended up calling out for help because the drugs took over my body, and I needed to push. The doctor came running in, yelling for supplies. I wound up being cut from the vagina and perineum almost to the anus and my baby was then vacuumed out. She was pink and vigorous. I was afraid to look at her. They said she was fine. I was not fine. I was traumatized.

Postpartum, I had what I now know to be birth trauma. PTSD–a normal response to such an intense situation. I had the symptoms, I just did not know what was wrong at the time. I was getting frequent intrusive memories and flashbacks of the experience. Anything that reminded me of the birth triggered horrible feelings in my body. I had a fight-or-flight response whenever I saw a pregnant woman or newborn baby, whenever anyone would ask me about my birth or talk about their birth–I could not discuss any of it without feeling horrible inside. I felt I could not talk about it or be asked about it at all. I felt wound up, hypervigilant, overprotective, and worried something terrible would happen to her–like danger could happen any time. I couldn't sleep. Even though I loved her completely and wholly, it was hard to look at her and not be reminded of my birth, and because oftentimes I was, I would cry or feel triggered into a panic. I could not even imagine going back to work and facing the scene. When I had to start thinking about returning to work, I began having nightmares. My adrenaline would pump up, and I would feel sick. I'd be hyper-alert and on-guard all of the time, as I was also afraid of the sensations in my body.

"You'll get over it," genuinely caring people would say, or they would ask, "What is the big deal? You have a healthy baby." That made me feel worse; like something was really wrong with me, so I felt more ashamed, guilty, alone, and isolated. I stopped telling anyone what I was feeling.

Throughout history, births were considered a miraculous family celebration (as they should be), and babies were born at home. Once births were moved into hospitals in the 1900s in parts of the modern world, birth slowly started to be considered and treated like a medical event. By simply looking at my own story, it's clear that we've created a very intrusive and almost violent way of bringing life into the world. It's no wonder birth trauma is more prevalent than ever.

The grassroots organization Improving Birth coined the term "obstetric violence"—which is playing out in labor and delivery units in certain parts of the world. The World Health Organization called for increased scrutiny of these disrespectful childbirth care practices, as women treated in this way feel assaulted and violated, and must be taken as seriously as rape. Women in vulnerable situations of childbirth are being stripped of their power, voice, and dignity, and are coerced or feared into unwanted invasive procedures. There is loss of control and privacy, and the interventions involve their most intimate selves. If the staff is cold, insensitive, unsupportive, and uncaring, or downright condescending and hostile, it only enhances the traumatic emotional pain felt by the laboring mom.

By no means am I condemning hospitals and doctors. I work with wonderful ones, and I support women birthing in all settings with all types of trained excellent providers. I am also not condemning modern medicine. I am eternally grateful for it when it is necessary and lifesaving. While I am a holistic practitioner who helps women planning natural births, part of holistic care is embracing medical and surgical interventions when occasionally needed when there are serious complications or emergency situations, as often they can save the lives of both mother and baby. There can still be trauma when a planned natural birth ends up in the operating room or outcome is devastating. But with awareness and sensitivity, we can validate, mitigate the traumatic impact, and more effectively heal.

Birth Trauma in Babies

When thinking of trauma, we largely conjure up images of disastrous and catastrophic situations. There is a significant amount of research, however, that shows us that any highly intense situation—especially where there is overwhelm, fear and helplessness—can have just as significantly a traumatic effect on our health.

And we generally know that the traumas that have the deepest roots in our lives are the traumas that happen the earliest, all the way back to experiences of young childhood—including birth and womb time—when we were fully conscious but not yet verbal.

This may sound overly dramatic, but it is now backed by science and solid research. Being born is a momentous and tender step in our life. We don't pay enough attention to the psychological impact of childbirth on newborns. We assume that babies are not aware and won't remember the pain of transition, made even more difficult by maternity and newborn care given without this sensitivity.

While it may not be written in our conscious memories, experiencing birth remains deep in our being, within our very cells and is certainly within our subconscious, influencing much of our behavior, reactions, and perspectives later on in life. How we relate, in our adult lives, to stress at home or at work, pressure from loved ones, and how we go about making our toughest decisions can very well be traced back to how we experienced birth when our response to stresses within our nervous system was developing.

Let's take a look at how a baby should experience birth and why they may have a traumatic experience instead. In looking at why a baby experiences trauma, we'll delve a bit into the possible causes and symptoms that come with birth trauma in babies. This is the starting point for why we should begin to rethink who babies are and what they're trying to tell us!

The Dynamics of a Normal and Healthy Birth

According to Dr. Graham Kennedy on EnhancingTheFuture.co.uk:

> *"The birth process is more than just the means through which we come into this world. It is the first major period of transition in our lives. This transition from our experience of being intimately connected with our mother, whilst in the womb, to gradually separating and individuating, once we leave the womb, affects us not only physically but also emotionally and psychologically. The effects of this transition can range from mild to severe depending on the nature of the birth."*

On the physical level, birth happens naturally by a complex series of biological events believed to be initiated by the baby. When the baby is ready, it is their biological priority and they navigate their way down the birth canal with the help from the contractions of mama's uterus, her instinctive pushing, gravity, and mobile positioning. An immediate connection to the mother and breastfeeding are crucial after birth to begin bonding and for the baby's healthy adjustment and development.

Birth itself is tough enough without even considering interventions. Going down the birth canal includes twisting, turning in the body as well as with the head and neck, not to mention all of the compression and pressure the baby feels. But we as a species have handled it just fine, born into a calm community of love and support, soothed in the warmth and comfort of mama's chest, quiet surroundings, soft lighting, breastfeeding, and baby-wearing.

If the baby feels overwhelmed and frightened at any time, this feeling can be kept locked into their bodies as trauma until they work it out of their system after birth. But, it can also be kept locked for a long period of time, developing into behavioral and learning difficulties in the child's later years.

We know from decades of research in neurology, embryology, and psychology, that newborns are born fully aware and conscious. They are exquisitely sensitive, and are even more vulnerable to acute or chronic stress and trauma than adults. Consciousness actually begins in the womb. We have known for years that drugs, alcohol, nicotine, poor nutrition, and certain infections in a mom can drastically affect the unborn baby–altering DNA and genetic expression, as well as physical, mental, and emotional development. What a mom eats, drinks, breathes, thinks, feels, and experiences goes right to the baby. So, do her stress hormones.

We are learning that trauma from high impact experiences during childbirth is not only stored as nonverbal memories within newborns, it impacts their life at a critical time in their development, affecting short- and long-term physical and mental health–their entire neurological system, from their learning capacity to mental orientation, emotional stability, and stress management. The fight-or-flight stress response creates a strong memory in babies and leads to similar responses to similar cues until resolved in their nervous system. 80% of children with sensory processing disorder, ADHD, developmental delays, and autism have a history of birth trauma. This is staggering.

Dr. Graham Kennedy goes on to point out:

> *"Babies are far more conscious and aware, even as newborns than we realize. They are also incredibly sensitive to what is going on in their environment. Unlike adults, babies do not have the option of fighting or fleeing as a response to threatening or overwhelming circumstances. As a result, the only option left available to them in these circumstances is to freeze. This makes them much more vulnerable to the effects of overwhelm and traumatization than adults, or even older children."*

The Damage of Today's "Technological" Birth

The typical hospital birth today will include an array of drugs and procedures just to get started! These are administered to the mother for inciting stronger, more frequent contractions, sedation for sleep, and anesthesia to numb the pain. But, a baby is, of course, susceptible to anything the mother has been given since its conception, all the way through to the breastfeeding stage.

In addition to being flooded with stress hormones that mom feels from her own fear, the manner in which she is treated and interventions she doesn't really want, a baby experiences actual trauma from the aggressive way they are often ushered from the comfort of the dark cozy womb attached to their mother, into the world.

Just think for a newborn, what is like to for them to:

- Get drugged to induce labor, to make contractions stronger and more intense around them
- Get drugged to numb the pain, sedate, or destroy their microbiome of essential healthy balance of bacteria within them
- Feel a hook to break the water bag protecting them
- Have an internal probe screwed on their head to monitor continuous heart rate and contractions
- Be pulled out by forceps, vacuum, or cesarean
- Have their umbilical cord immediately clamped off, cutting off their lifeline of blood volume and oxygen, (other nutrients,

antibodies, and stem cells to boost their immunity) as they transition to using their lungs instead as independent human beings; then they often have to be resuscitated
- Be born into a world of bright lights, rough handling by strangers who disregard their experience
- Get tubes stuck down their throat to suction them, have their ability to see blunted by antibiotic ointment in their eyes
- Be given a vitamin K shot and hepatitis vaccine injection, and poked for other blood tests
- Get probes put on them for screening procedures
- Be taken to the nursery away from their parents with strangers and left alone for hours in hospital isolettes/cribs,
- Be given formula and pacifiers instead of their mother's breastmilk and skin-to-skin comfort.

This is routine and standard in most US hospitals and some other parts of the modern world. I am not even including the effects of NICU treatment and procedures (even if necessary) or being strapped down for medical circumcision.

In his book *Babies Remember Birth*, leading birth psychologist Dr. David Chamberlain, wrote:

> *"Additional medication is put in the baby's eyes immediately after birth. For many years physicians used a caustic solution of silver nitrate. After much consumer pressure, they began to use a painless but vision-blurring antibiotic ointment. Babies are given antibiotics and other drugs during their hospital stay—perhaps even to counteract common hospital pathogens. Technology may mandate fetal scalp monitoring via an electrode screwed into the baby's scalp while still in the birth canal, or delivery via vacuum extractor, an increasing practice now that the use of forceps is officially discouraged."*

And, this doesn't include the effects of the environment the baby's born into. The light is too bright and too harsh in the delivery room and nurseries, and the noise level is also much too high. There are possible needle injections to administer a vitamin and possibly a vaccine, but also to draw a large blood sample for testing.

In this same book, Dr. David Chamberlain noted:

> *"Physical handling will be rushed and disorienting, while compulsive wiping, washing, weighing and measuring all irritate. If the baby is not already crying, a cry must be provoked (babies were often held upside down and slapped on their backs)."*

The standard birth today just doesn't encourage a safe, quiet, intimate, and private environment for mother and baby to flow naturally within it. This type of maternity care definitely does not promote trust or give the baby the message that it is safe, kind, or comfortable to be here. It certainly does not help to enable a tender bond to develop between mother and baby. It actually elicits their instinctual stress response of fight or flight. And when there is fear of harm, overwhelm, helplessness, and inability to fight or flee, their nervous system gets stuck in trauma. It's no wonder that some babies are so "fussy" or won't breastfeed with ease or are experiencing colic:

> *"While in the hospital, all mothers and babies are on professional turf where everything is regulated by hospital protocol designed not for patients but for staff. Even in the most lenient hospital environments, parents must expect to insist upon continuous contact with their baby, as well as privacy, or they will not get it. The mental and emotional damage done by birth technology to infants in the last century has followed our babies into childhood and right into adulthood and has made necessary the development of reconstructive therapies for body and mind." (Babies Remember Birth, Dr. David Chamberlain)*

- Why do we need these routine procedures and therapies, especially in healthy birth?
- What kind of effects is the standard birth having on our babies?
- What kind of effects come with birth trauma in babies?

- When looking at birth from a baby's perspective, it does indeed sound traumatic and unfathomable, but these practices are all too common and routine.

Common practices do not make sense and contribute to poor outcomes. As previously discussed, the US ranks near the top as compared to other modernized countries in terms of maternal and newborn morbidity and mortality, despite high rates of medical and surgical interventions. In the United States, 23% of all births performed in a hospital are induced; this means the mother is given drugs and chemicals to induce more frequent and intense contractions. Additionally, 65% of those women will also be given epidurals on top of that to cope with the unnaturally intense pain from the medications. Furthermore, over 30% of births in America wind up in a C-section, and this number is rising. These numbers no longer seem ordinary when compared to natural births, in which 95% of them will deliver healthy babies without intervention.

Although babies can't verbally explain their trauma to us, the symptoms they endure for their traumatic birth are the language with which we can begin to translate for them a solution. Think of an adult in a stressed or post-traumatic state—perhaps poor appetite, trouble sleeping, expressions of angst, irritability, and irregular breathing. Well, a baby is not so different. Don't mistake these symptoms as those of simply a "fussy" or "difficult" baby:

- Increased heart and respiratory rate
- Increased startle response, reactivity, jerky movements
- Irritability, fussiness, being inconsolable, excessive crying (here, a baby is usually labeled as "fussy" or "difficult"), or no cry at all
- Poor sleep or excessive sleep
- Feeding difficulties
- Bonding issues, decreased eye contact, glossed divergent eyes.

Dr. Graham Kennedy explained:

"Most parents and professionals consider it ordinary for infants to awaken during the night, cry for extended periods, have

gastrointestinal distress, or be irritable. Few parents or professionals have seen trauma-free babies, so few have experienced babies who are symptom-free.

In addition, few have glimpsed the human potential that is possible when babies are freed from the bonds of early trauma.'

The effects of early trauma do not have to be a life sentence. With appropriate therapeutic support, they can be fully healed. Nor is there an age limit beyond which these early traumas can be treated."

We've assumed, for a long time, that babies are little, cute, and albeit empty and emotionally unfeeling creatures when they come into the world. Dr. David Chamberlain, in Babies Remember Birth, explained:

"Leading researchers now sing the praises of infants. Harvard's Berry Brazelton calls them 'talented'; Hanus Papousek, a German pioneer in infant studies, calls them 'precocious'; famed pediatrician Marshall Klaus calls them 'amazing.' Professor T.G.R. Bower, one of the most innovative of all infant researchers, declares that newborns are 'extremely competent' in perception, learning, and communication."

And, the research to fully understand who these amazing beings are is still unfolding and is only now gaining momentum.

Prevention and Healing

In the meantime, how do we help our moms and babies heal from birth trauma or help them avoid it altogether? Let's take a look at how we can prevent birth trauma and how to heal it if you or your baby is already dealing with it.

Begin with preparation in pregnancy. Plan to have a natural birth. A healthy pregnancy and beautiful natural birth in a respectful supportive environment are sure ways of encouraging a healthy outcome without birth trauma for you or your baby. This takes preparation, especially today. Prepare in advance to promote a healthful and deeply fulfilling experience, while preventing any need for intervention that can lead to traumatic experiences. Don't just wing it.

This is why excellent childbirth education is a must, why planning for your birth is so important today, and it is a major reason why I created my Love Your Birth course. The lessons in the course come from my extensive experience guiding and empowering women and their families in my practice. They have led to the awesome birth experiences that I have been honored to witness for well over 20 years. In it, I go over crucial tips to help you develop a comprehensive plan and prepare for a natural birth, which significantly reduces risk of a traumatic birth experience for you and for your baby.

Get back in touch with the part of yourself that already knows how to do this. Our bodies know how to birth a baby—it's the same way we've been doing it for thousands of years before medical procedures and technology took over. So, a big part of preventing birth trauma would be a mindset shift—in fact, it's a return to what we already know. A first step in the gradual shift of your mindset would be to forgive yourself the conditioning you've been taught to rely on—that you must hand your body (and, essentially, your power) over to your doctor, hospital, modern medicine, and technology. We've been raised a certain way in this era of medical and technological advances.

Birth, for most healthy women, is a normal process that needs no intervention when all is well, but instead, sensitive support and encouragement. Choose your provider and setting wisely. Look for a midwife or doctor and birth setting with high rates of successful natural births, without routine unnecessary interventions, that completely allows you to have your voice, respects and supports your decisions and is sensitive to you and your baby's emotional experience of it all. And do hire a doula, or have a doula- like support person, who can be your coach for your big day.

A Return to Confidence

With this mindset shift comes a return to the confidence of knowing that we, as healthy women, have a feminine capacity to grow, birth, and breastfeed our babies. With confidence, you'll feel more capable of taking on the responsibility of your pregnancy and outlining what you want for your child's birth—not what the medical system deems it should be or believes it is. Confidence in pregnancy and birth comes from an understanding that healthy women birth like they breathe—naturally. What I mean is that you don't have to teach your organs to function, your heart to pump blood, or your lungs to fill with air—they are brilliantly designed to do that without your involvement.

However, this confidence is also best supported in a space where a woman can feel at peace and that she is being celebrated in a gentle and beautiful way. If a woman is stressed, if she's being monitored in a way that is invasive, where there's poking and prodding—especially without consent—then, this woman is definitely not going to labor well and most definitely not as quickly or easily as she otherwise would. She'll then need to be medicated to "get things moving," which will cause an accelerated and more intense labor, and that results in the need for pain relief medications.

Our current maternity care system is disconnected and medical treatment of birth is what's causing the need for more medical and surgical intervention and emergency situations in the first place. It leads to a cascade of further interventions and more serious problems like the high rates of maternal and newborn morbidity and mortality that plague the United States. This is why a woman's physical, mental, and emotional state and space are so important in avoiding birth trauma. In a space where a woman feels respected and heard, she will feel safe enough to birth in a way that is natural and healthy for herself and her baby.

Healing from the Trauma for Moms

Acknowledgment, Validation, Support

Now that we have a sense of what it takes to put in place a birth free of trauma, how do we heal it if we've already experienced it? If there's any trauma you've experienced or are experiencing now, know that it's not your fault!

Full healing is possible. I want you to feel that, imagine that for yourself, and know that it is true. I have not only felt it myself but have witnessed it in countless others just like you, who have sought my guidance for their trauma healing in the last two decades.

The foundation of healing any sort of trauma is acknowledgment, validation, and support. If you need more personal guidance, let a qualified professional know.

Acknowledgement and validation seem counterintuitive to our culture of suppression, but don't repress your feelings. Embrace every single one of them—joyful and mournful. Just as it is part of life to have light and dark, sun and rain, there is joy and pain. They are all sacred human experiences. Feeling all of your feelings makes way for processing them, but also the allowance to trust them—yes, I said trust them! And healing is in the feeling and expressing emotions healthfully, so they do not get stuck and cause physical and psychological health problems.

"Bad" feelings aren't bad in and of themselves—and you certainly should not feel guilty for having them (that definitely doesn't help create any path toward healing!). Bad feelings are actually guides toward helping you find what's upsetting you, to find what's imbalanced in your body. Your body is brilliant and does not lie. Our mind can make up all sorts of false stories, but your body tells the truth. It is wise to listen to its messages. In this way, holistic intervention looks a lot different than medical and surgical intervention.

As a midwife, holistic practices search through the painful feelings of birth trauma and look to see what they are telling us and what can be done to help relieve or remedy the root cause.

What can we change in terms of lifestyle habits that can help us cope with any of the feelings we're worried about? We look at how can we help your body, your mind, and your heart to heal. What is truly soothing for all of who you are?

The idea is to listen to what's really going on with you as a new mama. What are you eating and drinking? How are you sleeping? How can you get more quality sleep, eat foods and take supplements that support your wellbeing, and avoid what harms you?

Sometimes it simply goes back to needing that sense of support. Perhaps you need extra help if you are feeling overwhelmed. Maybe you need more regular outings with a good friend and a cup of tea. It may help to join a support group of mothers who have experienced birth trauma and connect with those who have healed from it. One day you can be that mentor for another suffering mama.

Maybe you need a daily walk by yourself or to take a dance or yoga class. Maybe you simply need more time to yourself, to unplug and be outdoors in nature, and to ensure quiet moments where you're simply breathing.

Maybe you need to feel and express certain emotions more deeply. Can you do that through song and dance, listening to sad and/or angry songs, and then something uplifting and moving it through your body? I have been in many healing workshops of small groups to several thousand dancing the dark emotions as well as dancing the joy. You fully felt, expressed, and innocently moved through your emotions in toddlerhood (remember the temper tantrums and jumping for joy?), so you can do it now, and music helps you remember how. I have over a thousand songs for this that I use myself and to help others. My healing advice also includes making sure you get a good laugh, a good cry, and several good soul-nurturing hugs every day!

Surgical/Medical Intervention

Medical and surgical interventions have their place as I always say, and when they are needed, they are something for which to cultivate immense gratitude. In cases of high risk where the mother and/or baby are in real danger, these interventions can absolutely make all of the lifesaving difference. But, please take note that these situations are emergency or high-risk situations, and when it comes to normal and healthy pregnancies and births, pharmaceutical drugs and surgery should not be the norm. They usually cause more problems, especially when all is well; and even when there are issues, they do not result in true healing. What is needed is a more comprehensive holistic approach.

When there is severe postpartum depression and a mother's feelings are so grave that she feels the need to harm herself or her baby, psychiatric care can be a complete necessity as part of a larger healing regimen. When there are symptoms of depression, anxiety, and other mental illness, I prefer to first build the foundation of the body's health and start with reading leading integrative psychiatrist Dr. Kelly Brogan's bestselling books *A Mind of Your Own*, as well as *Own Your Self* and use her natural and highly effective modalities..

Somatic Healing and Clarity Breathwork

According to decades of cutting-edge research in trauma, we are learning that the best way to heal trauma is not necessarily through the traditional practice of cognitive and medical therapy but somatic therapy. You literally have to reset the nervous system wired to the trauma response, release it from your body and shake it off! This sounds trivial, but the body, quite literally, physically stores its trauma, and it can impact our health, wellbeing, and just about every aspect of our lives.

If you've ever noticed an animal shake itself, as they all do, or a bird flap its wings profusely (usually after a particularly intense situation for them), that's because they are alleviating themselves of the initial and sudden stress that the situation created within their bodies. A deer in the wild, after escaping from a tiger and reaching safety, shakes off the trauma energy and resumes being in a calm state without carrying emotional baggage.

Babies, toddlers, and young children authentically feel, express, and move their emotions -joy as well as sadness and anger in full-blown temper tantrums. Then they get up and get back to playing. Cultural conditioning has caused many of us to shut down, tune out, repress, deny, escape from, and numb our uncomfortable and intense feelings.

When humans encounter the stress of an intense situation, the fight-or-flight response kicks in, and we often hold our breath or breathe more rapidly and shallowly. Any emotion felt at the time is stored as trapped energy in the body. Think of a horror movie you've watched, when you're suddenly surprised, scared, or horrified; the typical reaction is to take a quick and sudden gasp, not to breathe slowly and deeply into your lungs and focus on inner peace.

It might be worth asking your own parents, if you can, about the process of pregnancy and birth that they'd experienced in bringing you into the world. As you'll inevitably learn with trauma, it is not simply forgotten.

A return to our emotions is essential in giving birth. Needless to say, this is supposed to be a time of love and honor and joy—when a birth is led with these feelings, the chances of it being successful, natural, and healthy are that much higher.

We live in a society today that is in constant overdrive fight-or-flight mode without a means of release and reset. We are storing more and more stress energy in our bodies, and this one of the main causes of modern chronic physical and psychological illnesses. A great way to begin the somatic healing process is by Clarity Breathwork, and this process is what truly helped me move through and out of my own birth traumas, even the trauma of childhood abuse and major adult stresses.

Clarity Breathwork is a powerful and effective modality that uses a specific type of breathing to release the trapped trauma energy and psychic pain that is stored in your body, without having to think or talk much about it. It allows your nervous system to reset to optimal original settings. It enables your body to more easily release and even shake off whatever stress that it has been storing. It leaves you feeling an incredible sense of lasting relief. You will notice more ease, flow, and joy in your life and relationships. Its healing effects are so profound, I had to become a practitioner myself and share the gold.

Whatever trauma you've felt or are feeling, please know that your pain is real, you are not to blame, you are not alone, and there is support and healing for you. Every woman has the right to the pregnancy and birth that she has envisioned for herself and her baby. A woman who is treated with a sense of respect and dignity and whose choices are honored will not only labor well but will be far less likely to look back on her birthing experience with a sense of guilt, shame, failure, or deep emotional pain. It is possible to have a return to self and allow your body to experience pregnancy, birth, and life afterward in a safe, peaceful, sensual, and passionate way. It is possible to get back your inner calm and joy. This is your birthright!

Was your birth upsetting or traumatic? Do you have more questions about processing your birth and need help healing? Arrange some time to chat with me. I'd love to answer your questions and help you heal and get yourself back. I have a program specifically for you, that can also include this revolutionary natural healing modality called Clarity Breathwork.

For more information, check out the various podcasts I have been interviewed on about the subject of birth trauma as listed on my website, including The Wellness Mama.

What to Do During and After the Birth for Your Baby

Babies are actually more alert, cognizant, and sensitive than we realize. If we interrupt the birthing and postpartum process when all is well, with any kind of medical or surgical procedures, testing and interventions, the baby will feel terrified, unsafe, without agency, violated, and threatened. Then the trauma reaction ensues! As mentioned, interventions that can cause trauma can include drugs, internal electrodes on their head, forceps, vacuum, cesarean, immediate cord clamping, suctioning their airway, rough handling, or separation from their mom. All the more so when there are complications and interventions are truly needed.

We need to be sensitive to the baby's psychological experience when giving care during and after the process of delivery. In the womb and certainly as a newborn, a baby is fully aware and conscious and is even more vulnerable to trauma than an adult, as a baby's nervous system is still developing.

In addition to the prevention mentioned above, we can help minimize the risk of birth trauma by creating a homey and private atmosphere for both mom and her baby in all settings. That includes dim, soft lighting, and a quiet, peaceful, slow-paced environment. Also, if a mom feels loved, honored, supported, and cared for, if she feels calm, safe, intimate, and sensual, she'll not only labor well, but also will have yummy hormones that pass over to her baby, so her baby is bathed in them and feels this as well.

When I talk about gentle care, I'm talking about gentle handling, soothing and reassuring voice and touch, eye contact, being held, breastfeeding, and a lot of skin-to-skin contact with mom or her partner—this should begin after birth. Don't cut the cord immediately either. That is your baby's life line to oxygen, blood volume, essential nutrients, and immunity to help the baby transition to life outside the womb. Clamp it only after the pulsing stops or the placenta is birthed.

Babies also love relaxing music and bathwater. Who wouldn't like flower petals floating around, the ambiance of real or electric candles, and a delicious light scent of lavender or citrus? If you have a water birth, watch them open up, move their arms and legs, and look around when held in the birthing pool.

This is a sacred time for meeting, connecting to, and bonding with each other, so unplug from your phone and computer, and have someone else in charge of spreading the exciting news and taking pictures.

If a cesarean birth is needed, it can be gentle to simulate a family-centered natural birth as much as possible, so it feels like a huge personal celebration rather than an operation. These same concepts apply however a baby comes into the world.

Furthermore, any procedures or exams that need to happen after the baby's birthed can be done at mom's bedside while she's holding and soothing her baby, explaining what's going on if something is being done to either of them. A healthy baby needs to stay with their parents at all times and not be rolled away in an isolated crib, taken to the noisy and brightly lit nursery of strangers for any examination or intervention.

How Babies Can Heal from Birth Trauma

In today's technological world, as discussed, there are more stressful, scary, drug-induced labors, and surgical births than ever before, especially in the United States. A healthy birth has become an impersonal medical and/or surgical event, a potential crisis waiting to happen in an intensive care like setting in many hospitals; it is not a normal, beautiful part of life, the humane, cozy, family-centered celebration it once was.

At least there are some improvements happening here and there, such as:

- Fetuses are no longer exposed to toxic X-rays.
- Women's pubic hair is no longer shaved.
- Women are not forced to take an enema.
- Women are not strapped down and given drugs that make them act psychotic, prevent memory of their birth, and endanger their babies.
- Partners and newborn babies are now allowed in the room with mom.
- Babies are not forced to have formula instead of breastfeeding.

After the Traumatic Birth

In working with traumatized babies and infants, the most important thing in giving care is love. This may seem obvious but don't take this parental superpower for granted! As a parent, lead with your heart. It is full of wisdom and does not lie, but rather sends you in the right direction. When interacting with your baby, always have tenderness, comfort, and compassion in mind—for yourself and your baby! The more compassion you have for yourself, the easier you can extend it to others in abundance.

Practice "kangaroo care" while in the hospital, if intensive care is needed, and definitely at home. This simply involves holding your baby (clothed in a diaper only) against your skin and covering yourselves with a blanket. Its benefits are well-documented and can be done safely despite a baby's attachment to medical devices in the NICU, depending on baby's condition. Basic closeness, touch, and attention improve their health and healing immensely.

Your baby needs to know that even when life gets difficult—because it will—there'll always be love. You can provide ongoing reassurance that you are there for your baby. Talk to your baby in a soothing manner, and allow them to tell their story with their body and in the nonverbal way that they do. They have much to say without the ability to talk.

Their excessive crying or "fussiness" is not simply difficult baby behavior—they're trying to tell us something. Validate their scary experience and let them know that they're safe now. Sing to them. Rock them. Calm them.

Take a look at renowned midwife Karen Strange's resources on baby trauma healing. She is an expert and international educator in neonatal resuscitation and works fully from the baby's perspective. You can begin using these incredible tools of connecting she teaches with your baby in pregnancy.

Working with a Therapist

In treating traumatized babies, Dr. Graham Kennedy tells us that a therapist will be observing and interacting with the affected baby through movement as well as through "hands-on palpation using craniosacral therapy." Therapists skilled in somatic experience and cutting-edge trauma healing modalities for babies are ideal. You can find a list of some wonderful ones on Karen Strange's website.

As Dr. Graham Kennedy explained: "Working with babies involves holding a space in which they feel supported enough to begin to tell us the story of what happened to them, what they experienced and where it became difficult or even traumatic."

Usually, the movements the baby begins to make are similar to those they made in the womb during labor, but this time giving us the story of what happened to them. This reenactment can have a profound change on the baby's brain, rewiring them to experience what they would have experienced in labor were they to have had a stress-free and intervention-free experience.

There are many possible imprints and effects of birth trauma, but they can all be healed. This is well-backed by much literature, science, and research, especially as we are growing in our understanding of trauma, its impact, and how to heal from it when we get stuck in trauma responses. For example, down the line, you may notice your infant or young child having trouble starting or completing tasks (or both!). This may be an effect of their birth having been interrupted. This may have caused your baby trauma, it is stored in their bodies, and now they've learned to carry with them a certain passivity.

Babies born by forceps, vacuum, or cesarean may, later on, feel they have to be rescued, can't do it alone, support is painful, get angry with authority, being controlled, or manipulated, or they may not want to be here at all—and that can impact every aspect of their lives. Babies who were drugged from their moms getting pain medication may suppress their aliveness, have issues with addiction, feel spacey or out of it, and have trouble being conscious in their own lives.

Babies who spent time in an incubator away from their parents, feel separate and alone, have a deep longing for connection and touch, develop a psychic wall of protection, and are easily triggered by abandonment.

The trauma response is an important part of our lives and it is our brain's and body's way of protecting us at the time of perceived danger. It is a normal instinctual reaction in animals, including humans of all ages, and does not become a disorder unless it is interfered with and suppressed. It does, however, need to be treated with expertise for complete effective healing. If there is a traumatic response dysfunction, it is not a life sentence. You don't have to hold on to those scripts anymore and neither does your baby. Full recovery is possible. In later childhood through adult years, this can be completely resolved with Clarity Breathwork. I do sessions locally in my practice, and online for the global community.

Healing birth trauma in babies is one of the most caring and giving things we can do for our children.

Do you want to heal from trauma, inner stress and emotional pain that is negatively impacting your life? Let me help you! Read my book Trauma Release Formula, available on Amazon.

Home Sweet Homebirth Midwifery, PLLC Disclaimers and Policies

Affiliate and Promotion Disclaimer

The following information is disclosed by Home Sweet Homebirth Midwifery, PLLC ("we" or "us") to you in accordance with the Federal Trade Commission's 16 CFR, Part 680 and 698: "Affiliate Marketing Rule." Sections of this book or website www.homesweethomebirth.com (the "site") may allow you to purchase products and services online provided by other third-party merchants. Some of the links that we post on this site or book are "affiliate links." This means that if you click on the affiliate link and purchase an item through that link, we will receive an affiliate commission. For example, we are a participant in the Amazon Services LLC Associates Program, an affiliate advertising program designed to provide a means for us to earn fees by linking to Amazon.com and affiliated sites.

We are not responsible for the quality, accuracy, timeliness, reliability, or any other aspect of the products and services purchased through affiliate links, the information contained on any third-party sales page, or any other third-party links, products, or services we promote. In addition, the merchant for your purchase will have privacy and data collection practices that are different from ours. If you make a purchase from a merchant on their website or on a website that we have promoted or posted a link to on any of our online medium, the information obtained during your visit to that website or that merchant's online store, and the information that you submit as part of the transaction, such as your name, e-mail address, street address, telephone number, and credit card number, may be collected by that merchant. For more information regarding any merchant, the merchant's online store, their privacy policies, or any additional terms and conditions that may apply to your visit to a merchant's website, visit that merchant's website and click on that merchant's relevant pages and their informational links, or contact that merchant directly.

You release us and our affiliates from any damages that you may incur and agree not to assert any claims against them or us in connection with your purchase or your use of any of the products, services, or information contained on sales pages made available to you by third parties through our site or promoted on any of our online medium. Your participation, correspondence, or business dealings with any third party found on or through our site or promoted on any of our online medium, regarding payment and delivery of specific goods and services, and any other terms, conditions, representations, or warranties associated with such dealings, are solely between you and that third party. You agree that we will not be responsible or liable for any loss, damage, or other matter of any sort incurred as the result of any third-party transaction.

Testimonial Disclaimer

The following information is disclosed by Home Sweet Homebirth Midwifery, PLLC ("we" or "us") to you in accordance with the Federal Trade Commission's 16 CFR, Part 255: "Guides Concerning the Use of Endorsements and Testimonials in Advertising." Testimonials appearing in this book or website www.homesweethomebirth.com (the "site") are received via text, audio, or video submission. They are individual's actual experiences, reflecting the real-life experiences of those who have used our products and/or services. We do not claim that they are typical results that consumers will generally achieve. The testimonials are not necessarily representative of all of those who will use our products and/ or services. We are not responsible for any of the opinions or comments posted to this site. You understand that any testimonials or endorsements (herein "opinions") by our customers or audience represented on this site, or through our products, programs, other websites, content, landing pages, sales pages, or offerings, are solely opinions from individuals.

Similarly, any information contained on this site and on our other programs, content, and offerings are solely our opinion and, therefore, not representations, warranties, or guarantees of any kind.

WellBeing Disclaimer

This book or website www.homesweethomebirth.com (the "site") is for informational purposes only. Home Sweet Homebirth Midwifery, PLLC ("we" or "us") and our subsidiaries, owners, principals, directors, executives, employees, staff, or agents are only licensed healthcare providers or professionals in their state and/or area of expertise. The information contained on this site will not treat or diagnose any disease, illness, or ailment, and if you should experience any such issues, you should seek the advice and examination of your registered physician or practitioner as determined by your own judgment. You understand the information contained on this site is not a substitute for healthcare, medical, or nutritional advice of any kind. You understand and agree that you are fully responsible for your wellbeing, including your dietary, mental, and physical choices and decisions and that of your child. You agree to seek medical advice as determined by your own judgment before taking any action in connection to the information contained on this site or discontinuing the use of any medications as prescribed by your medical practitioner. We shall in no event be held liable to any party for any direct, indirect, punitive, special, incidental, or other consequential damages arising directly or indirectly from any use of this material, which is provided "as is" and without warranties. Your continued use of the site indicates your acceptance of the terms and modifications or future modifications.

REFERENCES

References

Advisory Committee on Immunization Practices
- Website: www.cdc.gov/vaccines/acip

Agency for Healthcare Research and Quality
- Website: www.ahrq.gov
- https://guideline.gov
- https://ahrq.gov/gam/index.html

American Academy of Family Physicians
- Website: www.aafp.org
- https://aafp.org/patient-care/clinical-recommendations/all/vaginal-birth-after-cesarean.html
- https://.aafp.org/afp/2015/0201/p197.html
- https://aafp.org/news/blogs/leadervoices/entry/new_aafp_guideline_adds_to.html
- https://aafp.org/news/health-of-the-public/20150113lac-vbac.html

American Academy of Pediatrics
- Website: www.pediatrics.aappublications.org
- https://pediatrics.aappublications.org/content/106/2/244.short?sso=1&sso_redirect_count=1&nfstatus=401&nftoken=00000000-0000-0000-0000-000000000000&nfstatusdescription=ERROR%3a+No+local+token

American College of Community Midwives
- Website: www.collegeofmidwives.org
- https://collegeofmidwives.org/collegeofmidwives.org/ GBS_2006/GBSprophylactic-VaginalFlush_07.pdf

American College of Nurse-Midwives
- Bailes, Alice,(2016) *ACNM Homebirth Practice Handbook: 3rd Edition*
- Website: www.midwife.org
- https://midwife.org/acnm/files/acnmlibrarydata/ uploadfilename/000000000318/Ultrasound-in-Midwifery-Practice-FINAL-11-24-18.pdf
- https://midwife.org/acnm/files/ACNMLibraryData/ UPLOADFILENAME/000000000090/VBAC-PS-FINAL-10-10-17.pdf
- https://midwife.org/acnm/files/ACNMLibraryData/ UPLOADFILENAME/000000000310/AMTSL-PS-FINAL-10-10-17.pdf

American College of Obstetricians and Gynecologists
- Website: www.acog.org
- https://acog.org/clinical/clinical-guidance/practice-bulletin/ articles/2018/11/early-pregnancy-loss

American Institute of Ultrasound in Medicine
- Website: www.aium.org

American Midwifery Certification Board (AMCB)
- Website: www.amcbmidwife.org

Anand, Margot, (2003). *The New Art of Sexual Ecstasy: Following the Path of Sacred Sexuality.* Harpercollins.

Association of Radical Midwives
- Website: www.midwifery.org.uk

Baby Center
- Website: www.babycenter.com
- https://babycenter.com/0_c-sections-giving-birth-by-cesarean-section_160.bc

Bardacke, Nancy (2012). *Mindful Birthing: Training the Mind, Body, and Heart for Childbirth and Beyond.* HarperCollins.

Bays, Brandon, (2012). *The Journey: A Road Map to the Soul. Atria Books.*
- Website: www.thejourney.com

Belly Belly
- Website: www.bellybelly.com.au
- https://bellybelly.com.au/birth/twilight-sleep/

Birth Trauma Association
- Website: www.birthtraumaassociation.org.uk

Birth Works International
- Website: www.birthworks.org

Boroson, Martin (2009). *One-Moment Meditation: Stillness for People on the Go.* Winter Road.

The Breast Crawl
- Website: www.breastcrawl.org

Breastfeeding Online
- Website: www.ibconline.ca

Breastfeeding Inc
- Website: www.breastfeedinginc.ca

Breastfeeding USA
- Website: www.breastfeedingusa.org
- https://breastfeedingusa.org/content/article/understanding-your-fertility-while-breastfeeding

Brogan, Kelly MD

- Website: www.kellybroganMD.com
- (2019). *Own Your Self: The Surprising Path beyond Depression, Anxiety, and Fatigue to Reclaiming Your Authenticity, Vitality, and Freedom.* Hay House Inc.
- (2016). *A Mind of Your Own: The Truth About Depression and How Women Can Heal Their Bodies to Reclaim Their Lives.* Harper Thorsons.
- https://kellybroganmd.com/human-studies-condemn-ultrasound/
- https://kellybroganmd.com/antibiotics-during-pregnancy-lets-revisit/
- https://kellybroganmd.com/steps-healthy-microbiome/
- https://kellybroganmd.com/guts-bugs-and-babies/
- https://kellybroganmd.com/rejecting-flu-vaccine-in-pregnancy/
- https://kellybroganmd.com/pregnancy-friendly-protection-truth-about-whooping-cough-vaccine-pertussis/
- https://kellybroganmd.com/guarding-our-youth-gardasil/
- https://kellybroganmd.com/hepatitis-b-vaccine-for-your-newborn/
- https://kellybroganmd.com/tiniest-ones-doctors-ignore-data-premies/
- https://kellybroganmd.com/cdc-youre-fired-autism-coverup-exposed/
- https://kellybroganmd.com/driving-epidemic-sudden-infant-death-sids/
- https://kellybroganmd.com/immunologists-letter-legislators/
- https://kellybroganmd.com/emfs-in-pregnancy/
- https://kellybroganmd.com/need-sleep-heres-one-reason/
- https://kellybroganmd.com/so-long-coffee-hello-turmeric-latte/
- https://kellybroganmd.com/antibiotics-side-effects-and-alternatives/
- https://kellybroganmd.com/thinking-epidural/
- https://kellybroganmd.com/surprising-tylenol-side-effects/
- https://kellybroganmd.com/in-honor-of-fear-and-pain/
- https://kellybroganmd.com/5-rules-for-eating-away-your-depression/

- https://kellybroganmd.com/b12-deficiency-brain-health/
- https://kellybroganmd.com/causes-postpartum-depression/
- https://kellybroganmd.com/postpartum-depression-is-brexanolone-the-answer/
- https://kellybroganmd.com/a-discussion-of-pussy-a-reclamation/
- https://kellybroganmd.com/vitalmindreset/?ref=245

Brule, Dan (2017). *Just Breathe: Mastering Breathwork for Success in Life, Love, Business, and Beyond.* Atria.
- Website: www.breathmastery.com

Buckley, Sarah MD (2008). *Gentle Birth, Gentle Mothering: A Doctor's Guide to Natural Childbirth and Gentle Early Parenting Choices.* Celestial Arts.
- Website: www.sarahbuckley.com
- https://sarahbuckley.com/ultrasound-scans-cause-for-concern/

The Business of Being Born
- Website: www.thebusinessofbeingborn.com

The Candida Diet
- Website: www.thecandidadiet.com
- https://thecandidadiet.com/anti-candida-diet/

California Earth Minerals
- Website: www.californiaearthminerals.com
- https://californiaearthminerals.com/media/damrau-diarrhea-trials--bentonite-kills-germs-in-your-body.pdf

Castro, Miranda (2015). Homeopathy for Pregnancy, Birth, and Your Baby's First Year. Macmillan.
- Website: www.mirandacastro.com

Centerpointe
- Website: www.centerpointe.com
- https:// centerpointe.com/planets/sleep-mastery/

Centers for Disease Control and Prevention (CDC)
- Website: www.cdc.gov
- https://cdc.gov/nchs/data/hus/hus17.pdf
- https://cdc.gov/groupbstrep/index.html
- https://cdc.gov/groupbstrep/guidelines/index.html
- https://cdc.gov/groupbstrep/clinicians/index.html?CDC_AA_refVal=https%3A%2F%2Fwww.cdc.gov%2Fgroupbstrep%2Fclinicians%2Fobstetric-providers.html
- https://cdc.gov/flu/pdf/freeresources/pregnant/flushot_pregnant_factsheet.pdf
- https://cdc.gov/vaccines/schedules/easy-to-read/child.html?s_cid=bb-vaccines-Child-HP06-NCIRD

Cesarean Rates
- Website: www.cesareanrates.org

Chamberlain, David (1989). *Babies Remember Birth: And Other Extaordinary Scientific Discoveries About the Mind and Personality of Your Newborn.* Ballantine Books.
- Website: www.pathwaystofamilywellness.org

Chelec Cafritz, Lauren (2019). *Breath Love.* Warren.
- Website: www.experiencebreath.com

Childbearing Year
- Website: www. childbearing-year.com
- https://childbearing-year.com/excerpts-High_Blood_Pressure.php

Childbirth Connection
- Website: www.childbirthconnection.org
- https://childbirthconnection.org/giving-birth/c-section/resources/

Childbirth and Postpartum Professional Association
- Website: www.cappa.net

Citizens for Midwifery
- Website: www.citizensformidwifery.org
- https://cfmidwifery.org/midwifery/faq.aspx

Cleveland Clinic
- Website: www.my.clevelandclinic.org
- https://my.clevelandclinic.org/health/treatments/12578-kangaroo-care

Coalition for Improving Maternity Services
- Website: www.motherfriendly.org

Cochrane
- Website: www.cochrane.org
- https://cochrane.org/evidence#sthash.zGI6cDP8.dpuf
- https://cochrane.org/CD003518/PREG_expectant-care-waiting-versus-surgical-treatment-for-miscarriage
- https://cochrane.org/CD007412/PREG_delivering-placenta-third-stage-labour
- https://cochrane.org/CD003766/PREG_continuous-support-women-during-childbirth

Cummings, Stephen MD & Ullman, Dana (2004). *Everybody's Guide to Homeopathic Medicines.* TarcherPerigee.

Davis, Elizabeth & Pascali-Bonaro, Debra (2010) *Orgasmic Birth: Your Guide to a Safe, Satisfying, and Pleasurable Birth Experience.* Random House.

Delong, Dana, Delong, Peter, & Solaris, Ashanna (2008). *Clarity Breathwork Training Manuals Levels 1–4.*
- Website: www.claritybreathwork.com

Diastasis Rehab
- Website: www.diastasisrehab.com

Dispenza, Joe DC (2015). *You are the Placebo: Making Your Mind Matter.* Hay House.
- Website: www.drjoedispenza.com

DONA International
- Website: www.dona.org

Emmons, Henry MD (2010). *The Chemistry of Calm: A Powerful, Drug-Free Plan to Quiet Your Fears and Overcome Your Anxiety.* Atria.

Emmons, Henry MD (2006). *The Chemistry of Joy: A Three-Step Program for Overcoming Depression Through Western Science and Eastern Wisdom.* Fireside.

England, Pam & Horowitz, Rob (1998). *Birthing From Within: An Extra-Ordinary Guide to Childbirth Preparation.* Partera Press.

Enkin, Murray MD (2000), et al. *A Guide to Effective Care in Pregnancy and Childbirth.* Oxford University Press.

Environmental Working Group (EWG)
- Website: www.ewg.org
- https://ewg.org/foodnews/dirty-dozen.php

Evidence-Based Birth
- Website: www.evidencebasedbirth.com
- https://evidencebasedbirth.com/the-evidence-for-doulas/
- https://evidencebasedbirth.com/gestational-diabetes-and-the-glucola-test/
- https://evidencebasedbirth.com/waterbirth/
- https://evidencebasedbirth.com/groupbstrep/

Faber, Adele & Mazlish, Elaine (2012). *Siblings Without Rivalry: How to Help Your Children Live Together So You Can Live Too.* W. W. Norton & Company.

Fitsri
- Website: www.fitsri.com
- https://fitsri.com/yoga/benefits-of-yoga

The Fitness Tribe
- Website: www.thefitnesstribe.com
- https://thefitnesstribe.com/yoga-benefits/

Food and Drug Administration
- Website: www.fda.gov
- https://fda.gov/radiation-emitting-products/medical-imaging/ultrasound-imaging#benefitsrisks

Freedman, Francoise Barbira (2004). *Yoga for Pregnancy, Birth and Beyond*. DK.

Frye, Anne (2010). *Holistic Midwifery: A Comprehensive Textbook for Midwives in Homebirth Practice, Vol.1: Care During Pregnancy*. Labrys Press.

Frye, Anne (2013). *Holistic Midwifery: A Comprehensive Textbook for Midwives in Homebirth Practice, Vol. 2: Care of the Mother and Baby from the Onset of Labor Through the First Hours After Birth*. Labrys Press.

Frye, Anne (2007). *Understanding Diagnostic Tests in the Childbearing Year: A Holistic Approach 7th Edition*. Labrys Press.

Gaskin, Ina May (2002). *Spiritual Midwifery 4th ed*. Healthy Living Publications.

Gaskin, Ina May (2003). *Ina May's Guide to Childbirth: "Updated With New Material."* Bantam.

Gaskin, Ina May (2011). *Birth Matters: A Midwife's Manifesta*. Seven Stories Press.

Gentle Birth Archives For Suboptimal Fetal Positions
- Website: www.gentlebirth.org/archives/position.html

The Greater Good Movie
- Website: www.greatergoodmovie.org/learn-more/science/

Alan Greene, MD
- Website: www.drgreene.com
- https://drgreene.com/the-most-important-90-seconds-in-every-pregnancy
- https://youtube.com/watch?v=Cw53X98EvLQ

Greenmedinfo
- Website: www.greenmedinfo.com
- https://greenmedinfo.com/disease/streptococcus-infections-group-b
- https://greenmedinfo.com/article/early-onset-neonatal-group-b-streptococcal-infections-new-zealand-1998-1999-we

Group B Strep Support
- Website: www.gbss.org.uk
- https://gbss.org.uk/info-support/group-b-strep-testing/what-does-my-test-result-mean/waterbirth/

Harvard Health Publishing
- Website: www.health.harvard.edu
- https://health.harvard.edu/staying-healthy/yoga-benefits-beyond-the-mat
- https://health.harvard.edu/blog/yoga-in-pregnancy-many-poses-are-safer-than-once-thought-201512298898

Harvard Magazine
- Website: www.harvardmagazine.com
- https://harvardmagazine.com/2016/06/harvard-study-shows-how-antibiotics-disrupt-babies-microbiomes

Healthline
- Website: www.healthline.com
- https://healthline.com/nutrition/13-benefits-of-yoga#section13

The Healthy Home Economist
- Website: www.thehealthyhomeeconomist.com
- https://thehealthyhomeeconomist.com/epidurals -wolf-sheeps-clothing/?utm_source =feedburner&utm_ medium=email&utm_campaign= Feed%3A+TheHealthy HomeEconomist+%28The+Healthy +Home+Economist%29
- https://thehealthyhomeeconomist.com/epidurals-wolf-sheeps-clothing/

Hooper, Anne (2003). *Pure Sex: The Intimate Guide to Sexual Fulfillment.* Duncan Baird.

The Huffington Post
- https://www.huffpost.com/entry/diet-mental-health_b_4257003

Human Milkbanking Association of North America
- Website: www.hmbana.org

Improving Birth Coalition
- Website: www.motherfriendly.org
- https://motherfriendly.org/MFCI

Improving Birth
- Website: www. improvingbirth.org
- https://improvingbirth.org/2014/07/trauma/

Integrated Genetics (Laboratory Corporation of America Holdings)
- Website: www.integratedgenetics.com
- https://integratedgenetics.com/patients/pre-pregnancy/ inheritest?p=tests/reproductive-health/sensigene-rhd

International Breastfeeding Centre
- Website: www. ibconline.ca

International Breathwork Foundation
- Website: www.ibfbreathwork.org

International Cesarean Awareness Network (ICAN)
- Website: www.ican-online.org
- https://ican-online.org/advocacy/
- https://ican-online.org/support/

International Childbirth Education Association
- Website: www.icea.org
- https://icea.org/wp-content/uploads/2016/01/Water_Birth_PP.pdf

I Read Labels For You
- Website: www.ireadlabelsforyou.com

Iyengar, Greeta S. et al (2010). *Yoga for Motherhood: Safe Practice for Expectant & New Mothers.* Sterling/Penn.

Josephson, Laura (2002). *A Homeopathic Handbook of Natural Remedies: Safe and Effective Treatment of Common Ailments and Injuries.* Random House LLC.

Khalsa, Gurmukh Kaur (2014), *Bountiful, Beautiful, Blissful: Experience the Natural Power of Pregnancy and Birth with Kundalini Yoga and Meditation.* St. Martin's Press.
- Website: www.goldenbridgeyoga.com

Katie, Byron (2002). *Loving What Is: Four Questions That Can Change Your Life.* Random House LLC.
- Website: www.thework.com

Kellymom
- Website: www. kellymom.com
- https://kellymom.com/hot-topics/low-supply/
- https://kellymom.com/ages/older-infant/fertility/

Dr. Graham Kennedy
- Website: www.enhancingthefuture.co.uk

King, Tekoa L. et all (2018). *Varney's Midwifery 6th Edition*. Jones & Bartlett Learning.

Kitzinger, Sheila (2003). *The Complete Book of Pregnancy and Childbirth (Revised)*. Knopf.

Kitzinger, Sheila (2003). *Rediscovering Birth*. Atria.

Klaus, Marshall H. MD, Kennell, John H. MD. & Klaus, Phyllis H. (2012). *The Doula Book: How a Trained Labor Companion Can Help You Have a Shorter, Easier, and Healthier Birth*. Da Capo Lifelong Books.

Kravitz, Judith (1999). *Breathe Deep, Laugh Loudly: The Joy of Transformational Breathing*. Free Press Ink.
- Website: www.transformationalbreath.com

La Leche League International
- Website: www.llli.org

Lamaze
- Website: www.lamaze.org
- https://lamaze.org/Connecting-the-Dots/blog/epidural-analgesia-a-delicate-dance-between-its-positive-role-and-unwanted-side-effects-part-one
- https://lamaze.org/Connecting-the-Dots/blog/epidural-analgesia-a-delicate-dance-between-its-positive-role-and-unwanted-side-effects-part-two
- https://lamaze.org/Connecting-the-Dots/epidural-analgesia-a-delicate-dance-between-its-positive-role-unwanted-side-effects-part-three

Lee, Tara & Attwood, Mary (2013). *Pregnancy, Health, Yoga: Your Essential Guide for Bump, Birth and Beyond*. Duncan Baird.

Lekos, Leslie & Westgate, Megan (2015). *Yoga for Pregnancy: Poses, Meditations, and Inspiration for Expectant and New Mothers*. Skyhorse.

Lesser, Marc (2010). *Accomplishing More by Doing Less.* New World Library.

Manga, Ela MD (2019). *Breathe: Strategizing Energy in the Age of Burnout.* Jacana Media.
- Website: www.drelamanga.com

Mayoclinic
- Website: www.mayoclinic.org
- https://mayoclinic.org/healthy-lifestyle/pregnancy-week-by-week/in-depth/prenatal-yoga/art-20047193

Mamanatural
- Website: www.mamanatural.com
- https://mamanatural.com/signs-of-miscarriage/
- https://mamanatural.com/pregnancy-after-loss/
- https://mamanatural.com/getting-pregnant-after-miscarriage/
- https://mamanatural.com/gentle-cesarean

MDEdge
- Website: www.mdedge.com
- https://mdedge.com/familymedicine/article/61032/womens-health/how-long-expectant-management-safe-first-trimester

Microbirth
- Website: www.microbirth.com

Midwives Alliance of North America
- Website: www.mana.org

Midwifery Education Accreditation Council
- Website: www.meacschools.org

Midwifery Today
- Website: www.midwiferytoday.com
- https://midwiferytoday.com/?s=ultrasound+pregnancy
- https://midwiferytoday.com/mt-articles/questions-prenatal-ultrasound/

Mother Earth Living
- Website: www.motherearthliving.com
- https://motherearthliving.com/health-and-wellness/heroic-herbs-for-new-moms

Mother's Milkbank
- Website: www.milkbank.org
- https://milkbank.org/milk-banking/milk-banking-faqs

National Center for Biotechnology Information
- Website: www.ncbi.nlm.nih.gov/
- https://ncbi.nlm.nih.gov/pubmed/24754328
- https://ncbi.nlm.nih.gov/pmc/articles/PMC2390856/
- https://ncbi.nlm.nih.gov/pubmed/16567202
- https://ncbi.nlm.nih.gov/pubmed/8018609
- https://ncbi.nlm.nih.gov/pubmed/10561636
- https://ncbi.nlm.nih.gov/pubmed/23076901
- https://ncbi.nlm.nih.gov/pubmed/21322437
- https://ncbi.nlm.nih.gov/pubmed/19926166
- https://ncbi.nlm.nih.gov/pmc/articles/PMC1949222/
- https://ncbi.nlm.nih.gov/pmc/articles/PMC3486619/
- https://ncbi.nlm.nih.gov/pubmed/25889554
- https://ncbi.nlm.nih.gov/pubmed/16018774
- https://ncbi.nlm.nih.gov/pmc/articles/PMC3424788/

National Center for Complimentary and Integrative Health
- Website: www.nccih.nih.gov
- https://nccih.nih.gov/health/yoga/introduction.htm#hed2

National Guidelines Clearing House
- Website: www.guideline.gov
- https://guideline.gov/summaries/summary/49115/clinical-practice-guideline-planning-for-labor-and-vaginal-birth-after-cesarean?q=vbacs

National Health Service
- Website: www.nhs.uk
- https://nhs.uk/news/pregnancy-and-child/nice-recommends-home-births-for-some-mums/

National Institute of Health and Care Excellence
- Website: www.nice.org.uk
- https://nice.org.uk/guidance/cg149
- https://nice.org.uk/guidance/cg149/chapter/4-Research-recommendations

National Institute for Health and Care Excellence (NICE)
- Website: www.nice.org.uk

National Partnership
- Website: www.nationalpartnership.org
- https://nationalpartnership.org/our-work/resources/health-care/maternity/what-every-pregnant-woman-needs-to-know-about-cesarean-section.pdf
- https://nationalpartnership.org/our-work/resources/health-care/maternity/vaginal-or-cesarean-birth-what-is-at-stake.pdf
- https://nationalpartnership.org/our-work/resources/health-care/maternity/hormonal-physiology-of-childbearing.pdf

National Public Radio
- https://npr.org/2017/12/22/572298802/nearly-dying-in-childbirth-why-preventable-complications-are-growing-in-u-s

National Vaccine Information Center
- Website: www.nvic.org

Natural Medicine Journal
- Website: www.naturalmedicinejournal.com
- https://naturalmedicinejournal.com/journal/2013-08/activated-charcoal-bottom-line-monograph

Jack Newman MD of International Breastfeeding Centre
- Website www.breastfeedingonline.com

New York Times
- https://well.blogs.nytimes.com/2013/12/16/restarting-desire-afterward/

North American Registry of Midwives
- Website: www.narm.org

Northrup, Christiane MD (2006). *Mother- Daughter Wisdom: Creating a Legacy of Physical and Emotional Health.* Bantam.

Northrup, Christiane MD (2010). *Women's Bodies, Women's Wisdom: (Revised Edition): Creating Physical and Emotional Health and Healing.* Bantam
- Website: www.drnorthrup.com
- https://drnorthrup.com/pains-deeper-meaning/
- https://drnorthrup.com/taming-yeast-beast/

Obstetrics and Gynecology
- https://journals.lww.com/greenjournal/toc/publishahead

The Obstetrician and Gynecologist
- https://obgyn.onlinelibrary.wiley.com/doi/pdf/10.1111/tog.12082

Odent, Michel, MD (1994). *Birth Reborn: What Childbirth Should Be.* Souvenir Pr Ltd.
- Website: www.wombecology.com

Organic Intelligence
- www.organicintelligence.org

Orgasmic Birth
- Website www.orgasmicbirth.com

Parenting.com
- Website: www.parenting.com
- https://parenting.com/pregnancy/planning/
- https://parenting.com/article/ask-dr-sears-breastfeeding-as-birth-control

Pathways to Family Wellness
- Website: www.pathwaystofamilywellness.org

Planned Parenthood
- Website: www.plannedparenthood.org
- https://plannedparenthood.org/learn/birth-control/breastfeeding

Price, Catherine (2018). *How to Break Up With Your Phone: The 30-Day Plan to Take Back Your Life. Ten Speed Press.*

Weston A. Price DDS
- Website: www.westonaprice.org

Psychology Today
- Website: www.psychologytoday.com
- https://psychologytoday.com/us/blog/mindful-anger/201706/4-ways-childhood-trauma-impacts-adults
- https://psychologytoday.com/us/blog/the-intelligent-divorce/201503/somatic-experiencing

Research Gate
- Website: www.researchgate.net
- https://www.researchgate.net/publication/26656780_Sexuality_breastfeeding_What_do_you_know

Denise L. Robinson et al., (1999). *Primary Care Across the Lifespan.* Mosby.

Romm, Aviva J. MD
- Website: www.avivaromm.com
- (2014). *The Natural Pregnancy Book: Third Edition: Your Complete Guide to a Safe, Organic Pregnancy and Childbirth with Herbs, Nutrition, and Other Holistic Choices.* Random House LLC
- (2002). *Natural Health After Birth: The Complete Guide to Postpartum Wellness.* Healing Arts.
- (2017). *Botanical Medicine for Women's Health 2nd Edition.* Churchill Livingstone.
- https://avivaromm.com/10-things-pregnant-women-knew/
- https://avivaromm.com/glucose-testing-pregnancy/
- https://avivaromm.com/dont-drink-glucola-gestational-diabetes/
- https://avivaromm.com/group-b-strep-gbs-in-pregnancy-whats-a-mom-to-do/
- https://avivaromm.com/flu-vaccine-in-pregnancy-whats-a-girl-to-do/
- https://avivaromm.com/simple-steps-relieve-pain/
- https://avivaromm.com/depression-in-pregnancy/
- https://avivaromm.com/7-herbs-anxiety/
- https://avivaromm.com/treating-bladder-infections-naturally/
- https://avivaromm.com/vaginal-ecology-down-there/
- https://avivaromm.com/prevent-treat-bacterial-vaginosis/
- https://avivaromm.com/vaginal-infection-remedy/
- https://avivaromm.com/adaptogens-beating-stress/
- https://avivaromm.com/elimination-diet/
- https://avivaromm.com/preventing-migraines-naturally/
- https://avivaromm.com/headaches-in-pregnancy/
- https://avivaromm.com/postpartum-herb-baths/
- https://avivaromm.com/simple-steps-relieve-pain/
- https://avivaromm.com/women-turmeric-depression/
- https://avivaromm.com/vaginal-seeding-after-cesarean/

Rosenberg, Marshall B. (2015). *Nonviolent Communication: A Language of Life: Life Changing Tools for a Healthy Relationship (Nonviolent Communication Guides).* PuddleDancer Press.

Ross, Julia (2003). *The Mood Cure*. Penguin Books.

Royal College of Obstetricians and Gynecologists
- Website: www.rcog.org.uk
- https://rcog.org.uk/en/guidelines-research-services/guidelines/gtg36/
- https://rcog.org.uk/en/patients/patient-leaflets/group-b-streptococcus-gbs-infection-pregnancy-newborn-babies/
- https://gbss.org.uk/wp-content/uploads/2018/06/2018_06_RCOG_Summary_Leaflet.pdf

Sarno, John MD (2001). *The Mindbody Prescription: Healing the Body, Healing the Pain*. Hachette Book Group.

Science Direct
- Website: www.sciencedirect.com
- https://sciencedirect.com/science/article/pii/S1028455916300675

Sears, Robert W. MD (2011) *The Vaccine Book: Making the Right Decision for Your Child (Sears Parenting Library)*.

Sears, William MD et.al (2013). *The Baby Book, Revised Edition: Everything You Need to Know About Your Baby from Birth to Age Two*. Hachette Book Group.

Sears, Martha & Sears, William MD (2018). *The Breastfeeding Book: Everything You Need to Know About Nursing Your Child from Birth Through Weaning*. Little, Brown Spark.
- Website: www.askdrsears.com
- https://askdrsears.com/vaccines
- https://askdrsears.com/topics/feeding-eating/family-nutrition/foods-to-boost-immunity/how-your-immune-system-works

Science and Sensibility
- Website: www.scienceandsensibility.org
- https://scienceandsensibility.org/blog/straight-talk-on-epidurals-for-labor

Penny Simkin
- Website: https://www.pennysimkin.com
- https://pennysimkin.com/weighing-the-pros-and-cons-of-the-epidural/

Sinclair, Constance (2004). *A Midwife's Handbook*. Elsevier Health Sciences.

Somatic Experiencing Trauma Institute
- Website: www.traumahealing.org

Dr. Elisa Song
- Website: www.healthykidshappykids.com
- https://healthykidshappykids.com/2016/12/02/kids-get-flu-vaccine/
- https://healthykidshappykids.com/2016/12/01/treat-childs-flu-naturally/

Spinning Babies
- Website: www.spinningbabies.com
- https://spinningbabies.com/learn-more/baby-positions/belly-mapping/

Stapleton, Amba & Don (2014). *Nosara Yoga Institute's Nosara Yoga Interdisciplinary Teacher Training 200-Hour Foundational Course Manual*

Star, Winifred L. et al (1999). *Ambulatory Obstetrics: Third Edition*. UCSF Nursing Press.

Karen Strange
- Website:www.karenstrange.com
- https://karenstrange.com/therapiesworkshops/
- https://static1.squarespace.com/static/57766acbff7c5070b30f351b/t/5924a0f33c44d8ddbb16793e/1495572726846/ArticlesLinks+%282%29.pdf

- https://static1.squarespace.com/
  static/57766acbff7c5070b30f351b/t/58771c55cd0f68c658
  7b3032/1484201045711/SimpleTools_for_Mothers.1.17.pdf

Thomashauer, Regena (2018) , *Pussy: A Reclamation.* Hay House Inc.
- Website: www.mamagenas.com
- http://mamagenas.com/get-right-with-your-darkness/

Time
- https://time.com/3847755/mothers-children-health-save-the-children-report/

Tolle, Eckhart (2009). *Practicing the Power of Now: Essential Teachings, Meditations, and Exercises from the Power of Now.* Yogi Impressions.

U.S. Department of Health and Human Services
- https://chemm.nlm.nih.gov/pregnancycategories.htm

Vaccine Adverse Events Reporting System (VAERS)
- Website: www.vaers.hhs.gov

University of Wisconsin System
- Website: www.fammed.wisc.edu
- https://fammed.wisc.edu/files/webfm-uploads/documents/
  outreach
- https://fammed.wisc.edu/files/webfm-uploads/documents/
  outreach/im/handout_headache_diary.pdf

Vincent, Peggy (2003). *Baby Catcher: Chronicles of a Modern Midwife.* Scribner.

Weed, Susun (1996) . *Wise Woman Herbal for the Childbearing Year.* Ash Tree Publishing.
- Website: www.susunweed.com
- https://childbearing-year.com/excerpts-High_Blood_Pressure.php

We the Parents
- https://wetheparents.org/natural-induction-science

Weil, Andrew MD (2004). *Natural Health, Natural Medicine: The Complete Guide to Wellness and Self-Care for Optimum Health*. Mariner Books.

Weil, Andrew MD (2017). *Eating Well for Optimum Health: The Essential Guide to Bringing Health and Pleasure Back to Eating*. Anchor.

Weil, Andrew MD (1999). *Breathing: The Master Key to Self Healing Audio CD*. Sounds True.
- Website: www.drweil.com
- https://drweil.com/health-wellness/body-mind-spirit/sleep-issues/natural-sleep-aids-tips/
- https://drweil.com/diet-nutrition/anti-inflammatory-diet-pyramid/dr-weils-anti-inflammatory-diet/
- https://drweil.com/health-wellness/body-mind-spirit/back-pain/rocker-bottom-shoes-for-back-pain/
- https://drweil.com/health-wellness/body-mind-spirit/colds-flu/banishing-sinus-infection-misery/
- https://drweil.com/health-wellness/body-mind-spirit/gastrointestinal/diarrhea/
- https://drweil.com/health-wellness/body-mind-spirit/mental-health/is-same-worthwhile-for-depression/
- https://drweil.com/health-wellness/body-mind-spirit/mental-health/st-johns-wort-for-depression/
- https://drweil.com/health-wellness/health-centers/women/urinary-tract-infections-uti/
- https://drweil.com/health-wellness/health-centers/women/vaginitis/
- https://drweil.com/health-wellness/body-mind-spirit/hair-skin-nails/eczema-treatment-and-symptoms/
- https://drweil.com/health-wellness/body-mind-spirit/autoimmune-disorders/psoriasis/
- https://drweil.com/health-wellness/body-mind-spirit/hair-skin-nails/seeking-natural-psoriasis-relief/

- https://drweil.com/health-wellness/body-mind-spirit/headache/migraine-headaches-without-aura/
- https://drweil.com/blog/bulletins/lower-blood-pressure-without-drugs/
- https://drweil.com/health-wellness/balanced-living/wellness-therapies/biofeedback/

Wellness Mama
- Website: https://wellnessmama.com
- https://wellnessmama.com/4936/improve-sleep-naturally/
- https://wellnessmama.com/205858/camping-benefits/
- https://wellnessmama.com/91682/choose-natural-bedding/

Weschler, Toni (2015). *Taking Charge of Your Fertility: The Definitive Guide to Natural Birth Control, Pregnancy Achievement, and Reproductive Health.* William Morrow Paperbacks.
- Website: www.tcoyf.com

Wickham, Sara (2001). *Anti-D in Midwifery: Panacea or Paradox? Second Edition.* Books for Midwives.
- Website: www.sarawickham.com

Winston, Sherri (2010). *Women's Anatomy of Arousal: Secret Maps to Buried Pleasure.* Mango Garden Press.

Wiley (Wiley's Obstetrics and Gynaecology hub)
- Website: www.obgyn.onlinelibrary.wiley.com
- https://obgyn.onlinelibrary.wiley.com/doi/pdf/10.1111/tog.12082

Rachel Wolchin
- Website: www.rachelwolchin.com

Women's Health Today
- Website: www.womenshealthtoday.blog
- https://womenshealthtoday.blog/2017/02/07/birth-trauma-psychological-trauma-of-childbirth-in-our-time/

World Health Organization
- Website: www.who.int/en
- https://who.int/bulletin/volumes/85/10/06-039289/en/
- https://who.int/bulletin/volumes/87/3/08-052597/en/

Yoga Garden of San Francisco (2015). *Prenatal Yoga Teacher Training Manual with Marisa Toriggino.*

Yoga International
- Website: www.yogainternational.com
- https://yogainternational.com/article/view/a-beginners-guide-to-mula-bandha-root-lock

Yoga Journal
- Website: www.yogajournal.com
- https:// yogajournal.com/lifestyle/yoga-moms-healing-pelvic-floor
- https://yogajournal.com/lifestyle/baby-love

Working With Anne

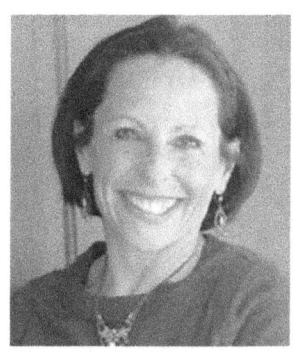

Anne Margolis is a Licensed Certified Nurse Midwife, Licensed Femme! Teacher, Certified Clarity Breathwork Practitioner, Yoga Teacher, and practitioner. She is a 3rd generation guide to mommas birthing babies in her family. Anne has helped thousands of families in her 24+ year midwifery practice and has personally ushered the births of over 1000 healthy babies into the world. She has also guided countless human beings to heal from emotional pain, inner stress, and trauma, tap into their strength and power, live fully and vibrantly, and reclaim their radiance, joyfulness, calm and overall sense of well-being.

Through her online childbirth course 'Love Your Birth', her online and in-person midwifery for pregnancy and postpartum support consultations, her birth professional mentoring, her holistic gynecology, Clairty Breathwork, and Femme! experience offerings she infuses wisdom, compassion, inspiration, and joy into the entire process of women's health care from teenaged years to menopause, as well as into facilitating incredible healing and wellness for both men and women of all ages.

Anne is a two-time number one national and international best-selling author of '*Natural Birth Secrets: An Insiders Guide How To Give Birth Holistically, Healthfully and Safely, and Love the Experience*', and also '*Trauma Release Formula: The Revolutionary Step by Step Program for Eliminating Effects of Childhood Abuse, Trauma, Emotional Pain and Crippling Inner Stress, to Living in Joy without Drugs or Therapy.*'

Visit her website for more information:
https://homesweethomebirth.com/ which has a wealth of free resources and advice.

If you loved this book, Anne would deeply appreciate a 5 Star Book Review.

The Love Your Birth Online Birthing Course

This is a one-of-a-kind program created by a seasoned holistic nurse midwife of over two decades who has seen everything! It contains simple tricks of the trade to make the journey to motherhood more holistically healthy and fulfilling. It's an insider's guide to the joys and challenges of giving birth in modern times.

Let her help you to have the most exquisite birth experience.

Anne has taken everything she's learned, trained, and supported women with locally for over twenty years in her private practice and she's poured all of her love, passion, knowledge, and experience into creating something truly special for you....LOVE YOUR BIRTH. The key to a positive birth is feeling confident, strong, relaxed, and empowered during the entire process, regardless of the twists and turns it may take.

She gives her full heart and all she knows in everything she does to support mommas and their families.

Visit her website for more information:
https://homesweethomebirth.com/

Chat With Anne

Do you have a personal health care question for a holistic midwife?

Concerns about a specific health-related issue?

Or do you need help planning your birth?

Look no further!

Anne has been a holistic midwife since 1995, worked in both supportive hospital-based practices and practiced homebirth midwifery and gynecology for over two decades! Her passion is to help women just like you!

Coaching Calls Can Include:

- Planning a pregnancy, fertility awareness, preconception holistic health
- Holistic Gynecology and Primary Care - preventing and treating common ailments and health problems naturally
- Planning a homebirth-like experience in the hospital
- Support and guidance to answer all of your questions during or after the online course training and create a birth you love
- Support and teaching tools for stress reduction, answering questions, and making informed decisions
- Questions about becoming a midwife or doula, starting, managing or growing your practice, self-care and preventing burnout

Visit her website for more information:
https://homesweethomebirth.com/

Other Books By Anne:

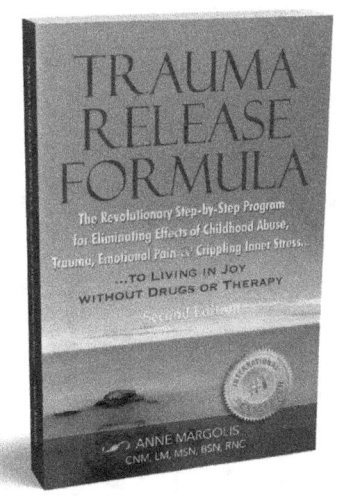

If you've experienced intense stress, emotional pain, or any type of trauma, this book is a must - it represents true hope that saved my life and the lives of countless others. Once you know the key that unlocks the emotional pain, suffering, your ongoing personal life, work and relationship issues, and ongoing stress-related physical symptoms and illness, and how to unlock it all, you experience such powerful healing.

Available from *https://homesweethomebirth.com/* and where all good books are sold!

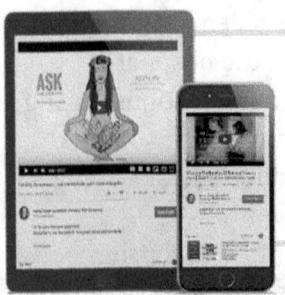

Want to learn more or have more questions?

Grab your free Book Bonuses below:
https://homesweethomebirth.com/nbsbookbonus

www.ingramcontent.com/pod-product-compliance
Lightning Source LLC
Chambersburg PA
CBHW071245220526
45468CB00001B/3